AGING
Volume 25

ALCOHOLISM IN THE ELDERLY
Social and Biomedical Issues

Aging Series

Aging
Volume 25

Alcoholism in the Elderly
Social and Biomedical Issues

Editors

James T. Hartford, M.D.
Associate Professor of Psychiatry
Chief, Geriatric Psychiatry
Department of Psychiatry
University of Cincinnati
College of Medicine
Cincinnati, Ohio

T. Samorajski, Ph.D.
Chief, Neurobiology Section
Texas Research Institute
of Mental Sciences;
Professor of Biology
Texas Woman's University;
Adjunct Professor of Neurobiology
and Anatomy
University of Texas Medical School
Houston, Texas

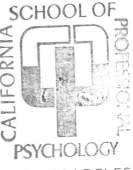

Raven Press ■ New York

Raven Press, 1140 Avenue of the Americas, New York, New York 10036

Made in the United States of America

Library of Congress Cataloging in Publication Data
Main entry under title:

Alcoholism in the elderly.

(Aging ; v. 25)
Includes bibliographies and index.
1. Alcoholism.   2. Aged—Alcohol use.   3. Alcohol—
Physiological effect.   4. Aging—Physiological aspects.
I. Hartford, James T.   II. Samorajski, T. (Thaddeus),
1923–   .   III. Series.   [DNLM: 1. Alcoholism—In old
age.   W1 AG342E v.25 / WM 274 A35715]
RC451.4.A5A427   1984   618.97'6861   83-22940
ISBN 0-89004-924-6

Preface

Although knowledge about aging has greatly increased, the problem of alcohol abuse in the elderly has been given little attention. In the large body of literature on alcohol abuse, the elderly alcoholic is, unfortunately, seldom included. One of the reasons for this omission is the difficulty in identifying the elderly alcohol abuser because of the tendency among older people to live alone, to be retired, and to have less social interaction. There is also a tendency to view alcohol abuse in the elderly as a benign activity and perhaps even to encourage it—with tragic results in many cases.

The despair and isolation that often accompany alcohol abuse are painfully familiar to those involved in the care of the elderly. Professionals in the fields of gerontology feel acutely responsible for evaluating and treating elderly alcohol abusers and are frustrated with the limited and superficial knowledge we have about this problem. We must identify this area as a priority for study and greatly increase our knowledge and understanding of the interrelated processes of aging and alcoholism.

The text is conceived as a systematic discussion of the problems of the elderly alcohol abuser. Our goal is to identify the problems of the older drinker, presenting symptoms, assessment, diagnostic, and treatment approaches. It is of vital importance that experts in alcoholism and experts in aging come together to develop advanced knowledge about the elderly alcoholic.

The book is divided into four broad areas: Sociology, Biology and Biochemistry, Diagnosis and Treatment, and Emerging Issues. The Sociology section deals with the evolutionary basis of alcoholism and epidemiological issues. In the Biology and Biochemistry section, animal models for alcohol and aging research are described. Other chapters of this section deal with changes in organ systems, neurotransmitter functions, biogenic amine metabolism, tolerance to alcohol, and brain cell membrane changes. Diagnosis and Treatment begins with a thorough discussion of age effects on alcohol metabolism, pharmacological issues, and medical issues in alcoholism in the elderly. These chapters are followed by discussions of neuropsychological and electrophysiological parameters, interaction of normal aging senile dementia and multi-infarct dementia with alcoholism, psychiatric aspects, and diagnostic treatment models. In the final section, Emerging Issues, Crook and Cohen comment on future directions for alcohol research in the elderly.

This text was developed with clinicians and researchers in the areas of aging and alcoholism in mind. It is hoped that through increased understanding of the problems faced by clinicians, researchers may be able to further define and develop new knowledge and understanding that can aid in the assessment and treatment of the elderly alcohol abuser. By reviewing pertinent research, those who treat elderly patients can develop greater understanding of alcohol abuse and greater appreciation of the magnitude of the problem in the elderly population. This information should be useful for teachers and students in the field of medicine, nursing, social work, and the allied health professions.

This work is without a doubt only a beginning. We do not present information as definitive or a comprehensive statement of fact, but rather as a thoughtful and honest account of what is currently known in the hope that further study based upon this work will provide us with much needed answers.

James T. Hartford, M.D.
T. Samorajski, Ph.D.

Acknowledgments

The editors are grateful to Charles M. Gaitz, M.D., Head, Gerontology Center, Texas Research Institute of Mental Sciences, who first introduced us to the problems of alcoholism in the geriatric population. We are also indebted to Joseph Schoolar, M.D., Director, Texas Research Institute of Mental Sciences, and Neil Burch, M.D., Head, Research Division, Texas Research Institute of Mental Sciences, for their encouragement of our investigative efforts. We wish to especially thank Susan Sansom for her patient work in helping with the minute details of editing this volume.

Finally, the editors express their sincerest thanks to the publisher for the continual cooperation and understanding of the problems encountered in the preparation of this book.

Contents

Diagnosis and Treatment

Emerging Issues

Contributors

Ernest L. Abel, Ph.D.
Research Scientist V
Research Institute on Alcoholism
1021 Main Street
Buffalo, New York 14203

H. James Armbrecht, Ph.D.
Research Chemist
Geriatric Research, Education, and
   Clinical Center
St. Louis Veterans Administration Medical
   Center; and
Assistant Professor of Medicine and
   Biochemistry
St. Louis University School of Medicine
St. Louis, Missouri 63125

Courtney Bissell
Research Associate
Texas Research Institute of Mental
   Sciences
1300 Moursund Avenue
Texas Medical Center
Houston, Texas 77030

Dan G. Blazer, M.D., Ph.D.
Associate Professor of Psychiatry
Head, Division of Social and Community
   Psychiatry
Duke University Medical Center
Durham, North Carolina 27710

H. Bruce Bosmann, Ph.D.
Martha Betty Semmons Professor of
   Geriatrics
Professor of Pharmacology and Cell
   Biophysics and of Internal Medicine
University of Cincinnati
College of Medicine
Cincinnati, Ohio 45267

Kenneth R. Brizzee
Head, Division of Biomedical Sciences
Delta Regional Primate Research Center
Tulane University
Covington, Louisiana 70433

Larry Brizzee
Research Associate
Texas Research Institute of Mental
   Sciences
1300 Moursund Avenue
Texas Medical Center
Houston, Texas 77030

Robert N. Butler, M.D.
Brookdale Professor of Geriatrics and
   Adult Development
Chairman, Gerald and May Ellen Ritter
   Department of Geriatrics and Adult
   Development
Mount Sinai Medical Center
1 Gustave L. Levy Place
New York, New York 10029

Gene Cohen, M.D., Ph.D.
Chief, Center for Studies of the Mental
   Health of the Aging
National Institute of Mental Health
Rockville, Maryland 20857

Thomas Crook, Ph.D.
Chief, Drug and Alcohol Program
Center for Studies of the Mental Health of
   the Aging
National Institute of Mental Health
Rockville, Maryland 20857

Carlo C. DiClemente, Ph.D.
Adjunct Professor, Psychology Department
University of Houston; and
Chief, Alcoholism Treatment Center
Texas Research Institute of Mental
* Sciences*
1300 Moursund Avenue
Texas Medical Center
Houston, Texas 77030

Robert E. Dustman, Ph.D.
Professor and Chairman, Division of
* Medical Psychology*
Department of Neurology
University of Utah College of Medicine;
Director, Neuropsychology Laboratory
Veterans Administration Medical Center
500 Foothill Drive
Salt Lake City, Utah 84148

Edmund H. Duthie, Jr., M.D.
Assistant Professor and Associate Chief
Section of Geriatrics and Gerontology
The Medical College of Wisconsin
Wood Veterans Administration Medical
* Center*
5000 W. National Avenue
Milwaukee, Wisconsin 53193

Steven H. Ferris, Ph.D.
Executive Director and Senior Research
* Psychologist*
Geriatric Study and Treatment Program
Millhauser Laboratories
Department of Psychiatry
New York University Medical Center
550 First Avenue
New York, NY 10016

Gary A. Flinn, M.D.
Research Psychiatrist
Geriatric Study and Treatment Program
Millhauser Laboratories
Department of Psychiatry
New York University Medical Center
550 First Avenue
New York, NY 10016

Gerhard Freund, M.D.
Chief, Endocrinology Service
Veterans Administration Medical Center;
Professor of Medicine and Neuroscience
Departments of Medicine and Neuroscience
University of Florida
College of Medicine
Gainesville, Florida 32602

Steven R. Gambert, M.D., F.A.C.P.
Professor of Medicine
Director, Division of Gerontology and
* Geriatric Medicine*
Department of Medicine;
Director, Center for Aging and Adult
* Development*
New York Medical College
Valhalla, New York 10595

David L. Garver, M.D.
Professor of Psychiatry, Pharmacology,
* and Cell Biophysics*
University of Cincinnati
College of Medicine
231 Bethesda Avenue
Cincinnati, Ohio 45267

Jack R. Gordon, M.D.
Head, Clinical Services Division
Texas Research Institute of Mental
* Sciences*
1300 Moursund Avenue
Texas Medical Center
Houston, Texas 77030

James T. Hartford, M.D.
Associate Professor of Psychiatry
Chief, Geriatric Psychiatry
Department of Psychiatry
University of Cincinnati
College of Medicine
231 Bethesda Avenue
Cincinnati, Ohio 45267

Francine Lancaster
Coordinator and Associate Professor of
* Biology*
Texas Woman's University
Texas Medical Center
Houston, Texas 77030

John W. Largen, Jr., Ph.D.
Cerebral Blood Flow Laboratory
Texas Research Institute of Mental
    Sciences
1300 Moursund Avenue
Texas Medical Center
Houston, Texas 77030

Christine L. Melchior, Ph.D.
Assistant Professor
Department of Physiology and Biophysics
Alcohol and Drug Abuse Research and
    Training Program
University of Illinois at the Medical Center
P.O. Box 6998
Chicago, Illinois 60680

John Stirling Meyer, M.D.
Chief, Cerebrovascular Research
Director, Cerebral Blood Flow Laboratory
Veterans Administration Medical Center
2002 Holcombe Boulevard
Houston, Texas 77211

Karl F. Mortel, Ph.D.
Research Associate
Cerebrovascular Research Laboratories
Veterans Administration Medical Center
2002 Holcombe Boulevard
Houston, Texas 77211

Margaret Newton, M.D.
Associate Professor
Section of Geriatrics and Gerontology
The Medical College of Wisconsin
Wood Veterans Administration Medical
    Center
5000 W. National Avenue
Milwaukee, Wisconsin 53193

Margaret R. Pennybacker, M.A.
Project Coordinator, Epidemiologic
    Catchment Area Project
Piedmont Health Study
Duke University Medical Center,
Durham, North Carolina 27710

Katherine Persson
Research Associate
Texas Research Institute of Mental
    Sciences
1300 Moursund Avenue
Texas Medical Center
Houston, Texas 77030

Barry Reisberg, M.D.
Clinical Director
Geriatric Study and Treatment Program
Millhauser Laboratories
Department of Psychiatry
New York University Medical Center
550 First Avenue
New York, NY 10016

Ronald F. Ritzmann, Ph.D.
Assistant Professor
Department of Physiology and Biophysics
Alcohol and Drug Abuse Research and
    Training Program
University of Illinois at the Medical Center
P.O. Box 6998
Chicago, Illinois 60680

Robert Rogers, M.A.
Research Associate
Cerebrovascular Research Laboratories
Veterans Administration Medical Center
2002 Holcombe Boulevard
Houston, Texas 77211

T. Samorajski, Ph.D.
Chief, Neurobiology Section
Texas Reseach Institute of Mental Sciences;
Professor of Biology
Texas Woman's University; and
Adjunct Professor of Neurobiology and
    Anatomy
University of Texas Medical School
Houston, Texas 77030

Joseph C. Schoolar, M.D., Ph.D.
Director, Texas Research Institute of
    Mental Sciences; and
Professor of Psychiatry and Pharmacology
Baylor College of Medicine
Houston, Texas 77030

Terry Shaw, Ph.D.
Associate Director
Cerebral Blood Flow Laboratory
Veterans Administration Medical Center
2002 Holcombe Boulevard
Houston, Texas 72211

Ole J. Thienhaus, M.D.
Fellow in Geriatric Psychiatry
Department of Psychiatry
University of Cincinnati
College of Medicine
231 Bethesda Avenue
Cincinnati, Ohio 45267

Kenneth M. Weiss, Ph.D.
Associate Professor of Geriatrics
Center for Demographic and Population
Genetics
University of Texas
Graduate School of Biomedical Sciences
Houston, Texas 77025

Richard E. Wilcox, Ph.D.
Associate Professor of Pharmacology and
Toxicology

Department of Pharmacology and
Toxicology
Alcohol and Drug Abuse Research
Program
College of Pharmacy
University of Texas
Austin, Texas 78712

Ronald W. Wise, Ph.D.
Research Chemist
Geriatric Research, Education, and
Clinical Center
St. Louis Veterans Adminsitration Medical
Center; and
Research Associate, Department of
Biochemistry
St. Louis Unviersity School of Medicine
St. Louis, Missouri 63125

W. Gibson Wood, Ph.D.
Evaluation Coordinator
Geriatric Research, Education, and
Clinical Center
St. Louis Veterans Administration Medical
Center; and
Assistant Research Professor of Medicine
St. Louis University School of Medicine
St. Louis, Missouri 63125

Foreword

Critical Issues of Alcoholism in the Elderly

Persons who suffer from alcoholism live to old age in greater numbers than ever, and some people become alcoholics only after growing old. The overall incidence of alcoholism in older people is lower than in younger ones, but in late life, the condition tends to be hidden because most older problem drinkers have retired from work. Certain groups of older people are highly prone to alcoholism; elderly widowers, for example, have the highest rates of alcoholism of all groups.

Alcohol abuse damages both the quality and the length of life; there is evidence that alcohol abuse shortens life expectancy by 10 to 12 years. The third leading health problem in the United States, alcoholism already has as many victims as do heart disease and cancer. Deaths directly caused by alcoholism are the result of cirrhosis of the liver; in addition, a substantial portion of highway and home accidents are the result of intoxication. The effects of alcohol may accelerate aging, and its clinical manifestations may cause severe types of heart disease, impair brain function, and lead to chronic male impotence by damaging the central nervous system and upsetting hormonal balance.

The indictment seems severe. Certainly there are pleasures to be gained when older persons drink in moderation. There is some evidence, for example, that moderate amounts of alcohol may actually help prevent heart disease by converting lipoproteins from low to high density. Yet the notion that alcohol is helpful in atherosclerosis is questionable—after all, alcohol is a drug that, in large doses, depresses the central nervous system. The pharmacokinetics of alcohol change with age, and the older person may be more susceptible to its damaging effects. In other words, impairment of intellectual function as a result of alcoholism may be added to already existing impairments caused by arteriosclerosis and senile brain disease. Alcoholism also affects muscular coordination and bodily equilibrium, increasing the incidence of falls and accidents among older persons. The wise physician will think carefully about therapeutic use of beer, wine, or whiskey.

Alcoholism in old age, then, is of two types in terms of duration: life-long and occurring in late life. The former used to cause death in middle-aged persons, but better medical management has helped many to live to old age. Some persons begin to consume alcohol in large quantities in late life because of grief, depression, loneliness, boredom, and even because of the minor aches and pains of old age. Alcoholism in nursing homes and homes for the aged is yet another problem.

This book provides a broad overview of the social, physiological, and psychological aspects of alcohol abuse. Recent approaches to diagnosis and treatment of alcoholism have important social and cultural implications. We need to learn much more about the problems of alcohol abuse and alcoholism in old age. The necessary teaching, the acquisition of new knowledge by research, and its application can only come about through a sensitive and knowledgeable survey of what is now known.

In view of the extraordinary prolongation of life that is characteristic of this century, and the unprecedented number of older persons who will be part of the population in the next, it is not too soon to develop a broad-based agenda to deal with the realities and abuse of alcoholism. This must reflect changes in public policy, liquor taxation, fundamental chemical research, treatment centers, and clinical and research training.

Robert N. Butler, M.D.

Alcoholism in the Elderly, edited by
J. T. Hartford and T. Samorajski.
Raven Press, New York © 1984.

Alcoholism: Perspectives for the 1980s

Joseph C. Schoolar

*Texas Research Institute of Mental Sciences; Departments of Psychiatry and
Pharmacology, Baylor College of Medicine, Houston, Texas 77030*

It is now three-quarters of a century since Sir William Osler said, "Know syphilis in all its manifestations and relations, and all things clinical will be added unto you." Anyone who practices medicine and is familiar with the varied manifestations and effects of the organism that causes the "great pox" can appreciate the aptness of Osler's remark. In modern medicine and society the statement is no less true for the problem of alcoholism. One would be hard pressed to think of a condition that involves so many fields: molecular biology, biochemistry, histology, physiology, pharmacology, pathology, neuroendocrinology, psychiatry—every subspecialty of medicine involved. Alcoholism affects the economic and social systems of our society as well: health-care delivery; the criminal justice system; industry, including production, research, and development; family unity and well-being—the list is almost endless.

Alcoholism and its sequelae constitute the third leading cause of death in the United States. Yet our attention to the problem, and consequently significant advances toward its solution, has, until recently, been lacking. This fact is underscored when one compares alcoholism with another major health problem, cardiovascular disease. While the deadly consequences of alcohol misuse continued to climb during the past decade, the incidence of fatal heart attacks decreased by more than 25%.

Why this impressive difference? Certainly, one reason is that the effort to reduce cardiovascular disease has been stronger, more comprehensive, and more focused than the attack against alcoholism. The emphasis on healthful styles of living is dramatically greater for cardiovascular disease than for alcoholism. Prevention of cardiac disability has, for many people, become a way of life.

With respect to factors known or suspected to contribute to cardiovascular disease, significant changes have occurred. There has been a shift in the pattern of cigarette smoking. Although the use of tobacco continues to rise in our country, more adults in the middle-age range have given up cigarettes. Nutritional habits are changing; integrated into our present thinking is recently acquired information about obesity and the effect of high-density lipoproteins. Enthusiasm for exercise has increased to the extent that there are now 30 million joggers in the United States. Millions of persons, professionals and lay people alike, have gone through cardiopulmonary resuscitation training, and they repeat that training regularly. Early detection for

1

heart disease, as well as for predisposing disorders like diabetes mellitus and hypertension, is practiced widely.

Although these changes cannot be tightly correlated to the reduction of cardiovascular disease, the trend is clear. Cardiovascular disease receives more research emphasis than does alcoholism. Although the former costs the nation less ($38 billion to $42 billion per year compared with $52 billion per year for alcoholism), 17 times more research funds are spent on heart disease than on alcoholism. The communication of research findings on heart disease has been more effective, even though issues of cure are at least as complex and the solution as elusive.

Were as much time, research, and total effort spent on conquering alcoholism, one wonders if the results would be equally positive. Efforts to prevent alcoholism and toward the treatment and dissemination and application of research findings are not as well advanced for alcoholism as are comparable efforts concerning cardiovascular disease. Physicians and psychologists who treat alcoholic patients recognize behavioral patterns that are indicators, but there are no predictive biological markers. Treatment intervention is less precise and definitive for the alcoholic.

Still, significant advances are taking place. At last, alcoholism is coming to be viewed as a treatable disease rather than as character failure (2). Scientists are investigating the causes of alcoholism and its effects with the aid of ever-increasing sophisticated laboratory technology. More comprehensive approaches to treatment are being developed, including the ramifications of systems theory. Treatment has come to be seen as an unremitting task, rather than a one-shot effort marked by pessimism.

Thus there is gratifying evidence that alcoholism as a field of research and treatment is broadening not only as a professional discipline but also with respect to effective public involvement. This larger frame allows new perspectives: heightened awareness of alcoholism and its effects, better education and training of lay and professional personnel, more emphasis on prevention, and a rather sudden upsurge of research in almost every facet of alcoholism—causes, effects, and treatment.

As to consciousness-raising, there is significantly more open discussion about alcoholism. The public media devote more attention to it, which often paves the way for new treatment programs. Certainly, the frankness of some nationally known people about their own problems with alcohol and the outcome of their treatment indicates a more rational view of alcoholism in our society.

Teaching is changing at all levels. More elementary and secondary schools are integrating alcohol education into their curricula, in greater depth, and with more imagination and valid psychological content. No longer is the topic dismissed after a canned speech and film, a sort of dutiful "quickie" performed without enthusiasm once a year. In some cases a referral service is the outgrowth of this more creative, useful approach.

Clinicians are changing too. Until a few years ago, the attitudes of physicians and health educators tended to be ossified at the negative pole. Until well into the 1970s, little time was given in medical schools to any sort of unified teaching about alcohol and drug abuse. Pharmacological issues were discussed in pharmacology class, pathophysiological effects in pathology, and the departments of internal medicine and psychiatry spent little time on alcoholism except as it related to their own special interests. Effort was scant and activity splintered; the topic was never treated in a unified manner and as a primary concern.

As a result, in large part, of the efforts of two of our national health institutes, the National Institution of Drug Abuse and the National Institute for Alcohol Abuse, fellows studying substance abuse now include faculty members of 60 medical schools, and these institutes have been active, by way of a task force, in promoting educational efforts in the field of alcohol and substance abuse. Disciplines represented on the task force include medicine, osteopathy, dentistry, nursing (including nurse practitioners), pharmacy, psychology, (physicians' assistants), social work, and of course, psychiatry. An association of librarians has been formed; monographs and curricula are available for the asking. I believe the impact of training young clinicians and scientists in this field will be incalculable.

As is true of all chronic diseases, one of our knottiest problems is prevention. Certainly, if existing strategies were to be improved and sustained, they would contribute to primary prevention. Demythologizing alcoholism, improving education programs and making them widely available, genetic counseling, family therapy, use of multiple treatment approaches, and the dissemination of research findings would all be useful. We do look forward to more effective prevention in our time.

Alcoholism is a significant issue for the elderly. Estimates of alcoholism in the over-65 age group range from 1 to 5% (1); 10 to 15% of elderly patients who seek medical help are estimated to "have a drinking problem that is in some way related to the presenting illness" (1). Their alcohol abuse may be of early or late onset; in either case they are apt to suffer greater adverse effects because of concomitant physical frailty. From this perspective, early prevention takes on an added importance.

Obviously, progress in combating alcoholism depends in significant measure on continued funding from all possible sources and for every aspect of a multifaceted approach. The fact that categorical and other allocated federal funds are dwindling calls for efforts to have these funds replaced and for creativity in developing other sources.

Private funding and voluntary contributions of all sorts are a vastly underutilized resource. Foundations and corporations are more readily supporting both research and treatment. These newer sources of support are sorely needed and welcomed. Interested and well-trained clergy function in many sectors as effective case finders, evaluators, and counselors. Industry is increasing its efforts toward early intervention and treatment for alcoholic employees. Humanitarian issues aside, early treatment of the alcoholic has been clearly demonstrated as economically profitable. And it is a significant step forward that treatment for alcoholism is increasingly included in insurance coverage; 33 states have legislation regarding the matter, and of the 33, 17 require insurance benefits on a parity with benefits for treatment of other illnesses (B. Montague, *personal communication*).

As we approach the end of this century, the perspective for alcoholism is one of potential and great challenge. How well we realize that potential is, for each of us, our own private challenge.

REFERENCES

1. Brody, J. A. (1982): Aging and alcohol abuse. *J. Am. Geriatr. Soc.*, 30(2):123.
2. Deluca, J. R. (1981): Introduction, *Fourth Special Report to the U.S. Congress on Alcohol and Health from the Secretary of Health and Human Services*, p. ix.

Alcoholism in the Elderly, edited by
J. T. Hartford and T. Samorajski.
Raven Press, New York © 1984.

The Evolutionary Basis of Alcoholism:
A Question of the Neocortex

Kenneth M. Weiss

*Center for Demographic and Population Genetics, University of Texas Graduate School
of Biomedical Sciences, Houston, Texas 77025*

What makes people drink? To a psychologist this may be a question of motivation or perception, to a sociologist it may have to do with social pressures and group dynamics, but to a biologist it is a much more curious question. Animal behavior is a finely tuned product of millions of years of evolution, and it is surprising to find that any animal would voluntarily disrupt its behavioral system. This is especially true if there may be some harm in doing so because there should be pressures of natural selection to eliminate animals who drink and any genes that they might carry to lead them to do so. Yet people drink. Are there genes for this kind of behavior? If there are, how did they arise and what has allowed them to persist? Also, as the elderly are past the age of reproduction, and, hence, in some sense beyond the reach of Darwinian selection, are there any ramifications regarding the kind of drinking patterns they might be expected to have?

There has been a wealth of research on alcohol use, especially on problems related to alcohol abuse. Many investigators have attempted to find genes related to alcoholism or alcohol metabolism. Others have studied the motivation of individuals who drink and the sociology of alcohol use. Generally, it has been concluded that drinking, especially problem drinking, is related to social stresses and anxiety. But little, if any, attention has been given to the more fundamental sense of the question "why do people drink?," namely, its evolutionary basis. It is our purpose here to look at this question and to hope to shed enough light on a very complex matter to reveal some of its shadow, if not all of its substance.

To an anthropologist (and this is one hat worn by the author), alcohol research has obviously been designed, and its questions framed, in the context of Western cultural values. Would someone from another kind of culture—say, an Australian aborigine—have thought that it was important to see whether by physically hurting caged mice (or wombats) they can be made to drink? Alcohol is the source of much trouble in the societies of the world, and as it is also associated with pleasure-seeking, it has fallen directly into the deeply imbedded western concept of "Original

---

The literature in this area is extensive; to save space and to be more useful to the reader, the bibliographic citations have concentrated on review or summary sources of fairly recent date.

Sin." Why else would it be controversial whether a hospital or nursing home patient be offered a glass of wine with dinner? Why such extensive efforts to document any of the microscopic advantages or disadvantages such drinking might have? There is a common feeling that even in nonabusers, to use drink to escape anxieties is somehow a negative thing. As a consequence, much of what is available in research on alcoholism is colored by stress on and concepts of social pathology, and the search for genes related to alcohol has taken on the nature of a search for rare pathological alleles.

In this chapter I attempt to view this question from as objective a viewpoint as possible, concerned with the biological nature and origins of the use of alcohol but not with any of its societal or biomedical implications for contemporary life. To study an issue from its biological evolutionary viewpoint, we must address several questions: (a) What is the specific trait being considered? Without clearly stipulating the trait of interest, we cannot be sure to recognize it when it arises nor to differentiate it from other traits. (b) Are there genes whose expression is related causally to the trait? (c) Are those genes manifest in the individuals who carry them in relation to the trait of interest, and can we specify which individuals carry them? Usually, to answer this question there must exist genetic variability, at least between species, but often we require variability within a species. (d) Are the genes expressed in the normal natural history of the animals bearing them? The evolutionary biologist has little interest in genes whose expression in the context of his investigation requires abnormal conditions unlikely to have arisen in nature. We would not, for example, expect to learn much about the evolution or function of the ABO blood group system by studying blood transfusions (though that was how the system was discovered), nor about the HLA system in relation to the rejection of organ transplants. We must discover what those gene products were doing over the past millions of years, in wild monkeys, mice, and men.

Alcohol use is a complex phenomenon. One of the major problems in alcohol research has been to define the trait under consideration, a point many of the workers themselves have freely acknowledged. However, in this survey of their work, I hope to show that (a) there *are* genetically based differences in the biological response to alcohol, (b) the search for genetic variability for the use of alcohol by animals *has* been successful, (c) genetic variation in relation to alcohol use in human beings *does* exist. However, this work is largely irrelevant to the evolution of alcohol use. Genes for that have *not* been found. They do not exist.

EVALUATION

The first order of business is to evaluate the evidence that there is, in fact, genetic basis for alcohol use and if there is, to understand what kinds of genes might be involved. We must compare the use of alcohol and its underlying genetics between human and nonhuman animals to be able to specify what, if any, similarities exist between our use and that of animals with whom we share common ancestry (and who share the laboratory with us). This will enable us to define alcohol use and the evolutionary question in a more meaningful way.

Drinking by nonhuman animals: "You can lead a horse to water, but...."

It would be very useful and important for us to be able to say precisely what natural use is made by animals in the wild. The expectation is that such use is minimal, but the evidence is notable by its absence. It is nearly impossible to study such a problem in natural habitats without the study itself affecting the behavior and undermining its relevance (for example, providing a predictable, observable source of alcohol whose use could be observed and an observation station). On the other hand, biomedical and psychological researchers have made extensive efforts to understand the use of alcohol by animals under laboratory conditions and to find any genetic basis that may exist for such use. (For summaries of this work the reader may consult references 18,46,54,22,69,40). This animal work has largely been aimed at developing animal modes for *human* alcohol use in the hopes that the analogy in animals would illuminate the phenomenon in man. This has colored the way the animals have been studied, of course, and affects what can be said about their natural behavior. Also, we are not descended from today's pigeons, mice, or even monkeys, nor have those animals been on an evolutionary track toward human-like patterns of drinking, so that what we find in animals may have nothing to do with us.

In general, it has been impossible to define alcohol use in sufficiently comprehensive terms that an adequate animal model of human use could be developed, and no available animal model contains all of the important elements of human use (12,69). It has been more than a minor nuisance that, unlike the people studying them, animals do not like to drink alcohol and avoid it when possible. For the physiologist interested in liver enzymes, any means to get ethanol into the body (such as by intubation) may suffice, but for behavioral research, it is necessary (in my opinion at least) to develop oral drinking by free choice when a nonalcoholic source of fluids is also available; single-candidate elections are not very informative about preferences. Yet it has taken considerable work and ingenuity to find, breed, choose, train, or coerce animals to drink (1,12).

In some experiments, animals under stresses like crowding (28,60), isolation (47), electric shock (39,40,32), or the like can be made to drink or to choose alcohol. Often, however, if the stressor is removed, the drinking that it conditioned also disappears over time, and the animal reverts to its prior preference for water (12). Animals will occasionally "work" for alcohol, such as by pressing laboratory levers (49,59), though usually this will take place only under deprivation or duress of some kind. This kind of drinking can be voluntary in the sense that water, which does not relieve the stress, is available, but it seems to me to be somewhat akin to the voluntary confessions of heretics before the Inquisitor: timely decisions in the right direction, and very adaptive, but hardly the kind for which we here seek explanation. In fact, animals forced by laboratory circumstances to select alcohol may attempt strategies to minimize their intake, such as by licking the alcohol delivery tube rather than by actually drinking from it (40), and it is not clear in any case that a pharmacological dose is being ingested in many of these experiments (46,39,40,36,12).

More benign experiments have elicited stress-free voluntary drinking among animals ranging from rodents to apes (12). In some studies, drinking is obtained by a reduction of dietary calories, whereas in others ethanol is made appealing by being offered in solution with pleasant flavors or sweeteners; usually the proportion of alcohol must be less than 10% or so even when it is in a palatable solution (1). This drinking is done with pure water also available, and it *has* been shown that the animal is specifically choosing the alcohol solution (69,60). However, it is not always clear that it is the alcohol, rather than its congeners, that is the goal. Still, enticements of this kind may not be totally artifactual in relation to human drinking, since many a human has had to be lured into a bar for the first time, encouraged to take fluids by being provisioned with salty food, or coaxed to inebriation by social pressures or by a host of tropical fruit juices, shapely glasses, and colored drinking tubes (straws)—not to mention a contrived candlelight atmosphere.

There may be a physiological basis for drinking in animals whether or not such a basis is inherited rather than conditioned. Replacement of calories missing from the diet by drinking in some animals may indicate that they sensed the caloric value of the alcohol, although other experiments have been constructed to show that in some circumstances the animal could not have associated the caloric value with the alcohol. Some animal strains most easy to get to drink may have more efficient liver metabolism of ethanol and of acetaldehyde than nondrinking strains (17). Differences have also been found in levels of alcohol dehydrogenase (ADH) and aldehyde dehydrogenase (ALDH), although these findings are not found consistently in all models (45). Because the pathways are better understood, and because of the relationship to disease, the study of liver-related effects of alcohol has been more extensive than that of neurochemical effects, but the latter have suggested differences in brain serotonin, dopamine, and other biogenic amine levels in drinking strains (46,49). Because acetaldehyde may affect neuronal membrane potential in the CNS, and because there may be differences in general brain activity patterns, it has not been clear whether susceptibility to or selection of alcohol is more likely to be due to liver or neurologic differences. But, as results regarding liver metabolites are less convincing than those involving the CNS, the latter seem at present to be more useful in explaining animal choice than the former (46,45,18).

There has been considerable effort to develop genetic strains of animals that choose to drink. This would obviously make better material than studying enzyme differences, which may or may not be primary in relation to alcohol use. This has been done successfully with a mouse strain known as "C57BL," whereas the "DBA" mouse seems genetically averse to drink. Similarly, by breeding via behavioral selection among offspring, Eriksson (17) has been able to develop strains of rats that choose, and strains that avoid, alcohol. Most rats and other animals, however, resist alcohol. Genetically based differences in various physiological measures have been found, generally in the neurochemical system, though it is premature to say how much of this explains the choice aspects of drinking (35). Eriksson (17) has also bred separate strains of rats tolerant and intolerant to alcohol by controlled strain intercrossing: this seems related to liver metabolism in these animals, and intoxication level differences for given ethanol concentrations seem also to be under genetic control (17). In studies of the quantitative genetics of behavioral correlates of alcohol drinking in animals, a wide variety of behavioral elements seem, on preliminary evidence, to be heritable (15,19). Such work is, however, in its infancy. Studies of crossing between drinking and nondrinking mouse strains have shown that the difference is genetically based, although the heritability is not complete (54), and subtleties in the environment are difficult to rule out. Alcohol-choosing strains seem to be metabolically restricted in the proportion of their total caloric needs, which their livers can metabolize from alcohol, as contrasted with humans in whom life can be supported for a long time by drinking in place of food as a source of calories (54). It may be that animals are physiologically unable to cause themselves serious pathology by drinking instead of eating. Indeed, the noxious effects of alcohol may prevent animals from drinking much alcohol as a rule, and a genetically higher toxicity reaction may partially explain the avoidance of, and protection from, alcohol seen in laboratory animals (54).

Thus, the search through the library of available laboratory animals has shown that genes leading to drinking *do* exist, and that these can be increased in frequency and expressed by controlled breeding. This requires, however, the manipulation and modularization of the environment, such as making food and liquid sources separate, separating and controlling the access mechanisms of water and of the ethanol solutions, dietary component regulation, and so on. Sinclair (60) has argued that an animal analog currently exists for each of the basic aspects of human drinking, such as inverse relation between drinking and the effort required to obtain drink, drinking to avoid stress, and so on. He takes this as implying that there is basic biological similarity between animal drinking and that of humans—i.e., that the animals can tell us what we need to know. However, we shall argue here that a major element in human drinking can have no animal analog. In any case, modularization of the environment clearly destroys the total-environmental nature of alcohol use, which is of obvious importance in human drinking, nor is there an animal model for the recreational use of alcohol to my knowledge. This is not to denigrate the importance of animal studies for understanding some specific and isolated elements of drinking, or the physiology that may underlie them. But we must be circumspect about claiming that any important drinking genes have been found in animals: we can hardly argue that rare and difficult-to-express genes have driven a major biological system, and we should be careful not to place our understanding of human alcohol use in the hands, or paws, of selected and manipulated animals who would prefer to be left alone with their water bottles. The exception is often irrelevant to the rule.

"When it comes to drinking, he behaves like an animal!"

We are all familiar with the use of alcohol in the civilized nations such as our own. However, to gain any real idea of the nature of human beings in regard to alcohol behavior we must take a broader look at the natural history of our species as a whole, especially to assess the way conditions may have been during the majority of our biological evolution when any genetic basis for alcohol use was evolving. To do this, we turn to the anthropological literature. There are today, or were at first contact with western observers, a diversity of human cultures representing those that archeological evidence shows were typical of what most of our ancestors experienced. These include small hunting-gathering bands, tribes, and chiefdoms of varying levels of social complexity, horticultural tribes, and a diversity of preliterature agricultural societies (57). There are many incidental and descriptive reports of alcohol use in these cultures, and these have been summarized in several places (2,30,31,44,16,13). In general, most agricultural societies had and used alcohol in some form or other. In some hunting-gathering groups alcohol was used, although in others there was no source and hence no use of it. The pattern is basically the same for other mind-affecting drugs. In North America, alcohol was little known until contact with whites, who introduced it. In a geographical survey, Mendelbaum (41) found that there was wide regional similarity in alcohol-use patterns, indicating that it was an integral part of the general cultural matrix in much the same way that religion, technology, and so on, are.

The pattern of alcohol use spans the spectrum from some cultures that have seen it as evil and eschewed drinking, to others that encouraged frequent drunkenness. However, anthropologists are generally agreed that under aboriginal conditions, chronic alcoholism or drink-related social pathologies were very rare. Some groups recognized that heavy drinking could lead to fighting and forced men to surrender their weapons before drinking, and certainly the release of sexual and aggressive tensions was a factor in drinking. But in many cultures alcohol was associated with other things such as ceremonial aspects of religion, curing disease, seeking lost objects, steeling warriors for battle, dealing with the spirit world, etc.

Thus, although there was little serious social pathology associated with alcohol (until the effects of conquest when alcoholism in the civilized sense became a serious problem), its use was common in preliterate societies when it was available. Human beings in the wild do not avoid alcohol or find it too noxious to drink. Indeed, if animals will "work" to obtain alcohol by pushing little pedals in their cages, the extent to which humans will go to intoxicate themselves is little short of astounding—and says something about the relevance of animal models. Though it involves a drug other than alcohol, the best case to my knowledge is that of the Yanomama Indians of Venezuela (10,61). An intoxicant snuff called "ebene" is prepared. A hollow, yard-long reed is placed in the nostril of one Indian by another, who forcefully blows ebene through the reed into his nose. This induces an immediate pain recoil, followed by an hour or so of intense mucus discharge, twitching, and choking, accompanied by nausea and vomiting. This is rewarded by a period of hallucinations and then a deep, but disturbed, stupor.

That is working for drugs, and we must ask *why* human beings in diverse cultures not only will use alcohol but will go to such lengths to make and take it. To answer partially, at least from a psychological or social point of view, the methodology of cross-cultural research has been employed. From reports of a large number of cultures (44), various attributes of the culture can be rated by a properly constructed numerical scale. For example, the frequency of drinking, severity of side effects, degree of drunkenness, and so on, can be scored, as can elements of social and kinship structure, childrearing practices, and the like. [The difference between the societies generally studied by anthropology and the civilizations of the world is that the former are structured largely around kinship, whereas civilization is a way of life organized around property, laws and government, and the use of organized armed forces to enforce hierarchical social structures—an objective rather than subjective means of social structuring (58). This can make a fundamental difference in human relations and experiences.] From quantitative measures such as these, multivariate statistical methods can be applied to determine sets of attributes, or factors, that are statistically explanatory of the various patterns of drinking observed. Several studies of this kind have been done (3,29,30,31). High general anxiety levels, especially as caused by subsistence uncertainty and the effects of acculturation, were found to be associated with drunkenness (33), but later analysis has shown that social structure itself, especially corporate kin groups, and not anxiety levels per se affect the ability of a society to control drunkenness and its frequency (21). Later work placed less emphasis on drunkenness and its control and has taken a more positive, or at least balanced, view of "normal" drinking, based on a much enlarged set of societies (6,11,4,5). In all of these studies there has been a statistical association between drinking and relief of anxiety, especially anxiety over the reliability of food supply. However, it is not obvious which societies have the least reliable food sources—indeed, hunter-gatherer societies have been characterized as the original "affluent" societies (55). Security over food sources is an elusive concept for an outsider to quantify in objective terms, and use of culture-form as an indicator of this may not be reliable. In any case, the studies have not agreed as to whether such food-related anxiety relief was primary or secondary; social structure, which is related to food acquisition and resource distribution, has appeared in Field (21) and the Barry, Bacon, and Child studies (2–6), to be a better explanation than anxiety itself for heavy drinking.

Although associated with relief of anxiety in our minds and statistically in other cultures, we must not lose sight of the fact that drinking can be done for pleasure and that it is considered a positive factor in most societies rather than a sin or pathology, and that it usually is an integral part of a functioning social structure rather than a destructive threat to social order. The study by Bacon et al. (4) found that it is not the *individual* level of anxiety that is a major explanatory variable for alcohol use, but rather the social structure itself in the degree that it supports feelings of dependency in its members (3). Their most important explanatory factor was one termed "integrated drinking." This is drinking that occurs in a ceremonial, approved context, is widely partaken, and where children as well as adults find supportive tolerance for dependency relationships. Although drinking may be frequent and even heavy in such societies, drink-related social problems are few, as indeed they are when integrated drinking occurs in western social subgroups such as Jews (62). At first contact, 75% of preliterate societies that had alcohol used it in an integrated way, whereas only about 9% of those to whom alcohol was introduced by a dominant outside culture (i.e., usually us) did so.

We should beware not to romanticize the primitive past as pristine and without problems as much as we should avoid condemning our own society out of hand. Cross-cultural studies are undoubtedly affected by the biases of the anthropologist studying the various groups (who have often been Europhobes), and by the "softness" or vagueness of the variables used to quantify cultural characteristics. The effects of acculturation are difficult to assess and often underplayed by ethnologists studying a group, and there are many problems with attempts to apply western psychology, with its Freudian background, to non-western cultures. However, it is important to recognize that the nearly universal use of alcohol, even heavy use, by human cultures was usually of a positive and benign kind. Furthermore, considering the many causes of mortality and short life expectancy, alcohol-related chronic disease could only occasionally have occurred, at most, and drinking was not a health problem. The small, kinship-based cultures in which human existence has been experienced until the past few centuries may have had a village square, but they did not have Skid Row.

Human drinking: nature or nurture?

Animals generally avoid drinking, but when they do drink, genes may play a role. Humans generally drink—but are there any genes involved? The first level at which an answer to this question can be sought is the family, i.e., by looking for genetic variants related to alcohol use, segregating in Mendelian fashion from parents to offspring. There have been many attempts to use family data to assess what role, if any, genes may play in human drinking; these are summarized in (45,26,63). Usually, because of difficulties in defining a clear and objectively specifiable trait, such studies have been confined to heavy drinking, addiction, or sociopathological drinking. After all, as "normal" drinking is done by most people, it would be difficult to find genes related to it—or else one might conclude that all of us have them except for Mormons, who all must somehow be descended from ancestors with a dysfunctional mutant gene! Among the many family studies of alcoholism that have been done, there has been found a consistent excess frequency of alcoholism in close relatives of alcoholics (14,26,23). However, this excess does not clearly follow a specific Mendelian pattern (e.g., single dominant gene) and on the strength of the evidence, could also be explained in terms of cultural inheritance.

To help sort out environmental from genetic factors, studies of alcoholism or heavy drinking have been done among special kinds of samples: twins, half-siblings, and adoptees. Monozygous twins have a higher concordance rate for alcoholism than do dizygous twins (34,48,38). Furthermore, half-siblings and adoptees have alcoholism patterns that correspond more closely to their biological parents, whether or not they lived with them, than to adoptive parents (24,25,56,8,9). It may be that if everyone were exposed to the opportunity to become alcoholic, a large part of the determination of who would do so is genetic in nature (63); even so, the number of genetic loci involved, their mode of action, and their frequencies are totally unknown.

There were early reports that alcoholism was a single sex-linked disorder; this was based on inheritance patterns as well as an apparent association with sex-linked color blindness. Though some later studies supported this, others have found results incompatible with sex-linkage (e.g., alcoholic sons of alcoholic fathers). At most, a fraction of alcoholism may be of this type. Other attempts to locate genes for alcoholism on chromosomes by linking alcoholism to known single-gene traits such as the ABO blood group system or its related secretor locus have failed to produce reliable results (26,66). There is some suggestion of an association between cirrhosis of the liver and the HLA system, but to date such genes as have been associated with alcoholism are all probably associated with alcohol-related pathology rather than with drinking as the primary variable (45).

Another strategy for detecting the existence of genetic variation is to assess it at the racial level, and there are indeed well-known results from such work. There are differences in the frequency of ADH variants between Mongoloid people (including Amerindians) and Caucasians, and there are probably also ALDH differences. Mongoloid people have a high frequency of a fast ADH response, and they also have a high frequency of facial flushing in reaction to low alcohol doses (52,53,67,68). However, although some work indicates an intraindividual association between these variants (43), this has not clearly been shown to be general enough that we could be sure that there is a genetic connection. Nor do we know if this has any important general relationship to actual social drinking patterns.

It is not clear whether we ought to look for alcohol-related genes in connection with liver metabolism or neural physiology, or to neither of these. Although the social behavioral aspect of drinking relates to its psychotropic effects, these could result from different levels, say, of acetaldehyde, or from differing responses of the neuronal membrane to alcohol metabolites . . . or to entirely different biochemical pathways. Current indications seem to suggest that there are neurological differences between alcoholics and nonalcoholics, e.g., in electroencephalogram (EEG) patterns and perhaps in some catecholamine levels, whereas liver-related differences are not always found (51). Monozygous twins have EEG patterns that respond in a very similar way to alcohol loading, unlike dizygous twins or siblings; this perhaps indicates that there may be a neurological basis for susceptibility to alcoholism that is genetic in nature (51). As we noted earlier, animals who drink may differ in both liver and neuroendocrinological variables, but it is, at present, not possible to say much about the neuroendocrinological factors either in human or in animal alcohol use (45,26). In any case, would such genetic correlates be related to the causes of alcoholism—or even to the cause of initial drinking—or are they merely the results of its use in those individuals who carry the primary genetic variants?

Alcoholism is a frank disorder that is relatively easy to diagnose, and sociopathology has symptoms (indeed, is defined by them) such as higher divorce rates, criminal records, driving accidents or offenses. Thus, it is relatively easy to acquire data on alcoholism. But alcoholism is only the tail of a very broad distribution of alcohol use in western populations, and, indeed, many heavy drinkers never become alcoholics. It is not at all obvious that the study of this kind of extreme can reveal much about genes that control alcohol use as a general phenomenon. After all, the average drinker seems not to bear any genes for alcoholism. Unless it is the alcoholic who makes the rest of the population drink, which does not seem likely, we must step away from the consideration of this extreme and consider the evolutionary history of alcohol use at a more fundamental, if genetically less specific and more speculative, point of view.

EVOLUTION

We have surveyed a great deal of work done to characterize the use of alcohol and underlying genes. Yet this work is almost wholly irrelevant to the problem of evolutionary explanation, which a drinking animal presents. To see that this is so, and to attempt to find a solution, we must turn to a more general consideration of the natural history of mammals and of man. The solution, as we shall see, contains no alcohol.

The nature of animals: water, water everywhere

A wild animal has only a few things to do in life: eat, reproduce, and survive. Most animal behavior is directly concerned with these objectives, and, indeed, the explanation for the evolution of the advanced warm-blooded species, birds and mammals, probably has greatly to do with their plasticity to evolve a wide range of complex behaviors, especially social behavior. The repertoire of behavior elements includes territoriality, social grouping, dominance structures, divisions of labor, ritual display, vocal calling, interindividual recognition, stereotyped competition between males, and so on (7). Predator and prey alike have for hundreds of millions of years been involved in a highly complex behavioral arms race. In higher animals, the demands of this struggle have led to an increased level of intelligence and social structure, and there must be an evolutionary explanation for this (65).

To satisfy the demands of existence, birds and mammals have evolved very specific and exquisitely sensitive neural apparatus, including the ability to consider a wealth of stimuli from their environment and to pass sophisticated judgments on how to respond to them (lower animals can do this to a great extent, too, of course, but reflex and stereotypy play a greater role in their responses). Along with this, one of the hallmarks of most animals is *alertness*. Alertness to the presence of food and water is important, and it is possible that the taste mechanisms themselves evolved as means of vigilance against plant toxins prior to ingestion—which may explain the distaste animals have for alcohol. Even more important is the ability to assess and respond quickly to an array of unexpected but threatening contingencies. A moment's inattentiveness by a bird or mammal could lead to its capture by a predator, to the capture of one of its defenseless young, or to the loss of its mate or territory to a conspecific interloper. These contingencies require constant vigilance, which is an animal's profession.

As a bit of an aside, so crucial is the need for alertness in animal life that it has been difficult to provide a convincing scenario for the evolution of *sleep*. Sleep potentially puts an animal at high vulnerability, and for it to evolve under such risks there would need to be strong countervailing positive benefits from sleep. Physiologists have themselves lost much sleep searching for such a benefit, and most explanations are postfacto constructs. Interestingly, however, the natural history of sleep corresponds more closely to differences in ecological niche than to differences in physiology or metabolism. Sleeping is done in chosen places and at times that for a given kind of animal are secure, and when procuring mates or food is not necessary. Wakefulness and activity at such times would serve no useful purpose but would needlessly expose the animal to potential detection and capture by predators. Predators rarely catch sleeping prey. To a great extent, sleep is alert inanimation, but, unlike intoxication, it is not torpor.

Given these considerations, it would be somewhat surprising if one were to find that wild animals would knowingly subject themselves to conditions in which they sensed a loss of control or ability to perceive dangers in their surroundings. Yet, this is just what would be required if voluntary use of alcohol for its pharmacological effects had evolved in nature, and we have seen that genes leading to drinking in animals *do* exist at least in the laboratory. Why do these genes exist? Did they arise by natural selection in relation to alcohol?

For natural selection to have had anything to do with the genes we find in animals, those genes must have been expressed. This presents difficulties. First, laboratory animals often must be genetically manipulated by highly selective breeding to produce reliable, clearly genetically based, drinking strains. The genes are rare and were found only by screening many animal strains. Hence, drink-prone genotypes must only rarely have occurred in the wild ancestors of today's laboratory animals. For example, if such genes are recessive (as they seem to be, since they occur in inbred animals) so that they will only be expressed in the homozygous state, and if their frequency in wild animals, from which the inbred strains were originally developed, were, say, one in a 100 (they probably are much less), only one animal in 10,000 would have had the prodrinking genotype.

A second problem is that in order for such genes to be expressed, in addition to the availability of the genotypes in nature, there must have been a natural pharmacologically potent source of alcohol, and this must have been available at sufficient concentration, amount, and reliability for psychotropic alcohol use to be discovered and learned. Although small amounts of ethanol are common, large amounts probably occurred only very rarely, perhaps only seasonally, and in food that was eaten for its nutritional value not its intoxicating properties. In most natural situations, food is eaten long before it can become so fermented as to be intoxicating.

The expressed genes for drinking, in the form of the inebriated animal, must then have been screened by natural selection. For such genes to rise in frequency or to persist in the population, the inebriate must have had some advantage over his tea drinking compatriots in the search for food or the competition for territory or mates, and so on. It is difficult to imagine what this might have been. Although sexual inhibitions may be reduced, so is sexual performance, and in any case sexual access to mates in animals has nothing to do with shyness at parties but with highly ritualized displays and competition (65). This demands alertness. Similarly, maintaining territory depends on stereotyped display and fighting ability and the quick recognition of rivals, which would be diminished under the effects of alcohol. Finally, in its diminished state of alertness the animal who had tasted of the "forbidden fruit," rather than leaving it for the ants, would have fallen preferentially to the harvesting of predators. The wages of such sin would be the loss to the species of the genes that led to drinking.

In the absence of direct evidence one can, of course, be facile about offering explanations of what "could" or "could not" have occurred in the course of evolution. The literature is certainly laden with such untrammeled stories. Certainly it is conceivable that here and there some individual animals, or species, in the past would have been aided by drinking alcohol. Its calories could have helped them in hard times, if by some means fermented material was available when other food sources were limited or unavailable (which seems to me to be unlikely). Small doses could have bolstered courage and aided in outdoing a sober but less resolute rival, and so on. However, these seem to me to be very unlikely, or at most to have been rare, for some objective rather than purely speculative reasons: (a) we do not observe this in current animal behavior; (b) after millions of years of opportunity for selection for drinking to have made its mark, we find that genes leading to drinking are infrequent; and, (c) opportunities to obtain sufficient alcohol must have been unusual. One is reluctant to attribute positive selective advantage for something that leads to disorientation in animals so highly specialized for complex behavior. The burden of proof for anyone who would suggest that the genes for drinking we currently find in the laboratory have evolved in relation to drinking is a heavy one.

The nature of human beings: "For you know not why you go, nor where"

Human beings are mammals with a mammalian limbic system and are subject to predation, loss of territoriality, and so on. Yet we drink. How are we different from other animals? It is not utterly pretentious for an anthropologist to attempt to capture the essential nature of human beings in a few lines, so I will attempt it. Human beings evolved from ape-like ancestors over a period of about 5 to 10 million years because food resources were available to a diurnal primate who could get about on its back legs in the heat and tropical sun of open country (probably the African savanna). While anthropologists earn their living by debating the specific sequence of selective events that might explain this, essentially it is agreed that the evolution of bipedalism and tool use *predated* the evolutionary development of the powerful neocortex. Early hominids were active mainly while the lions slept, but they still were physically defenseless and relied on tools for their survival (unlike other animals who use tools only for occasional purposes). Without tools, hominids, including ourselves, cannot outrun, outclimb, outfight, or outbite any prey they might want or any predator that might want them. Once this tool-based pattern was laid down, however, the rapid ballooning of the neocortex occurred in response to it, to the point that about 100,000 years ago it had become what, for a mammal body plan, can only be described as a grotesquely enlarged organ.

Some anthropologists point to tool use, then, as the reason why a better brain may have evolved; others, however, attribute this to the complex social and communicational life of our primate relatives or to the requirements of coordinated hunting-gathering, food-sharing, and protection of ultradefenseless young. It has been argued that the last pulse of evolutionary growth of the brain occurred in response to the use of language for tribal organization and marking of territories (37) in marginal habitats. This has been challenged by Falk, who, based on studies of primate and fossil hominid cranial endocasts, feels that early human-like thought capability, including language, was part of our early development of bipedalism and so on (20).

All of these explanations are essentially related. The gist of the way in which human beings evolved to accomplish all of the above tasks was, in anthropological terms, that we evolved the ability to *symbol*. This is the crux of the difference between animal and human cognition. Human beings can conceive of more abstract entities and have more conscious control over imagery of things not currently providing input stimuli. From what we know, only human beings have such concepts as morning, a flood, grandfather, and three. Perhaps a squirrel can imagine "morning" in some sense, but if so only in a rudimentary way that no more makes it a human being than the way we can climb trees makes us squirrels. Animals may wonder if they will find a mate; people wonder if they are beautiful.

The origins of symboling capability were doubtlessly gradual and based in the mundane. But the brain, once evolved, could be turned to other uses. It was, as Gould (27) terms it, an "exaptation." The neocortex, which could be used to envision an axe within a stone so that it could be fashioned, could also be used by Michaelangelo to envision the Pietà within a block of Carrara marble. We can also do more: we can envision the nonphysical, or even things that may not exist. This allows us to have (or create) religion as a major part of our environment, as real to us as the forest, to conceive of souls and spirits, of hexes, of "what people think of me," and of an elaborate bestiary of evil circumstances, people, creatures, deeds, and eventualities to be anxious about.

Understanding that the human brain is an exaptation for much or even most of human culture is one of the most fundamental yet woefully missing concepts in the social sciences. Its absence underlies a monumental amount of misguided effort to explain in materialistic and evolutionary terms things that do not demand special pleading. For example, self-sacrifice seems unbiological, irrational, and antievolutionary, and sociobiologists have gone to great pains to construct special genes for the purpose and special selective forces to favor those genes, including the need to evoke a rational calculus of relationships to be employed before generous behavior is performed (65). Yet there need be no such genes, and a human sacrifice is not necessarily irrational when not done for a close relative. To the seeker, He whose company may be attained by the *jihad* may be as real as is a coffee cup behind a cupboard door.

This discourse on symboling is not as irrelevant as it may seem to be. Human drinking is a highly social behavior and is clearly done in a context of human culture. Even just moderate drinking for pleasure is often done in a highly cere- monial, ritual, or at least symbolically social way, both in our own culture and, as we have seen, in the preliterate societies. The kinds of anxieties that are relieved by drinking are also uniquely human. An animal needs to be alert to or anxious about potential dangers that demand an immediate and physically competent re- sponse. Humans, imbedded in a thoroughly symbolic world, are concerned with things more abstract, against which there may be *no* defensive action or against which vigilance is irrelevant. What can one do against a fear of drought, cancer, retirement, or the wrath of God? If one feels trapped by the "System," there is no one to bite or claw. Religion may be an opiate for the people, as Marx remarked, but for many of them a more substantial form of relief is preferred, at least as an adjuvant therapy. You can run away from a wolf, but not from a witch.

Given the unique human kinds of anxieties and expectations, as contrasted with animal concerns, it is not surprising that drinking as a response might occur, for if the neocortex can create a dragon, under drink it can slay it. On the other hand, we do possess the full mammalian limbic system, and it is this that, figuratively as well as literally, underlies the neocortex. What is surprising to me is that a human being is capable of willfully disorienting himself and overriding the primal dictates of the limbic system to be alert and arousable. I believe that the answer to this problem, too, lies in the neocortex. The same organ that can imagine a wealth of worry can also imagine a sense of safety. Our societies, preliterate as well as civilized, are structured to delimit intraspecific rivalries, and even warfare has its rules of conduct. Our division of labor allows us to provide for sentries, and our neocortex permits us to believe (rightly or wrongly) that they are on guard. This system does not always work, as many a wronged husband, king, or soldier has learned to his woe—but it works generally. Finally, it is ironic that we may also share something fundamental with our little laboratory friends: we know from experience that our cages are safe. Biologists long ago noted the relevance of the similarities between human beings and other domestic animals.

Although humans are nearly unique in their willingness to drink, there are no genes that evolved in relation to this. The drinking behavior of individuals in cultures that were *never* exposed to alcohol prior to contact with agricultural civilizations was not materially different from that of those in civilizations who had had alcohol in their ancestry for 10,000 years and the opportunity to have evolved genes for imbibing. In another light, any natural selection that may have occurred against drinkers in those many millennia seems obviously not to have reduced the frequency of genes compatible with drinking. That is because those genes have to do with being human, not with drinking, and every human being has them; they cannot be selected for or against among individuals. There may be genetic variants differently affected by alcohol, but genes effecting drinking evolved long before alcohol was discovered: they created human beings.

Alcohol use by the elderly

At last we come to the general problem addressed by this book, which is alcohol use in the elderly in our society. From a biological point of view, there is little that needs to be added. The metabolic response to alcohol seems qualitatively little different in older individuals from what it was when they were younger, though our knowledge about this is quite limited (42). In the course of our evolution as a species, mortality was such that the elderly were rather rare and provided fairly little material on which the forces of evolution could act (64). Evolution is indifferent to what those who have finished rearing their young may or may not do. It is unlikely that, in their few numbers, the elderly made a substantial difference to the fitness of their grown offspring or other close relatives (64), and even today, when many people are able to function in society for a long time postreproductively, the elderly have made most of the contribution to the genetic fitness of their offspring that they will make. They are *hors concours* evolutionarily. If sensing this is a source of depression in the elderly, it can also be a source of some relief in that the elderly no longer need to compete at the intense level required of their younger compatriots. Furthermore, of course, it is uniquely human that they can make a social contribution to society because we are concerned with more than just the necessities of biological life, and social or symbolic contributions are not inherently restricted; it is this that can provide great psychological satisfaction—exactly because of our highly developed neocortex.

Drinking among the elderly generally declines as compared with younger people. The frequency of heavy drinkers is lower, partly because many heavy drinkers do not live as long as lighter drinkers, but even among former heavy drinkers the amount of drinking wanes with age (42). The body may be less able to tolerate the same dose levels as formerly, or the individual may worry about causing ill-health by heavy drinking. He or she may simply be bored with drinking or tired of dealing with its ill-effects. But if drinking heavily is a function of anxiety and stress, much of anxiety and stress is based on the biological drives for territory, mates, and competition within the species, and these problems are reduced with age. Thus, there is a natural life-cycle reduction of the kinds of anxieties that lead people to drink, anxieties that are felt by the youthful individual attempting to wrest a territory for himself, or the mid-lived trying to maintain it. Those individuals able to integrate their knowledge of their elder status into their thoughts, and to accept it, may have less reason to drink for that kind of escape.

This may explain the lowered drinking among the elderly, especially heavy drinking, but then why do many elderly people drink? The primary reason, as with society at large, is obviously just pleasure and relaxation. This is an association with decades' standing, and there is no reason it should cease. Certainly, in the elderly there are also therapeutic reasons to drink, such as the relief of minor pain. There are powerful social factors, too, which are life-cycle related: the death of friends, the marital stresses of retirement, the moving away of children, boredom after retirement, and so on. These are well documented. There is also, of course, the fear of impending illness and death, a purely human symbolic kind of fear, which we can be sure does not affect rats or mice. Fear of, and depression at, incapacitation or serious illness, or of death, may lead to anxieties that can be relieved by the effects of alcohol, and it is unseemly to classify these anxieties in any sense that connotes that they may be unreasonable or pathological. There is no defense against these fears and no amount of alertness can stay them. Wisdom, fatigue, and religion may provide countervailing forces, but for some these may not suffice.

We are discussing genetic and evolutionary concepts in relation to drinking and of course are not, in any sense, trying to play down the importance of problem drinking in older individuals, in whom reactions to psychotropic drugs account for a majority of those treated for adverse drug reactions (50). However, to the extent that anxiety relief lies behind this use of alcohol, it is important to understand the internal, symbolic rationality (from the perspective of the drinker) that is its basis.

CONCLUSION

We have argued the general irrelevance of genes related to animal alcohol use, and to human physiological response to alcohol, in regard to the willingness of human beings to drink. Drinking is a cultural and social phenomenon. Neurological genetic variation, which behavior genetic studies have shown may be related to alcoholism, is not important in explaining the cultural phenomenon of drinking. Similarly, in regard to liver enzyme variants, it should be recognized that the liver contains a complex, easily inducible detoxification system that responds to alcohols. That there is genetic variation in this system is probably a sign either of past selection pressures in some environments or (more likely) a general interindividual variability in the ability to respond to different xenobiotic toxins, which, in general, increases the likelihood that a successful defense exists (much as immunological diversity exists). Nothing in relation to drinking ethanol at pharmacological concentrations need be involved in the evolution of such variability.

Human drinking often, even intentionally, stresses our detoxification system to its physiological limits. It is not surprising that under such stresses genetic variants are revealed, but it is not at all clear that these would have been detectable under natural exposure levels from a small bit of ethanol in a damaged fruit picked from a tree by a monkey. The manifestation of variants under heavy loading by alcohol does not imply that those variations were produced by evolution in regard to that stress at a high, much less markedly lower, level.

The animal and human evidence thus seems, from this perspective, unrelated to the reasons humans drink. The search for a particulate genetic solution to a general problem may relate to specific aspects of that problem, such as chemical addiction, but will not explain the general phenomenon itself. Human drinking is fundamentally a question of the neocortex, but at the present, that is an organ whose evolution we understand only generally and whose structure remains a mystery.

ACKNOWLEDGMENTS

This work was done partially with the support of the National Institute on Aging, grant AG 01028 and the National Cancer Institute, grant CA 19311, which are gratefully acknowledged. I thank Mine Kuban Yucel for her help in searching the literature. This is Demographic Epidemiology of Aging and Disease, paper number 15.

REFERENCES

1. Altshuler, H. (1981): Animal models for alcohol research. In: *Currents in Alcoholism*, Vol. 8, edited by M. Galanter, pp. 343–357. Grune and Stratton, New York.
2. Bacon, M. K. (1974): The dependency-conflict hypothesis and the frequency of drunkenness: Further evidence from a cross-cultural study. *Q. J. Stud. Alcohol*, 35:863.
3. Bacon, M. K. (1976): Alcohol use in tribal societies. In: *Social Aspects of Alcoholism*, edited by B. Kissin and H. Begleiter, pp. 1–36. Plenum Press, New York.
4. Bacon, M. K., Barry, H., and Child, I. (1965): A cross-cultural study of drinking. II. Relations to other features of culture. *Q. J. Stud. Alcohol*, Suppl. 3:29–48.
5. Bacon, M. K., Barry, H., Child, I., and Snyder, C. (1965): A cross-cultural study of drinking. V. Detailed definitions and data. *Q. J. Stud. Alcohol*, Suppl. 3:78–111.
6. Barry, H., Buchwald, C., Child, I., and Bacon, M. K. (1965): A cross-cultural study of drinking. IV. Comparisons with Horton ratings. *Q. J. Stud. Alcohol*, Suppl. 3:62–77.
7. Brown, J. (1975): *The Evolution of Behavior*. Norton, New York.
8. Cadoret, R., Cain, C., and Grove, W. (1980): Development of alcoholism in adoptees raised apart from alcoholic relatives. *Arch. Gen. Psychiatry*, 37:561–563.
9. Cadoret, R., and Guth, A. (1978): Inheritance of alcoholism in adoptees. *Br. J. Psychiatry*, 132:252–258.
10. Chagnon, N. A. (1968): *Yanomamo: The Fierce People*. Holt, Rinehart, and Winston, New York.
11. Child, I., Bacon, M. K., and Barry, H. (1965): A cross-cultural study of drinking. I. Descriptive measurements of drinking customs. *Q. J. Stud. Alcohol*, Suppl. 3:1–28.
12. Cicero, T. J. (1979): Animal models of alcoholism? In: *Animal Models in Alcohol Research*, edited by K. Eriksson, J. D. Sinclair, and K. Kiianmaa, pp. 99–117. Academic Press, London.
13. Cooper, J. M. (1963): Stimulants and narcotics. In: *Handbook of South American Indians. Vol. 5: The Comparative Ethnology of South American Indians*, edited by J. H. Steward, pp. 525–558. Cooper Square Publishers, New York.
14. Cotton, N. S. (1979): The familial incidence of alcoholism. *J. Stud. Alcohol*, 40:89–115.
15. Drewek, K. J. (1979): Inherited drinking and its behavioral correlates. In: *Animal Models in Alcohol Research*, edited by K. Eriksson, J. D. Sinclair, and K. Kiianmaa, pp. 35–49. Academic Press, London.
16. Driver, H. (1969): *Indians of North America* 2nd ed., University of Chicago Press, Chicago.
17. Eriksson, K. (1979): Inherited metabolism and behavior towards alcohol: critical evaluation of human and animal research. In: *Animal Models in Alcohol Research*, edited by K. Eriksson, J. D. Sinclair, and K. Kiianmaa, pp. 3–20. Academic Press, London.
18. Eriksson, K., Sinclair, J. D., And Kiianmaa, K. (1979): *Animal Models in Alcohol Research*. Academic Press, London.
19. Erwin, V., and McClearn, G. (1981): Genetic influences on alcohol consumption and actions of alcohol. In: *Currents in Alcoholism*, Vol. 8, edited by M. Galanter, pp. 405–420. Grune and Stratton, New York.
20. Falk, D. (1980): Language, handedness and primate brains: Did the Australopithecines sign? *Am. Anthrop.*, 82:72–78.
21. Field, P. B. (1962): A new cross-cultural study of drunkenness. In: *Society, Culture, and Drinking Patterns*, edited by D. Pittman and C. Snyder, pp. 49–77. John Wiley, New York.
22. Fitz-Gerald, F. L. (1972): Voluntary alcohol consumption in apes. In: *The Biology of Alcoholism. Vol. 2: Physiology and Behavior*, edited by B. Kissin and H. Begleiter, pp. 169–192. Plenum Press, New York.
23. Goodwin, D. W. (1979): Alcoholism and heredity. *Arch. Gen. Psychiatry*, 36:57.
24. Goodwin, D. W., Schulsinger, F., Hermansen, L., Guze, S. B., and Winokur, G. (1973): Alcohol

problems in adoptees raised apart from alcoholic biological parents. *Arch. Gen. Psychiatry*, 28:238–243.

25. Goodwin, D. W., Schulsinger, F., Moller, F., Hermansen, L., Winokur, G., and Guse, S. B. (1974): Drinking problems in adopted and nonadopted sons of alcoholics. *Arch. Gen. Psychiatry*, 31:164–169.

26. Goodwin, D. W., and Guse, S. B. (1974): Heredity and alcoholism. In: *The Biology of Alcoholism. Vol. 3: Clinical Pathology*, edited by B. Kissin and H. Begleiter, pp. 37–52. Plenum Press, New York.

27. Gould, S. J. (1982): Darwinism and the expansion of evolutionary theory. *Science*, 216:380–387.

28. Hannon, R., and Donlon-Bantz, K. (1976): Effect of housing density on alcohol consumption by rats. *J. Stud. Alcohol*, 37:1556–1563.

29. Heath, D. B. (1975): A critical review of ethnographic studies of alcohol use. In: *Research Advances in Alcohol and Drug Problems*, edited by R. Gibbins, Y. Israel, H. Kalant, R. Popham, W. Schmidt, and R. Smart, pp. 1–92. John Wiley, New York.

30. Heath, D. B. (1976a): Anthropological perspectives on alcohol: An historical review. In: *Cross-cultural Approaches to the Study of Alcohol: An Interdisciplinary Perspective*, edited by M. Everett, M. Waddell, and D. Heath, pp. 41–102. Mouton, The Hague.

31. Heath, D. B. (1976b): Anthropological perspectives on the social biology of alcohol: An introduction to the literature. In: *Social Aspects of Alcoholism*, edited by B. Kissin and H. Begleiter, pp. 37–76. Plenum Press, New York.

32. Holmes, P. W., and Smith, B. L. (1973): Ethanol consumption by pigeons under stress. *Q. J. Stud. Alcohol*, 34:764–768.

33. Horton, D. (1943): The functions of alcohol in primitive societies: A cross-cultural study. *Q. J. Stud. Alcohol*, 4:199–320.

34. Kaij, L. (1960): *Alcoholism in Twins*. Almqvist and Wiksell, Stockholm.

35. Kakihana, R., and Butte, J. (1979): Biochemical correlates of inherited drinking in laboratory animals. In: *Animal Models in Alcohol Research*, edited by K. Eriksson, J. D. Sinclair, and K. Kiianmaa, pp. 21–33. Academic Press, London.

36. Lester, D., and Freed, E. (1972): A rat model of alcoholism? In: *Nature and Nurture in Alcoholism*, edited by F. Seixas, G. Omenn, E. Burk, and S. Eggleston. Ann. N.Y. Acad. Sci.

37. Livingstone, F. B. (1973): Did the Australopithecines sign? *Curr. Anthrop.*, 13:25–29.

38. Loehlin, J. C. (1972): An analysis of alcohol-related questionnaire items from the national merit twin study. *Ann. N.Y. Acad. Sci.*, 197:117–120.

39. Mello, N., and Mendelson, J. (1965): Operant drinking of alcohol on a rate-contingent ratio schedule of reinforcement. *J. Psychiatr. Res.*, 3:145–152.

40. Mello, N., and Mendelson, J. (1971): The effects of drinking to avoid shock on alcohol intake in primates. In: *Biological Aspects of Alcohol*, edited by M. Roach, W. McIsaac, and P. Creaven. University of Texas Press, Austin.

41. Mendelbaum, D. G. (1965): Alcohol and culture. *Curr. Anthrop.*, 6:281–294.

42. Mishara, B., and Kastenbaum, R. (1980): *Alcohol and Old Age*. Grune and Stratton, New York.

43. Mizoi, Y., Hishida, S., and Ijiri, I. (1979): Individual differences in facial flushing and blood acetaldehyde levels after alcohol ingestion. In: *Animal Models in Alcohol Research*, edited by K. Eriksson, J. D. Sinclair, and K. Kiianmaa, pp. 475–480. Academic Press, London.

44. Murdock, G. P. (1963): *Outline of World Cultures*. Human Relations Area Files, New Haven, Connecticut.

45. Murray, R. M., and Gurling, H. M. D. (1980): Genetic contributions to normal and abnormal drinking. In: *Psychopharmacology of Alcohol*, edited by M. Sandler, pp. 89–105. Raven Press, New York.

46. Myers, R. D., and Veale, W. L. (1972): The determinants of alcohol preference in animals. In: *The Biology of Alcoholism, Vol. 2: Physiology and Behavior*, edited by B. Kissin and H. Begleiter, pp. 131–168. Plenum Press, New York.

47. Parker, L., and Radow, B. (1974): Isolation stress and volitional ethanol consumption in the rat. *Physiol. Behav.*, 12:1–3.

48. Partanen, J., Bruun, K., and Markkanen, T. (1966): *Inheritance of Drinking Behavior*. The Finnish Foundation for Alcohol Studies, 14:1–159.

49. Penn, D., McBride, W., Lumeng, L., Gaff, T., and Li, T. (1978): *Pharmacol. Biochem. Behav.*, 8:475–481.

50. Peterson, D., and Thomas, C. (1975): Acute drug reactions among the elderly. *J. Gerontol.*, 30:552–556.
51. Propping, P. (1977): Genetic control of ethanol action on the central nervous system. *Hum. Genet.*, 35:309–334.
52. Reed, T. E. (1978): Racial comparisons of alcohol metabolism: background, problems, and results. *Alcoholism: Clin. Exp. Res.*, 2:83–87.
53. Reed, T. E., Kalant, H., Gibbins, R., Kapur, B., and Rankin, J. (1976): Alcohol and aldehyde metabolism in Caucasians, Chinese, and Amerinds. *Can. Med. Assoc. J.*, 115:851–855.
54. Rogers, D. A. (1972): Factors underlying differences in alcohol preference of inbred strains of mice. In: *The Biology of Alcoholism, Vol. 2: Physiology and Behavior*, edited by B. Kissin and H. Begleiter, pp. 107–130. Plenum Press, New York.
55. Sahlins, M. (1972): *Stone Age Economics*. Aldine, Chicago.
56. Schuckit, M., Goodwin, D., and Winokur, G. (1972): A study of alcoholism in half siblings. *Am. J. Psychiatry*, 128:1132–1136.
57. Service, E. (1971): *Primitive Social Organization*. Random House, New York.
58. Service, E. (1976): *The Origins of the State and Civilization*. Norton, New York.
59. Sinclair, J. D. (1974): Rats learning to work for alcohol. *Nature*, 249:590–592.
60. Sinclair, J. D. (1979): Comparison of the factors which influence voluntary drinking in humans and animals. In: *Animal Models in Alcohol Research*, edited by K. Eriksson, J. D. Sinclair, and K. Kiianmaa, pp. 119–137. Academic Press, New York.
61. Smole, W. J. (1976): *The Yanomama Indians: A Cultural Geography*. University of Texas Press, Austin.
62. Snyder, C. R. (1958): *Alcohol and the Jews: A Cultural Study of Drinking and Sobriety*. Yale Center of Alcohol Studies Monograph, 1, Free Press, Glencoe, IL.
63. Vogel, F., and Motulsky, A. G. (1979): *Human Genetics*. Springer-Verlag, New York.
64. Weiss, K. M. (1981): Evolutionary perspectives on human aging. In: *Other Ways of Growing Old*, edited by P. Amoss and S. Harrell, pp. 25–58, 251–153. Stanford University Press, Stanford, CA.
65. Wilson, E. O. (1975): *Sociobiology*. Harvard University Press, Cambridge.
66. Winokur, G., Tanna, V., Elston, R., and Go, R. (1976): Lack of association of genetic traits with alcoholism. *J. Stud. Alcohol*, 37:1313–1316.
67. Wolff, P. H. (1972): Ethnic differences in alcohol sensitivity. *Science*, 175:449–450.
68. Wolff, P. H. (1973): Vasomotor sensitivity to alcohol in diverse Mongoloid populations. *Am. J. Hum. Genet.*, 25:193–199.
69. Woods, J., Ikomi, F., and Winger, G. (1971): The reinforcing property of ethanol. In: *Biological Aspects of Alcohol*, edited by M. Roach, W. McIsaac, and P. Creaven, pp. 371–388. University of Texas Press, Austin.

Alcoholism in the Elderly, edited by
J. T. Hartford and T. Samorajski.
Raven Press, New York © 1984.

Epidemiology of Alcoholism in the Elderly

*Dan G. Blazer and **Margaret R. Pennybacker

*Department of Psychiatry and Division of Social and Community Psychiatry; and
**Epidemiologic Catchment Area Project, Piedmont Health Study, Duke University
Medical Center, Durham, North Carolina 27710

Clinicians, as well as public health administrators, who wish to comprehend late-life alcoholism within the context of society do well to avail themselves of the epidemiologic perspective. Unfortunately, the availability and quality of population data on late-life alcoholism are sparse and frequently inconclusive. Therefore, need for an epidemiologic approach to the study of alcohol disorders in the elderly is emphasized in this chapter. Studies reviewed from the literature are used not only to document the cumulative experience to date, but also to illustrate methodology shortcomings. Directions for improved research design and implementation are also discussed.

Epidemiology is the study of the distribution of disease in a population. Two essential components of the epidemiologic method are case definition and case finding. Criteria must be determined by which individuals can be included in or excluded from the sample cases. Once the criteria have been established, a method of drawing samples from a population must be selected for the purpose of case finding.

DEFINITION OF A CASE

To determine the number of older people who suffer from alcohol abuse or dependence, criteria for defining a person as a case or noncase must be established. Studies of alcohol use among older people have used different criteria to identify cases. Some studies have attempted to diagnose alcoholism while others have examined "problem drinking" or the drinking practices of older people. The results of studies using different criteria are not strictly comparable, and the rates found have varied greatly.

There are a number of special problems that are encountered when attempting to select the criteria used to identify cases of alcoholism among the elderly. Criteria that have frequently been used to define alcoholism or problem drinking are (a) quantity and frequency of consumption; (b) social problems or problems in role performance due to drinking; (c) tolerance and withdrawal symptoms; and (d) physical health problems.

Those research criteria most often used to define cases have as their norm the younger population and are particularly problematic in their focus on the quantity and frequency of alcohol consumption. Older alcoholics tend to drink daily but to consume smaller amounts than younger alcoholics. And although they consume smaller amounts of alcohol, older drinkers may have problems because of the interaction of medications with alcohol and the presence of chronic illnesses (17).

Smart and Liban (19) suggest that factors other than volume and frequency of consumption are important in predicting problem drinking among the elderly. The degree of isolation, of family involvement, and physical health impairments can help predict problem drinking. Zimberg (22) advocates a "social problems" definition. He claims that older people should be considered alcoholic whenever their drinking causes problems with their families, physical or mental health, employment, finances, or the law, and they are either unwilling or unable to modify their drinking habits to eliminate their problems. The Fourth Special Report to the United States Congress (27) also calls for a pragmatic definition of alcoholism. Problems with a spouse, adult children, others in the social environment, health problems, and accidents due to alcohol use should be the criteria for identifying older alcoholics.

However, many of the social problems frequently used are less likely to apply to older people, for they are less likely to be married or employed and therefore less likely to report marital and job problems related to alcohol use. Older drinkers often maintain a "low profile" and are less likely to cause public disturbances resulting in legal problems (27).

The diagnostic criteria of tolerance or withdrawal symptoms for alcohol dependence may not apply to older drinkers. Withdrawal symptoms may be found only among drinkers who maintain consistently high blood alcohol levels (17). The requirement for withdrawal symptoms may exclude many older drinkers who suffer alcohol-related problems in spite of low levels of consumption.

Alcohol is related to dysfunction at multiple levels simultaneously, for aging cells, organ systems, and organisms (i.e., the whole person) respond differently to alcohol (3). Younger people have higher metabolic rates, faster rates of elimination, fewer nutritional problems, and generally better health (26); therefore, they can consume larger quantities of alcohol without adverse effects. The end result is that a large number of older people who have severe problems resulting from the use of alcohol may be missed by applying the criteria commonly used to identify cases of alcoholism.

CASE FINDING

Older people also pose special problems for case finding in both community surveys and surveys of clinical and institutional settings. Treatment cases may be different from those found in community surveys. Wing et al. (21) note that for every treated case of a psychiatric disorder, there are many untreated ones in the general population. Untreated cases tend to be milder, of shorter duration, or occur in people who resist seeking treatment from the health-care system.

Zimberg (25) claims that older people with alcohol-related problems do not enter the health-care system in a conventional manner. They are rarely found in alcohol detoxification centers because the low quantities of alcohol they consume rarely require detoxification. There is also evidence that older people avoid programs designed for alcoholics such as Alcoholics Anonymous (AA). Only 3% of the people admitted to federally funded alcohol treatment programs are 65 or older (27).

Older alcoholics avoid seeking care until a crisis forces them to seek treatment (11). They are also less likely to encounter the legal system through arrests for public disturbances or drunk driving. In addition, the isolated elderly may have a particularly high incidence of alcoholism (12).

When the elderly with alcohol-related problems do enter the health-care system, alcoholism is frequently undiagnosed. This is possibly the biggest barrier to effective treatment of alcoholism among the elderly (26). Physicians often fail to diagnose alcoholism in the elderly because they confuse perceived symptoms of aging with symptoms of alcoholism. When older people with alcohol-related problems seek medical care, alcoholism is rarely the presenting condition (22). Physicians tend to see and treat the patients' physical problems and fail to recognize or ignore problems with alcohol (15). These patients attempt to hide their problem drinking by denying that a problem exists. Glassock (7) suggests that a "conspiracy of silence" exists between the patient, his or her family, and the health-care provider to keep the patient's drinking problem quiet to avoid the stigma associated with drinking problems.

Community surveys also fail to identify elderly alcoholics because of underreporting symptoms and failure of some surveys to find isolated or transient older people (20). In sum, people seen in treatment may differ substantially from untreated cases in the population, and the methods of case finding employed by many studies, combined with strict case definitions, may miss a substantial number of older alcoholics.

CLINICAL RELEVANCE

When treating older patients, the physician should use standard criteria for diagnosing alcoholism only as a starting point (17). Because elders may be in a position of increased vulnerability because of the stresses of aging and the interaction of medical problems and medications with alcohol, a high index of suspicion is essential for an accurate diagnosis.

Zimberg (25) has identified two types of elderly alcoholics: those who are reacting to one or more of the stresses associated with aging, and those who have a long history of alcohol abuse and continue to drink excessively in late life. A study of treated elderly alcoholics has shown that two-thirds of the patients were early-onset alcoholics and one-third were the late-onset type (13). Late-onset alcoholism is more likely to be identified by family members because of the obvious behavior changes associated with the onset of excessive drinking. Unfortunately, the majority of problems related to alcohol in late life arise in those persons who have a life-long pattern of alcohol abuse. Family members, not to mention the patient, tend to overlook the relevance of alcohol to the physical and psychosocial dysfunction that develops.

The results of the studies of alcoholism among the elderly vary greatly owing to the variety of criteria used to define a case, differences in the samples studied, and differences in data collection procedures. The rates of elders with alcohol-related problems range from 1 to 24% in the community studies and 0 to 63% in the clinical studies (Table 1).

Community surveys have examined the drinking patterns and practices of older people rather than attempting to diagnose alcoholism. For example, Cahalan and Cisin (5) found that 20% of the males and 2% of the females aged 60 or older in their sample were heavy drinkers. Eight percent of the males and 1% of the females were found to be problem drinkers (4). In a community survey done in New York State, Barnes (2) found that 24% of the males aged 60 to 69 were heavy drinkers. Bailey et al. (1) found that 22% of the people aged 65 to 74 and 12% of those 75 or older in their New York City sample were alcoholics. In contrast, Smart and Liban (19) found that 10.6% of people aged 60 or older in a Canadian sample had at least one symptom of alcohol dependency, while 3.5% had at least one alcohol-related problem symptom.

The majority of the studies of alcoholism in the elderly have used patient samples. Schuckit and Miller (16) found that 18% of the geriatric patients on the acute medical wards of a Veterans Administration hospital were alcoholics. McCusker et al. (10) studied patients admitted to the medical wards of a Harlem hospital and found that 63% of the males aged 50 to 69 and 56% of the males aged 70 or older abused alcohol. Thirty-five percent of the females aged 50 to 69 were alcoholics, but none of the females aged 70 or older were. Veterans hospitals and public mental hospitals, however, would be expected to attract a larger percentage of overt alcohol problems throughout the life cycle than would private mental hospitals or general medical facilities. Zimberg (23) found the rate of alcoholism among elderly patients he studied to be much lower at 17%. Simon et al. (18) found that 28% of the aged mentally ill patients they studied had a serious drinking problem on admission. In the nursing homes studied by Blose (3), 40 to 60% of the white male patients had alcohol-related problems.

Because large-scale epidemiologic studies of the incidence and prevalence of alcoholism among elderly community residents have been unavailable to date, it is impossible to estimate accurately the number of elderly alcoholics. Yet the rates are far from being insignificant and suggest a major public health problem.

ETIOLOGIC FACTORS

A discussion of the etiologic factors of alcoholism in the elderly is aided by the distinction made by Zimberg and others between early- and late-onset disorders. Rosin and Glatt (13) refer to the early-onset type as "primary" alcoholism. They

TABLE 1. Prevalence of alcoholism and alcohol problems among the elderly

Reference	Percent prevalence	Sample	Criteria
Cahalan and Cisin (5)	20 Males 2 Females	National community	Heavy drinkers
Cahalan (4)	8 Males 1 Female	National community	Problem drinkers
Barnes (2)	24 Males	NY State community	Heavy drinkers
Bailey, Haberman, and Alksne (1)	22 Aged 65–74 12 Aged 75+	NYC community	Alcoholic
Smart and Liban (19)	10.6 3.5	Canadian community	≥1 Dependency symptom ≥1 Problem symptom
Schuckit and Miller (16)	18	Medical ward patients in a VA hospital	Alcoholic
McCusker, Cherubin. and Zimberg (10)	63 Males aged 50–69 35 Females aged 50–69 56 Males aged 70+ 0 Females aged 70+	Medical ward patients in a Harlem hospital	Alcohol abuse
Simon, Epstein, and Reynolds (18)	28	Mentally ill patients	Serious drinking problem on admission
Zimberg (22)	17	Community mental health center inpatients	Alcohol-abuse problem on admission
Blose (3)	40–60	White male nursing home patients	Alcohol-related problems

suggest the causes of this disorder are personality and behavior factors. Late-onset alcoholism or "reactive" alcoholism is believed to be due to "environmental influences" such as bereavement, retirement, loneliness, infirmity, or marital stress. Glatt (8) identifies three precipitating factors in late-onset alcoholism: (a) habitual drinking patterns prior to late life; (b) personality factors; and (c) environmental factors. The personality factors include anxiety and worry whereas environmental factors include loss and loneliness. He notes, however, that personality factors probably play less of an etiologic role in late-onset alcoholism. Because of the cross-sectional nature of most of the studies of alcoholism in late life, the causal order of events is usually not clear. In addition to being a reaction to stressful life events, alcoholism may, in fact, cause stressful events such as marital discord and social isolation.

The lack of longitudinal studies of alcoholism also makes it difficult to project the extent of the problem in the future. Cross-sectional studies compare the drinking practices of one age group with those of other age groups at one point in time. Although there is evidence that many alcoholics abstain or decrease their drinking in late life, not all do. The possibility of cohort effects should not be ignored when attempting to explain why older people drink less. Older persons who entered adulthood during the prohibition and the economic depression prior to World War II may have had lower rates of alcohol use throughout their lives. The fact that larger numbers of people in successive cohorts consume alcoholic beverages, coupled with Glatt's finding that late-onset alcoholics drink moderately prior to old age, suggests that more elders may be at risk for developing late-onset alcoholism in the future. Research has consistently shown that males drink more than females; but as social roles and norms for women change, females are increasing their rate of alcohol use while the rate for males remains fairly stable. Women make up a larger proportion of the elderly, and they may be at greater risk for alcoholism in the future. Sheer numbers (1,500 people reach age 65 in the United States each day) indicate that alcoholism and alcohol-related problems among the elderly will be greater in the future.

TREATMENT

It is estimated that 85% of all alcoholics and problem-drinkers are not receiving formal treatment services, and the elderly comprise a disproportionately small number of those who do receive treatment (27). Nine percent of the alcoholics treated in a Washington State alcohol treatment program were aged 60 or over, proportionately less than their demographic representations in the community (14).

Zimberg (22,24) and Pascerelli (12) report good treatment outcomes for both early- and late-onset elderly alcoholics. Seventy-three percent of elderly alcoholics completed an alcohol treatment program, as compared with 40% of younger alcoholics. The older group required a shorter time in treatment (14), which emphasizes the need for effective case-finding techniques. Older drinkers, as mentioned, tend to avoid traditional treatment groups for alcoholics such as AA. Treatment of the late-life alcoholic may be among the most cost-efficient and effective interventions in the psychiatric care of the elderly.

Glassock (7) notes that there are few treatment programs designed to address the needs of the elderly and that there is a need for self-help groups tailored specifically for these people. Because alcohol-related problems often involve the patient's family and seldom come to public attention, effective outreach programs might be designed to reach the older alcoholic through his or her family, friends, or existing programs for senior citizens. Because they tend to avoid the usual sources of care, there is a need for outreach programs and new case-finding techniques (25). Epidemiologic studies can provide the data base for launching such programs by documenting the nature and extent of alcohol-related problems in our elderly population.

NEED FOR RESEARCH

Although the problem of alcoholism among the elderly has received more attention in recent years, and the extent of the problem is now better understood, reliable estimates of the number of older people who are alcoholics or who suffer from alcohol-related problems cannot yet be determined. Large-scale studies of random samples of elderly community and institutional residents are needed to determine adequately the scope of the problem.

The Epidemiologic Catchment Area (ECA) program, sponsored by the National Institute of Mental Health (NIMH), presents a unique opportunity to answer many questions about older alcoholics. The ECA program is designed to directly estimate the incidence and prevalence of psychiatric disorders among people living in the community and in long-term care institutions. The frequency of alcohol abuse and alcohol dependence, along with a number of other *DSM III*[1] diagnoses of the American Psychiatric Association, are determined by the survey. Five sites geographically distributed across the country are participating and will have a combined sample of more than 15,000 community residents and 2,500 institutional residents. Rigorous methods of case finding are being employed to guard against underrepresentation of hard-to-reach groups. Although the survey design includes all adults aged 18 and older, three survey sites also have oversamples of the elderly.

The core data collection instrument of the ECA program is the Diagnostic Interview Schedule (DIS), which was developed by NIMH. The DIS was designed to yield computer-generated diagnoses of specific psychiatric disorders based on symptom self-reports using *DSM-III*, Feighner, and research diagnostic criteria (RDC) criteria.

The inclusion of questions on specific social problems, tolerance and withdrawal symptoms, physical symptoms, and quantity and frequency of intake of alcohol will permit calculations of rates using varying definitions of alcoholism. The number of older people who suffer from significant alcohol-related problems, but who might be missed by more rigorous diagnostic definitions, can therefore be estimated.

---

[1]*Diagnostic and Statistical Manual of Mental Disorders.*

Another valuable feature of the study for the understanding of the nature of alcoholism in the elderly is that it links symptom and diagnostic information to health services utilization data. Those groups with reported need who are not currently receiving care will be identified. Data on the sources of care used by the elderly and the barriers to treatment for underserved populations will be examined.

The information gathered on lifetime and current symptoms, coupled with age of onset, will allow the identification of two types of alcoholics, early- and late-onset. The proportion of each type in the community and in institutions can then be determined. Some survey sites are also gathering data on stressful life events which can be related to late-onset alcoholism.

The design is longitudinal in that the first personal interview is followed by a short telephone interview 6 months later and an additional personal interview 1 year after the initial interview. Although the length of the data-collection period is too short to assess the effects of differential drinking patterns associated with different cohorts of individuals, it will present some clues as to the causal order of events leading to late-life alcoholism.

Data gathered in the ECA program will complement other epidemiologic studies presently being conducted, such as case-control studies of elderly alcoholics in treatment facilities and the Scandinavian genetic studies (9,6). The significant improvement in case-finding techniques, coupled with such a large probability sample from the community, will permit the testing of etiologic hypotheses previously inaccessible to researchers and clinicians. Though any epidemiologic study is inherently flawed, and certain crucial data inevitably escape detection, epidemiologists should possess a data base within the next three years that will be far superior to any available to date. If the estimates derived from analysis of the ECA data approximate those of previous studies, then greater confidence can be given to more indirect and less rigorous methods of inquiry. If not, then many of our present assumptions about late-life alcoholism must be revised.

REFERENCES

1. Bailey, M. B., Haberman, P. W., and Alksne, H. (1965): The epidemiology of alcoholism in an urban residential area. *Q. J. Stud. Alcohol*, 26:19–40.
2. Barnes, G. M. (1979): Alcohol use among older persons: Findings from a western New York State general population survey. *J. Am. Geriatr. Soc.*, 26:244–250.
3. Blose, I. L. (1978): The relationship of alcohol and the elderly. *Alcoholism*, 2:17–21.
4. Cahalan, D. (1970): *Problem Drinkers*. p. 98. Jossey-Bass, San Francisco.
5. Cahalan, D., and Cisin, I. H. (1968): American drinking practices: Summary of findings from a national probability sample. *Q. J. Stud. Alcohol*, 29:130–151.
6. Cloninger, C. R., Bohman, M., and Sigvardsson, S. (1981): Inheritance of alcohol abuse. *Arch. Gen. Psychiatry*, 38:861–868.
7. Glassock, J. A. (1982): Older alcoholics: An underserved population. *Generations*, Spring 192:23–24,64.
8. Glatt, M. M. (1978): Experiences with elderly alcoholics in England. *Alcoholism*, 2:23–26.
9. Goodwin, D. W., Crane, J. B., and Guze, S. B. (1969): Alcoholic "blackouts": A review and clinical study of 100 alcoholics. *Am. J. Psychiatry*, 126:191–198.
10. McCusker, J., Cherubin, C. F., and Zimberg, S. (1971): Prevalence of alcoholism in a general municipal hospital population. *N.Y. State J. Med.*, 71:751–754.

11. Myerson, D. J. (1978): Organic problems in the aged: Brain syndromes and alcoholism—as the alcoholic grows older. *J. Geriatr. Psychiatry*, 11:175–189.
12. Pascerelli, E. F. (1974): Drug dependence: An age old problem compounded by old age. *Geriatrics*, 29:109–115.
13. Rosin, A. J., and Glatt, M. M. (1971): Alcohol excess in the elderly. *J. Stud. Alcohol*, 32:53–59.
14. Schuckit, M. A. (1977): Geriatric alcoholism and drug abuse. *Gerontologist*, 17:168–174.
15. Schuckit, M. A., Atkinson, J. H., and Miller, P. L. (1980): A three-year follow-up of elderly alcoholics. *J. Clin. Psychiatry*, 42:412–416.
16. Schuckit, M. A., and Miller, P. L. (1976): Alcoholism in elderly men: A survey of a general medical ward. *Ann. N.Y. Acad. Sci.*, 273:558–571.
17. Schuckit, M. A., and Pastor, P. A. (1978): The elderly as a unique population: Alcoholism. *Alcoholism*, 2:31–38.
18. Simon, A., Epstein, L. J., and Reynolds, L. (1968): Alcoholism in the geriatric mentally ill. *Geriatrics*, 23:125–131.
19. Smart, R. G., and Liban, C. B. (1981): Predictors of problem drinking among elderly, middle-aged and youthful drinkers. *J. Psychoactive Drugs*, 13:153–163.
20. Van der Kolk, B. A. (1978): Organic problems in the aged: Brain syndromes and alcoholism—introductory remarks on alcoholism. *J. Geriatr. Psychiatry*, 11:171–174.
21. Wing, J. K., Bebbington, P., and Robins, L. N. (1981): Theory-testing in psychiatric epidemiology. In: *What Is a Case?*, edited by J. K. Wing, P. Bebbington, and L. N. Robins, pp. 1–9. Grant McIntyre, London.
22. Zimberg, S. (1974): The elderly alcoholic. *Gerontologist*, 14:221–224.
23. Zimberg, S. (1974): Two types of problem drinkers: both can be managed. *Geriatrics*, 29(8):135–138.
24. Zimberg, S. (1978): Diagnosis and treatment of the elderly alcoholic. *Alcoholism*, 2:27–29.
25. Zimberg, S. (1978): Treatment of the elderly alcholic in the community and in an institutional setting. *Addict. Dis.*, 3:417–427.
26. U.S. Department of Health, Education and Welfare, Public Health Service, Alcohol, Drug Abuse, and Mental Health Administration (1978): Third Special Report to the U.S. Congress on *Alcohol and Health*, Rockville, MD.
27. U.S. Department of Health and Human Services, Public Health Service, Alcohol, Drug Abuse, and Mental Health Administration (1981): Fourth Special Report to the U.S. Congress on *Alcohol and Health*, Rockville, MD.

Alcoholism in the Elderly, edited by
J. T. Hartford and T. Samorajski.
Raven Press, New York © 1984.

Animal Models for Alcohol and Aging Research: Methodological Issues

Ernest L. Abel

Research Institute on Alcoholism, Buffalo, New York 14203

Currently there are about 20 million Americans over the age of 65 (4). This represents about 10% of the population of the United States, and the proportion of the elderly continues to accelerate at a pace that exceeds the population growth of the country as a whole. At the turn of the century, Americans over the age of 65 accounted for 4% of the population. In 1972, this proportion had increased to 10%. By the year 2032, it is expected to rise to 17 to 20% (4). With medical advances in the treatment of problems such as cancer and cardiovascular diseases, the trend toward increased life expectancy will, no doubt, continue unabated for many years to come. Associated with the increase in the population of the elderly are a number of important social and medical considerations hitherto largely ignored. For example, the impact of growing numbers of the elderly on family life, the many adjustments that must be made by society to the elderly in terms of community services, the many adjustments that must be made by the elderly themselves to new social and occupational crises, and so on, are just now beginning to receive attention.

Inherent in the biological aging process itself is the biomedical problem of deteriorating health and mental function. Among the many biomedical events associated with aging are various physiological changes that influence drug responsiveness such as decreases in drug metabolizing activity due to changes in hepatic enzyme reactions, decreases in drug elimination rate due to changes in renal function, altered drug distribution due to reduced fluid volume and mass in the body, and altered responsiveness of the central nervous system. Because of changes in nerve cell functioning associated with aging, for instance, the elderly may be more susceptible to many of alcohol's effects such that a given amount of alcohol may have a much greater effect on the elderly than on younger adults. Thus, although they may drink less, the elderly may be more likely to have drinking problems because of age-related complications.

There is, in fact, evidence that the elderly are a particularly at-risk population for alcohol-related problems. Drunkenness has been reported to be responsible for the majority of arrests in Americans over 60 years of age (5), and alcohol has been found to be a contributing factor in suicide among the elderly (14). In this context, it should be noted that people over 65 account for about 25% of the annual suicides in the United States (4).

Many investigators assume that the elderly alcohol abuser is the younger alcohol abuser who has survived to old age. Yet, mounting evidence indicates that many of the elderly develop problem-drinking behavior who have not had such difficulties as younger adults. On the basis of their study of elderly patients seen in alcoholism and geriatric units, for example, Glatt and Rosin (9) contend that many elderly alcoholics are actually nondrinkers or moderate drinkers until they reach old age, at which time they begin heavy drinking to deal with the emotional stresses associated with aging.

In their recent overview of the neurobiological interactions between aging and alcohol abuse, Freund and Butters (8) identified three "challenges for the future" in alcohol-related research. These were: (a) to describe and compare alcohol-related alterations at different ages for all levels of biological organization; (b) to determine the causal relationship, if any, between alcohol or aging and the pathogenesis of impaired behavior; and, (c) to determine risk factors that predispose individuals to become more affected than others by alcohol abuse and aging.

Each of these "challenges" encompasses a vast array of additional questions, the answers to which may elucidate the overall problem of how alcohol and the aging process interact. Because of the myriad interactions between alcohol use and abuse and the aging process in humans, it is difficult, if not impossible, to conduct meaningful research on this target population, even if researchers were not constrained by ethical considerations. The only viable alternative is to conduct relevant research in animals and to extrapolate the findings from such research to humans. The validity of such extrapolation will, of course, depend in large measure on the methodological rigor with which such studies are conducted.

One of the main advantages of animal studies is the potential for exercising "control" over those variables that would be difficult, if not impossible, to control in humans, e.g., use of other drugs, overall health, physical stress. Animal studies also permit more intensive and methodological examination of important parameters such as dosage, actual blood alcohol levels, and acetaldehyde levels. Studies in animals also permit dissociation of alcohol's pharmacological actions from its nutritional properties to some extent. These and other issues are discussed more fully in following sections. Another basic advantage of animal studies is the shortened life-span of these subjects, especially in the case of rats and mice—two of the most widely used species in the laboratory.

The basic disadvantage, of course, is that observations in rats and mice may not be relevant to humans. However, as Johnson (12) has commented, "there are many aspects of rodent aging...from the molecular level to the level of the whole organism, which are so similar to human aging that it is hard to believe that rodent models are not valid." Johnson then goes on to catalog an impressive list of similarities between humans and rodents to support this statement. Thus, whereas the question of validity must always be asked, it is reassuring that the answer is more positive than negative with respect to the value of animal experimentation vis à vis the human condition.

METHODOLOGICAL ISSUES INVOLVED IN DEVELOPING ANIMAL MODELS TO STUDY ALCOHOL AND AGING

Dose-Response Studies

The need for dose-response studies should be obvious. A given dose of alcohol may or may not have an observable biobehavioral effect for many reasons. The dose may be too low to produce any observable effect, for example. Only by exploring a range of different doses is it possible to examine alcohol's, or any drug's, effects in a meaningful way. Studies that fail to evaluate dosages in relation to actual blood alcohol levels in aging studies, however, may be misleading (see below).

Route of Administration

The means by which alcohol is introduced into the animals is important. The three most frequently used methods are the liquid diet method, placing alcohol into the drinking water, and direct administration by intubation or injection.

Voluntary consumption of alcohol in drinking water is by far the least methodologically rigorous procedure for several reasons. The first is that animals will rarely consume enough alcohol in their drinking water to achieve blood alcohol levels above 100 mg%.

A second reason is that animals of different ages differ in their voluntary consumption of alcohol. In general, the older the animal, the less alcohol it will consume (1,10,11,18). The concentration of the alcoholic solution is an important variable affecting this relationship. As indicated by Fig. 1, at concentrations below 10%

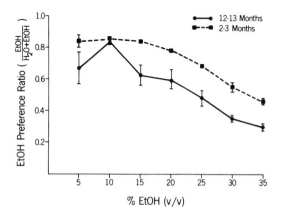

FIG. 1. Differential effects of age on preference for ethanol (EtOH) in mice. *Points* represent mean, *bars* represent SEM. (From Abel, ref. 1, with permission.)

vol/vol, differences in consumption between older and younger animals are not as great as when the concentrations are higher (see also Wood, ref. 18).

One of the reasons older animals may differ from younger animals in voluntary consumption of alcohol is a difference in taste sensitivity for alcohol (10). Another reason is that older animals achieve as high a blood alcohol level as younger animals, even though the former may consume less alcohol. A third possibility is that older animals achieve higher blood acetaldehyde levels than younger animals. As yet, none of these possibilities have been tested. In any case, placing alcohol in drinking water to introduce it into the animal has little value for exploring alcohol's effects on aging, and it creates too many methodological problems to result in unequivocal interpretations of any data resulting from such a procedure.

The liquid diet method is a widely used procedure wherein alcohol is placed into a commercially available diet such as Sustacal® or BioServ®, and this is provided to the animal as its only source of food and fluid. This procedure can result in blood alcohol levels above 100 mg%, and the diet is relatively easy to prepare and administer and can be used for chronic studies of alcohol administration. Although animals of different ages may not consume the same amount of diet, this problem can be circumvented to some extent by "pair-feeding," i.e., one group is allocated the same quantity of diet as that consumed by the group with which it is matched. The disadvantage of this method is that animals differ widely in their patterns of consumption; therefore, all animals will not be exposed to the same amount of alcohol at the same time. Differences in consumption patterns could mean that severity of withdrawal might not be due to age-related biochemical effects but to period since last exposure. This might especially occur if animals are pair-fed, since the pair-fed group often consumes much of its diet as soon as it is presented, whereas the ad-lib group eats sporadically during the 24-hr feeding period.

The third method involves the direct administration of alcohol into the animal. This method has the advantage of allowing more accurate determinations of dose-response effects, since all animals are given the same dose at the same time. Blood alcohol levels and the time course of blood alcohol disappearance can also be determined with greater uniformity. Another advantage is that dosages can be adjusted so that animals of different ages achieve the same alcohol levels. In this way, one can determine if differences between animals are due to differences in biological sensitivity to alcohol or to differences in blood alcohol levels. For example, Abel and York (2) observed that a given dose of alcohol impaired Rotarod performance in older animals to a greater extent than in younger animals. However, when older and younger animals were treated so that their blood alcohol levels did not differ significantly, age differences were no longer significant (2).

Nutritional Considerations

Alcohol contains 7.1 calories per gram. Ingestion of these calories means that animals (and humans) are able to satisfy some of their caloric needs from alcohol alone. However, these calories are "empty," i.e., they do not supply other nutrient requirements. In long-term studies, this may mean that animals that eat less because of alcohol ingestion may become undernourished. Alcohol's pharmacological actions would thus be confounded with its nutritional effects.

One way of dealing with the problem of undernutrition is the pair-feeding technique already mentioned. With this procedure, a control group is only allotted the same amount of food and water consumed the previous day by the animals with which it is paired. This procedure permits comparison of the effects of alcohol plus food and water reduction with that of food and water reduction alone. Comparisons would thus be made between the different pair-fed groups at the different ages being tested. If differences were observed, interpretation of data would have to take into account the role of nutritional factors in assessing alcohol's effects on the aging process.

With respect to nutritional factors, there is also the question of aging's effects on absorption of nutrients. Although this is not a consideration in acute studies involving alcohol administration, in long-term studies age-related effects on absorption of nutrients could be a confounding factor, especially since alcohol itself also affects absorption of nutrients from the intestine (3).

Elderly adults frequently complain of abdominal problems related to diet and appetite (7), and several studies have shown that absorption of nutrients from the intestine is impaired (7,13). Aging also affects absorption of nutrients in laboratory animals (19), and the combination of alcohol consumption and aging may result in undernutrition. While pair-feeding could control alcohol-related decreases in food intake, the problem of nutrient absorption has not been addressed. Whereas special diets have been prepared for pregnant laboratory animals, comparable attention has not yet been devoted to the need for special diets for aging animals.

Blood Alcohol Levels

In aging studies, it is essential to determine blood alcohol levels. Animals of different ages may differ in their responses to alcohol not because of differential sensitivity, but because of different blood alcohol levels resulting from the same dosage. For example, Abel and York (2) administered 1 g/kg alcohol to rats aged 2 to 3, 11 to 12, or 18 to 20 months of age. Blood alcohol levels were approximately 70, 80, and 100 mg%, respectively, for the three ages (see Fig. 2).

One reason for these differences in blood alcohol levels is an age-related decrease in body water content and a decreased lean body mass related to total body mass (17,16). As a result of the lower body water content in older animals, there is a smaller volume of distribution so that higher blood alcohol levels occur.

One way of dealing with this problem, proposed by York (20), is to estimate body water content and to inject animals on this basis. For example, York (20) "freeze-dried" rats 5 to 7, 14 to 16, and 24 to 26 months old to determine their body water content. He then injected a comparable group of animals on the basis of these body water estimates and was able to achieve roughly comparable blood alcohol levels for animals of different ages. Animals of different ages so injected did not differ in their hypothermic response to alcohol.

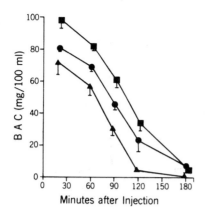

FIG. 2. Disappearance of ethanol (1.0 g/kg, i.p.) from the blood in young (▲, 2–3 months), middle-age (●, 12–14 months), and old (■, 18–20 months) rats. *N* = 10/group. *Vertical lines* refer to SEM. BAC, blood alcohol concentration. (From Abel, ref. 2, with permission.)

TABLE 1. *Ethanol hypnosis in rats of different ages*

Age group (months)	Weight (g)		Onset of hypnosis (min)		Sleep time (min)		Blood ethanol at waking (mg/100 ml)	
	Mean	SE	Mean	SE	Mean	SE	Mean	SE
Young (2–3)	183	3	1.88	0.06	177	10	268	8
Middle (12–14)	363	9	2.04	0.14	296	19	207	10
Old (18–20)	441	23	2.07	0.09	>454	36[a]	213	10

[a]For animals from which blood samples were taken sleep time = 384 min (SE = 50.7). From Abel, ref. 2, with permission.

These observations suggest that one reason for the differences between young and old animals in their responses to alcohol is not an age-related one, but, rather, a basic difference in blood alcohol levels.

On the other hand, there are data that do suggest greater age-related tissue sensitivity to alcohol's actions. Abel and York (2) reported that 18- to 20-month-old rats took significantly longer to regain their righting reflex than 2- to 3- or 11- to 12-month-old rats following an injection of alcohol (4 g/kg) [see also Abel (1) and Ernst et al. (6)]. However, blood (and presumably brain) alcohol levels were lower in older animals at the time of awakening (Table 1). This observation suggests that the central nervous system of the older animals was more sensitive to the effects of alcohol. Similarly, Abel (1) reported that 12- to 13-month-old mice "slept" longer than 2- to 3-month-old mice following injection of alcohol (4 g/kg, i.p.), but that blood alcohol levels at time of awakening were not significantly different (Fig. 3).

At the molecular level, Sun and Samorajski (15) observed a possible correlation of these observations of increased brain sensitivity in older animals. In their study, (Na^+-K^+)-adenosine triphosphatase (ATPase) activity was inhibited by alcohol to a greater extent in synaptosomes from older mice (26–29 months) compared with younger mice (3–8 months) and in brains from older humans obtained at autopsy.

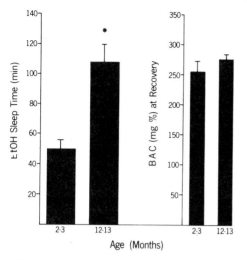

FIG. 3. Differential effects of ethanol (EtOH) on sleep time in mice of different ages and blood alcohol concentrations (BAC) at time of awakening. Bars represent SEM. $p < 0.05$. (From Abel, ref. 1, with permission.)

This enzyme is responsible for regulation of membrane polarization in the nervous system, and its activity is highly dependent on the structural integrity of nerve cell membranes (15). Since there is generally a progressive and irreversible alteration of nerve cell structure associated with aging, one might predict that the behavior of older animals and men would be affected to a much greater degree by an equivalent amount of alcohol than would younger animals. To demonstrate such a differential effect behaviorally, however, it is necessary to equate blood alcohol levels as previously discussed.

SUMMARY AND CONCLUSIONS

The elderly constitute a special biomedical group because of age-related changes in physiological functioning. One such change is the response to alcohol, which may be greater in older people than in their younger counterparts, despite equal amounts of consumption. The reasons for such differences are being explored through the use of "animal models." However, before such models can be of heuristic value, a number of methodological issues must be addressed. Hitherto, little attention has been devoted to these issues, especially in the case of long-term studies. Until these issues are resolved, conclusions will remain equivocal, and the value of animal studies for the understanding of alcohol's actions in the human will be diminished.

REFERENCES

1. Abel, E. L. (1978): Effects of ethanol and pentobarbital in mice of different ages. *Physiol. Psychol.*, 6:366–368.

2. Abel, E. L., and York, J. L. (1979): Age-related differences in response to ethanol in the rat. *Physiol. Psychol.*, 1:391–395.
3. Barone, E. R., Pirula, R. C., and Lieber, C. S. (1974): Small intestinal damage and changes in cell population produced by ethanol ingestion in the rat. *Gastroenterology*, 66:226–234.
4. Butler, R. N. (1975): *Why Survive? Being Old in America.* Harper and Row, New York.
5. Epstein, L. J., and Simon, A. (1970): Antisocial behavior of the elderly. *Calif. Mental Health Res. Dig.*, 8:78–79.
6. Ernst, A. J., Dempster, J. P., Yee, R., St. Denis, C., and Nakano, L. (1976): Alcohol toxicity, blood alcohol concentration, and body water in young and old rats. *J. Studies Alcohol*, 37:347–356.
7. Fikry, M. E., and Aboul-Wafa, M. H. (1965): Intestinal absorption in the old. *Gerontologia Clinica*, 7:171–178.
8. Freund, G., and Butters, N. (1982): Alcohol and aging: Challenges for the future. *Alcoholism: Clin. Exp. Res.*, 6:1–2.
9. Glatt, M., and Rosin, A. J. (1964): Aspects of alcoholism in the elderly. *Lancet*, 2:472–473.
10. Goodrick, C. L. (1967): Alcohol preference of the male Sprague-Dawley albino rat as a function of age. *J. Gerontol.*, 22:369–371.
11. Goodrick, C. L. (1975): Behavioral differences in young and aged mice. Strain differences for activity measures, operant learning, sensory discrimination, and alcohol preference. *Exp. Aging Res.*, 1:191–207.
12. Johnson, H. A. (1971): The relevance of the rodent as a model system of aging in man. In: *Development of the Rodent as a Model System of Aging*, edited by D. C. Gibson, pp. 3–6. N.I.C.H.D., Rockville, MD.
13. Meyer, J., Sorter, H., Oliver, J., and Necheles, H. (1943): Studies in old age. VII. Intestinal absorption in old age. *Gastroenterology*, 1:876–881.
14. Petrilowitsch, N. (1968): Problem areas in older persons as reflected in suicidal patients. In: *Problems of Psychotherapy Among Older Persons.* Karger, New York.
15. Sun, A. Y., and Samorajski, T. (1975): The effects of age and alcohol on ($Na^+ + K^+$)-ATPase activity of whole homogenate and synaptosomes from mouse and human brain. *J. Neurochem.*, 24:161–164.
16. Vestal, R. E., McGuire, E. A., Tobin, J. D., Andres, R., Norris, A. H., and Mizey, E. (1977): Aging and ethanol metabolism. *Clin. Pharmacol. Therap.*, 21:343–354.
17. Wiberg, G. S., Samson, J. M., Maxwell, W. B., Coldwell, B. B., and Trenholm, H. L. (1971): Further studies on the acute toxicity of ethanol in young-old rats: Relative importance of pulmonary excretion and total body water. *Toxicol. Appl. Pharmacol.*, 20:22–29.
18. Wood, U. G. (1976): Age-associated differences in response to alcohol in rats and mice: A biochemical and behavioral review. *Exp. Aging Res.*, 2:543–562.
19. Yeh, S. D. J., Soltz, W., and Chow, B. F. (1965): The effect of age on iron absorption in rats. *J. Gerontol.*, 20:177–180.
20. York, J. L. (1982): The influence of age upon the physiological response to ethanol. In: *Alcoholism and Aging. Advances in Research*, edited by W. G. Wood and M. Elias, CRC Press, Boca Raton, FL.

Alcoholism in the Elderly, edited by
J. T. Hartford and T. Samorajski.
Raven Press, New York © 1984.

Biology of Alcoholism and Aging in Rodents: Brain and Liver

*T. Samorajski, *Katherine Persson, *Courtney Bissell,
*Larry Brizzee, **Francine Lancaster, and †Kenneth R. Brizzee

*Texas Research Institute of Mental Sciences, Houston, Texas 77030;
**Texas Woman's University, Houston, Texas 77030; and †Delta Regional Primate
Research Center, Tulane University, Covington, Louisiana 70433

The effects of alcohol consumption and aging are similar in several ways. Impaired cognitive behavior, for example, is characteristic of both aging and alcohol abuse. Death of neurons is another feature common to aging and alcoholism, although the locus and severity of loss may differ in these two conditions. Similarities or differences of behavior or morphology, however, do not necessarily imply or exclude interactions between aging and alcohol consumption at molecular levels of organization (9,10). A multitude of causal mechanisms may be funneled into identical or different possible responses.

Inherent in the aging process itself are various molecular changes that influence responsiveness to drugs. Subtle changes with age in neuronal sensitivity, hepatic enzyme activity, kidney function, and reduced lean body mass may influence responsiveness to alcohol (1). Each of these issues complicates the question of how aging and alcohol interact. One way to deal with this problem is to determine the age levels at which interactions between aging and alcohol ingestion might occur.

One might predict that the behavior of older animals and of human beings would be affected more than that of younger ones by an equivalent amount of alcohol. Because of the long life and great individual differences among human subjects, it is difficult, if not impossible, to answer questions related to human aging and alcohol use and abuse. The only way to approach the answers is to conduct relevant research with appropriate "animal models" and draw inferences from the results to human conditions.

We undertook the present study with young, mature, and old mice and rats to determine the extent to which chronic administration of alcohol (ethanol) might affect brain and liver functions. Most investigators agree that excessive use of alcohol affects the nervous system and liver more markedly than it does other organs of the body. The C57BL/6J mouse strain was chosen for the first experiment since these rodents are highly inbred and are frequently used for alcohol studies and because they prefer ethanol to water (40). Rats (Sprague-Dawley strain) were also used (experiment 2) to facilitate the morphologic studies.

Rodent studies indicate that long-term exposure to alcohol leads to permanent neuroanatomical and functional deficits, which, in many respects, are similar to changes associated with aging (9,10). A major objective of this study, therefore, was to observe the pattern of behavior and the morphologic and biochemical changes in the brain and liver of mice and rats of different ages exposed to chronic ethanol administration. A clearer understanding of these changes may not only yield greater insight into the nature of alcohol and aging interactions, but may also contribute to the development of indices that may be useful for the assessment of brain and liver damage associated with aging and alcohol abuse. Finally, the study of multiple age changes in the brain and liver of rodents may help to elucidate treatment strategies that may be useful for human application.

METHODS

A total of 72 male C57BL/6J mice (Jackson Laboratories, Bar Harbor, ME) aged 10, 17, and 24 months (experiment 1) and 12 male Sprague-Dawley rats (National Institute of Aging) aged 6 and 28 months (experiment 2) were used in the study. Mice were housed 12 to a cage, rats one to a cage, and maintained in light- and temperature-controlled rooms. The animals were distributed into equal groups at each age level according to weight. Their physical appearance was examined daily, and they were weighed once weekly throughout the experimental period.

The experimental animals (mice and rats) were maintained on nutritionally complete liquid diets containing 6 to 7% vol/vol of ethanol, with ethanol supplying 37% of the available calories (45). Control animals were pair-fed an equivalent diet in which sucrose was substituted isocalorically for ethanol. The duration of ethanol treatment was 6 months because of evidence (27,44,45) that this period of treatment with 6 to 7% vol/vol of ethanol results in altered brain structure and function in rodents despite a nutritionally adequate diet.

Behavior and liver function tests (hexobarbital narcosis) were conducted after 2, 4, and 6 months of alcohol administration to assess treatment duration effects on mice of different ages. Tests were conducted after a 6- to 14-day alcohol-free period to eliminate or minimize withdrawal effects. Blood ethanol and acetaldehyde levels were determined after 4 months of ethanol treatment followed by 1 day for dryout. Mice were then challenged with an acute (2 mg/kg) dose of ethanol. Survival ranged from 83% (young controls) to 25% (old ethanol-treated mice) at the conclusion of the 6-month treatment period.

After the last test, all animals were sacrificed. Their brains and livers were removed and processed for biochemical and morphological studies. At the time of sacrifice, animals had been withdrawn from alcohol for 15 days. Behavior, biochemical, and morphological tests and evaluations were selected on the basis of previously published reports of significant changes with either aging or chronic alcohol administration (3,8,20,31,34,36).

RESULTS

Experiment 1—Mice

Blood Ethanol and Acetaldehyde Levels

Quantitations of blood ethanol and acetaldehyde levels were done by gas chromatography as previously described (18,19). Ethanol uptake and ethanol and acetaldehyde clearance rates were calculated from regression lines fitted to the data. The slopes of the regression lines were compared by one-way analysis of variance (ANOVA). Samples of blood for analysis were obtained only at one treatment interval (4 months of ethanol administration) to minimize the animals' stress.

Blood ethanol levels after a single dose of ethanol (EtOH) (2 mg/kg; 40% ethanol) administered to the 14-, 21-, and 28-month-old control and alcohol-treated mice (4 months plus a 1-day dryout) are shown in Fig. 1. Blood levels varied considerably between the three age groups of acute and chronically treated mice. In general, older mice (21 and 28 months) that had been treated previously with ethanol (4 months) tended to have lower blood alcohol levels than did acutely treated mice. The difference was significant ($P < 0.05$) at 21 months. There was a more rapid decrease in blood ethanol levels in the younger mice (14 months) during the 120 minutes after injection compared with the older (21 and 28 months) mice. This is probably caused by faster ethanol metabolism in younger animals (28).

Blood acetaldehyde levels after a single dose of ethanol (2 mg/kg) administered to the 14-, 21-, and 28-month-old control and alcohol-treated mice (4 months plus a 1-day dryout) are shown in Fig. 2. There was no significant difference in acetaldehyde clearance between acute and chronically treated mice at any of the three

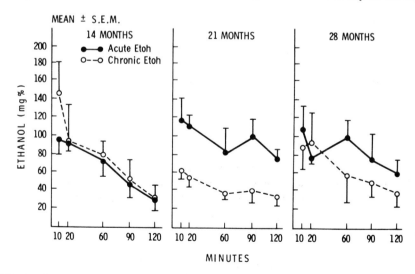

FIG. 1. Blood ethanol concentrations after a single oral dose of ethanol, 2 mg/kg, administered to 14-, 21-, and 28-month-old ethanol-treated (10% vol/vol for 4 months) and ethanol-free mice.

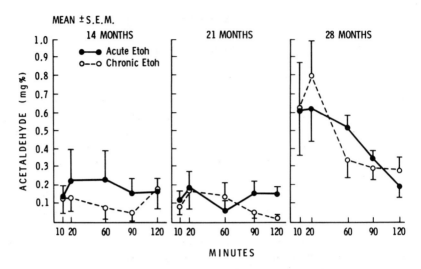

FIG. 2. Blood acetaldehyde concentrations after a single oral dose of ethanol, 2 mg/kg, administered to 14-, 21-, and 28-month-old ethanol-treated (10% vol/vol for 4 months) and ethanol-free mice.

age levels. There was, however, a significantly higher ($P<0.01$) acetaldehyde level in the 28-month-old acute and chronically treated mice during 60 minutes after ethanol ingestion when compared with the two younger groups. The higher acetaldehyde levels in old mice may be the result of greater activity of an ethanol-oxidizing system or mitochondrial change.

Elevated acetaldehyde levels could contribute to the neurologic, hepatic, and cardiac complications of older alcoholic patients (17). Interestingly and perhaps parodoxically, the three age groups (14, 21, and 28 months) of chronically treated mice, compared with their age-matched controls, had similar acetaldehyde levels after a single dose of ethanol (2 mg/kg; 40% ethanol). Higher than normal acetaldehyde levels in alcoholics have been reported for human subjects (17).

Locomotor Activity Performance

Spontaneous locomotor activity is an effective, simple, and widely used instrument for quantifying basic behavior. Mice readily learn to run in activity wheels, and deviations in daily scores may be taken as an indication of their health (31). In this study, spontaneous locomotor activity was measured for 5 consecutive days at the end of the first test period (2 months of ethanol), second test period (4 months of ethanol), and third test period (6 months of ethanol). Each test period was preceded by a 6-day ethanol washout. A summary of the results is shown in Fig. 3.

The most significant finding was the higher activity of the oldest ethanol-treated group when compared with that of the oldest control group of mice. In all three test periods (2, 4, and 6 months), the oldest ethanol mice were consistently and significantly ($P<0.05$ to $P<0.001$) more active than their corresponding controls.

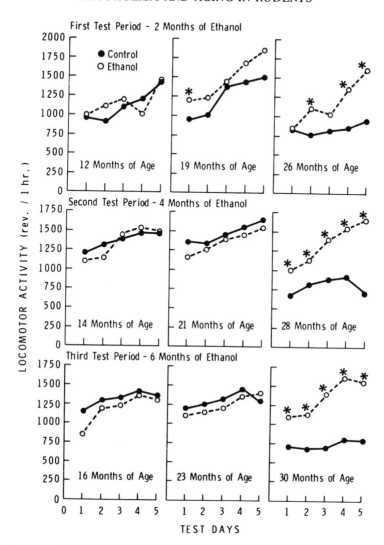

FIG. 3. Residual effects of 10% (vol/vol) ethanol after 2, 4, and 6 months of treatment on spontaneous locomotor activity as a function of age. Each value is a mean of 4 to 12 animals. (* = P<0.05 by ANOVA.)

The two younger ethanol- and placebo-treated groups did not differ from each other except for the first day's comparison of the 19-month-old mice. Mice in the oldest control group were also less active (P<0.05) than the two younger groups at each of the three test intervals. The increase in locomotor activity of the ethanol-treated mice may have been caused by excitability induced by ethanol withdrawal (6–11 days). Perhaps ethanol withdrawal-hyperexcitability lasts longer in older mice. Unfortunately, few data are available on the duration, cause, and consequence of ethanol withdrawal-hyperexcitability in older animals.

Hexobarbital Narcosis

Since hexobarbital is metabolized primarily by hepatic microsomal enzymes, differences in sleeping time produced by hexobarbital may be used as an approximation of possible ethanol-induced residual differences in liver functions (31). Mean sleeping time after administration of hexobarbital in an intraperitoneal (i.p.) dosage of 120 mg/kg to control and ethanol-treated male mice at three different test periods (2, 4, and 6 months of placebo or ethanol diet, plus 13 days of ethanol washout) are shown in Table 1.

Pretreatment of three different age groups of mice with ethanol did not produce any significant change in the duration of narcosis at any of the test intervals. There was, however, a pattern of prolonged hexobarbital narcosis with age for both alcohol-treated and control mice. Increased sleeping time with age was evident from longitudinal as well as cross-sectional group comparisons.

Time from injection of hexobarbital to narcosis decreased with age from a mean of 14 min at 12 months of age to 8 min at 30 months, suggesting an increased sensitivity of neurons or increased penetration of hexobarbital into the brain. There were, however, no significant differences between alcohol-treated or control mice at any of the intervals tested. The results of this study, which included a 13-day alcohol-free period before testing, show that consumption of alcohol by mice of three different age groups for periods of 2, 4, or 6 months did not result in permanent damage or accelerated aging of the liver microsomal system, as revealed by the hexobarbital test.

TABLE 1. *Aging and residual effects of long-term treatment with ethanol[a] on hexobarbital[b] narcosis of male C57BL/6J mice*

Age at test period (months)	Duration of barbital narcosis (min)			
	Control	Ethanol treatment		
		2 months	4 months	6 months
First test				
12	36 ± 3	36 ± 3	—	—
19	42 ± 7	42 ± 8	—	—
26	44 ± 6	56 ± 8	—	—
Second test				
14	52 ± 9	—	43 ± 6	—
21	61 ± 7	—	53 ± 3	—
28	62 ± 7	—	75 ± 23	—
Third test				
16	53 ± 9	—	—	56 ± 2
23	52 ± 6	—	—	60 ± 7
30	81 ± 12	—	—	74 ± 12

Values represent the mean ± SEM of results from groups of 7 to 12 mice.
[a]Ethanol = 6.2% vol/vol.
[b]Hexobarbital = 120 mg/kg.

Biochemistry

Superoxide dismutase activity (SOD EC 1.15.1.1)

Peroxidative damage has been implicated as a principal cause of age-related damage to cell constituents (14,15). The enzyme superoxide dismutase (SOD), which degrades the superoxide anion (O_2^-), is considered important in defense against the influence of these radicals. As the nervous system is a highly oxygenated tissue, inhibition of its SOD activity would result in an accumulation of cytotoxic O_2^- radicals.

The effects of acute and chronic ethanol administration on rat brain SOD activity have been studied (21). Intraperitoneal injections of ethanol lead to an inhibition of SOD activity. This may allow accumulation of cytotoxic O_2^- radicals, which may account for some nervous system disorders during acute alcohol administration. Changes in SOD activity in relation to aging have been reported also in organs of aging rats, mice (26), and humans (13). Comparisons of specific SOD activities in liver and brain demonstrated a significantly reduced activity in liver of aging rats but no change in the brain.

Since the brain and liver may differ broadly in degree of age- and alcohol-dependent damage to structure and function, we decided to compare age- and alcohol-related alterations in this enzyme's activity in the two organs. SOD has been reported to appear in the same molecular form in human brain and liver (4). SOD activity was measured according to the nonenzymatic method described by Fried et al. (11). We postulated that if ethanol accelerated the aging process in such organs as the liver and brain, we might observe a corresponding acceleration of age-associated SOD changes. This report presents information on brain and liver SOD activity after chronic administration of ethanol (6 months) to mice of three different age levels.

The specific activities of SOD in homogenates of liver and two different regions of the brain (cortex and striatum) are shown in Table 2. No age-dependent SOD changes appeared in the two regions of brain studied or in the liver. This is at variance with previous reports. Vanella et al. (41) found a significant decrease in copper/zinc SOD activity [which represents 92% of whole dismutase activity; (23)] in rat cerebral cortex. Reiss and Gershon (26) reported considerably reduced activity in liver of aging rats and mice, but no reduction in the brain of these animals.

With regard to alcohol effects on SOD activity in the brain and liver, the situation is even more confusing. Our results (Table 2) indicate that there may be an age-dependent increase in SOD activity in the brainstem (at 30 months) and thalamus (at 23 and 30 months) of ethanol-treated mice. Ledig et al. (21) reported that when ethanol was fed as the sole fluid, brain SOD activity decreased progressively. Perhaps the withdrawal of ethanol for 15 days in our experiment prior to sacrifice produced a rebound phenomenon in the SOD activity levels, leading to elevated recovery values. Recovery to control levels after ethanol withdrawal has been reported (21). A similar situation may exist with regard to our finding of no sig-

TABLE 2. *Aging and long-term (6 months) treatment effects of ethanol on SOD activity ($\mu g/mg$ protein) in the brain and liver of mice*

| | Age | | | | | |
| | 16 months | | 23 months | | 30 months | |
Region	Control	EtOH	Control	EtOH	Control	EtOH
Brainstem						
$\bar{X}$	11.6	12.9	12.5	10.4	12.2	17.9
SEM	±1.3	±1.7	±2.2	±1.6	±1.5	±4.2
(N)	(12)	(11)	(8)	(6)	(10)	(5)
Brain thalamus						
$\bar{X}$	14.9	18.8	18.2	26.1	18.3	31.8
SEM	±1.6	±4.6	±3.8	±2.4	±3.2	±4.0
(N)	(7)	(6)	(4)	(4)	(5)	(2)
Liver						
$\bar{X}$	11.2	11.2	12.2	14.9	13.8	9.4
SEM	±1.6	±1.4	±2.3	±2.7	±1.1	±1.4
(N)	(9)	(8)	(6)	(5)	(6)	(3)

nificant differences in liver SOD levels between ethanol-treated and ethanol-free control animals. Another possibility is that alcohol intoxication may not affect liver SOD activity. Undoubtedly, some of the discrepancies between the few published reports concerning age- and alcohol-related effects on brain and liver SOD activity are caused by unrecognized differences in experiments, which, once identified, may clarify current arguments.

Cholinergic receptor binding

Much research has indicated that neurotransmitter substances may be involved in aging (8,13,29) and alcohol abuse (5,12,16,32). Acetylcholine (ACh) is of particular interest because it has been implicated in geriatric memory dysfunction (2) and in long-term ethanol exposure, including the amnestic condition of Korsakoff (6). Cholinergic fibers link many regions of the brain, including the cerebellum, midbrain, basal ganglia, septal nucleus, hippocampus, and cerebral cortex (33)— structures in which pathologic changes occur in human alcoholics (42) and ethanol-ingesting rodents (27).

For these reasons, we were interested in determining whether or not the cholinergic response to alcohol in brain regions might be influenced by subject age. Three different age groups of mice (16, 23, and 30 months of age) were used. Specific binding of ^{3}H-quinuclidinyl benzilate (^{3}H-QNB) to postsynaptic muscarinic receptors was performed with homogenates of cerebellum and basal ganglia by the method of Yamamura et al. (47).

Values for the number of ^{3}H-QNB binding sites (total specific binding in femto-mole/mg protein) ±SEM for control and ethanol-treated animals at 16, 23, and 30 months of age are shown in Table 3. The changes in relation to age and ethanol treatment were variable. At 16 months, binding in the striatum of ethanol-treated

TABLE 3. Aging and long-term ethanol effects on cholinergic muscarinic ³H-QNB binding (fmol/mg protein) in various regions of the mouse brain

	Age					
	16 months		23 months		30 months	
Region	Control	EtOH	Control	EtOH	Control	EtOH
Striatum						
$\bar{X}$	1,151	1,432	1,253	1,009	1,159	678
SEM	±285	±385	±271	±226	±276	±261
(N)	(9)	(8)	(8)	(6)	(7)	(3)
Cerebellum						
$\bar{X}$	1.63	1.62	1.77	1.81	1.70	1.48
SEM	±.08	±.13	±.07	±.14	±.16	±.18
(N)	(10)	(8)	(8)	(6)	(7)	(3)

Values represent the mean ± SEM. Numbers in parentheses indicate number of separate experiments (animals) used to obtain the reported results.

animals when compared with age-matched controls was increased (20%); it decreased at 23 months (20%) and also at 30 months (42%). None of the differences reached statistical significance. No alteration in receptor binding was observed in the cerebellum, but cholinergic activity may not be high enough to detect age- or alcohol-induced changes in this region of the brain.

Binding values in relation to age also were variable. Control animals of the three age groups had similar values, but ethanol-treated animals had progressively lower values with age, decreasing by about 50% between 16 and 30 months of age. The results of the present study suggest, therefore, that the effect of aging on the striatal and the more limited cerebellar cholinergic system is relatively minor in the mouse, although somewhat different results have been reported by others (22,43).

Most researchers agree that ethanol increases the number of muscarinic receptors in brain regions that are susceptible to alcohol damage (striatum and mammillary bodies), although the degree of change reported is quite variable (24,25,39). Unfortunately, weight is specified more often than age to characterize the animals used. From such criteria it may be presumed that most investigators use very young animals. Undoubtedly, age, in addition to other variables (species, strain, duration of ethanol administration and withdrawal), also contributes to the effects of ethanol on cholinergic function (7). In agreement with published data, our youngest mice (23 months) responded to ethanol administration (6 months) plus ethanol withdrawal (10 days) by an increase in ³H-QNB binding. Progressively older animals, however, showed a decrease when compared with their age-matched controls. We concluded that this age-associated reversal in response to ethanol is due to the destruction of various critical components (postsynaptic receptors) associated with cholinergic muscarinic binding.

Experiment 2—Rats

Weight Changes, Survival, Liver and Brain Morphology

Weight and survival data

The first phase of this study was to determine the effect of our nutritionally balanced ethanol and control diets on body weight and survival of two groups of male Sprague-Dawley rats, 6 and 28 months of age, respectively.

Animals of similar age were divided into two groups (control and ethanol) according to weight and individually housed during the experimental period (6 months of liquid diet). As in the previous studies with mice, control rats were pair-fed an equivalent diet in which sucrose was substituted isocalorically for ethanol (7% vol/vol comprising 36.5% of available calories).

The data for body weights of the surviving rats are shown in Fig. 4. In general, the ethanol-treated rats tended to weigh more than their corresponding controls. It may also be noted that at the end of the treatment period, all four groups of surviving rats were of approximately the same mean weight (400 ± 36 g). Survival after 6 months of liquid diet among the four groups was as follows: three of three young controls, four of four young ethanol-treated, one of two old controls, and two of three old ethanol-treated. The survival ratio and the health status of the remaining old rats were surprisingly good in view of their advanced age (34 months) at termination of the alcohol-treatment phase. The animals in all four groups were kept on their respective control or ethanol diets until sacrificed by cardiac injection. Samples of brain (motor cortex and ventrolateral area of the caudate putamen) and liver were removed and processed for light and electron microscopy as previously

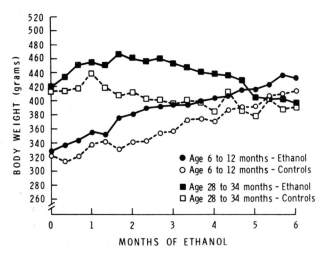

FIG. 4. Treatment effects of 10% ethanol (vol/vol) and isocalorically balanced liquid diets on body weight of young rats aged 6 to 12 months and of old rats aged 28 to 34 months. Each value is the mean of 2 to 4 rats that survived the treatment period.

described (3). Both qualitative and quantitative comparisons of mitochondrial, lipofuscin granules, and nerve endings were undertaken.

Liver morphology

It is generally accepted that the liver mitochondrial system is the main pathway for acetaldehyde oxidation (46). Since blood levels of acetaldehyde were elevated in older mice when compared with younger mice during ethanol administration, we decided to examine rat liver sections with both light and electron microscopy for evidence of tissue damage.

The level of alcohol administration to the rats and mice in this study (6%–7% vol/vol, 36% of total caloric intake) was sufficient to produce fatty liver in both young and old rats (Figs. 5 and 6). The fat droplets were often large and mainly confined to the centrolobular zone. The ultrastructural appearance of a liver hepatocyte taken from the central portion of a lobule of a young rat is shown in Fig. 7. Numerous mitochondria, clumps of glycogen granules, and parallel arrays of granular endoplasmic reticulum are generally seen in hepatocytes in approximately the same quantity and distribution regardless of age or ethanol treatment. A few hepatocytes of the old ethanol-treated rats appeared to have a less organized cellular matrix, a more extensive array of rough endoplasmic reticulum, and larger mitochondria than did similar cells from age-matched old control rats (Figs. 8 and 9). A comparison of mitochondrial density in hepatocytes of young and old alcohol-treated and alcohol-free rats is shown in Table 5. Mitochondrial density was not significantly different in the representative samples examined.

Brain morphology

A preliminary study of numerical density of various structures in the ventrolateral portion of the caudate-putamen (striatum) is shown in Table 4. Although there were not enough animals per group for statistical analysis, suggestive trends emerged. The older animals (control and ethanol-treated) generally showed a decreased number of neuronal nuclei (neurons) and an increase in the number of glial nuclei (glia). The younger group showed few overall effects of ethanol treatment.

There is, however, some suggestion of a differential effect of chronic ethanol treatment on neurohistologic changes in the old rats: a decrease in neurons and an increase in glia in the old ethanol-treated rats versus old control rats. The number of capillary fragments does not appear to change with age or ethanol treatment. Older aged rats have been known to develop neuronal loss and gliosis with little change in the numerical density of capillary fragments (3).

The ultrastructural appearance of medium-sized neurons in the ventrolateral caudate-putamen of young and old ethanol-treated and ethanol-free rats is shown in Figs. 10 to 13. Young and old control and ethanol-treated rats exhibited large, irregular, dense bodies (lipofuscin granules) in neuronal perikarya. These bodies seemed to be somewhat larger and more numerous in neurons of the old rats than in that of the young rats. Another striking feature of the neuronal bodies was the

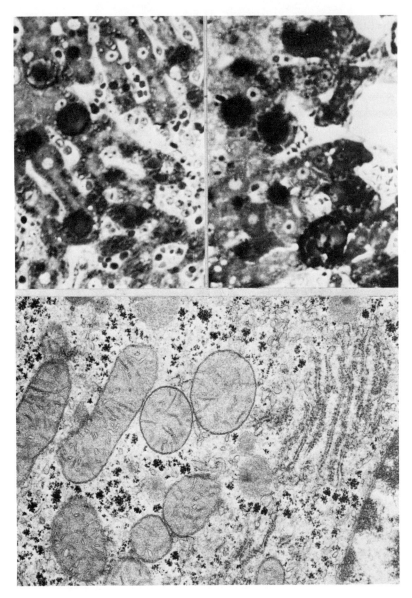

FIG. 5. (Top left) Fat droplets in liver centrolobular zone of 12-month-old rat on 10% ethanol (vol/vol) for 6 months. Toluidine blue. ×225. **FIG. 6. (Top right)** Fat droplets in liver centrolobular zone of 34-month-old rat on 10% ethanol (vol/vol) for 6 months. Toluidine blue. ×225. **FIG. 7. (Bottom)** Mitochondria, glycogen granules, and granular endoplasmic reticulum in hepatocyte of centrolobular zone of 12-month-old control rat. ×5,200.

larger size of the mitochondria in both young and old ethanol-treated rats when compared with their age-matched controls. Degenerating nerve endings were also occasionally observed in the neuropil of the alcohol-treated rats (Fig. 11). No

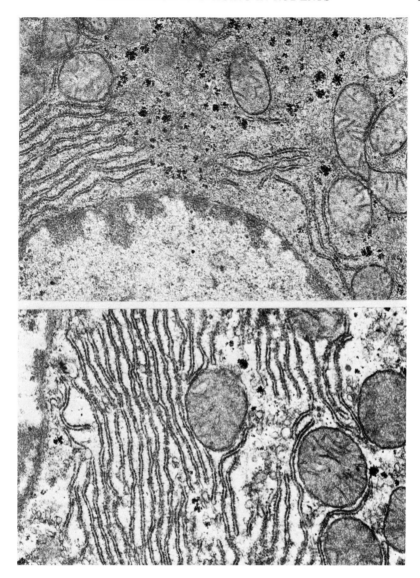

FIG. 8. (Top) Electron micrograph showing typical appearance of organelles in hepatocyte in liver centrolobular zone of 34-month-old control rat. ×5,200. FIG. 9. (Bottom) Electron micrograph of hepatocyte in liver centrolobular zone of 34-month-old rat on 10% ethanol (vol/vol) for 6 months. More than usual rough endoplasm is seen in age-similar control livers; the cellular matrix contains more water and slightly enlarged mitochondria. ×25,200.

structural differences were seen in glial elements in relation to age and/or alcohol administration.

The result of quantitative studies on the numerical density of mitochondria and lipofuscin is shown in Table 5. The number of animals per group was not large

TABLE 4. *Effects of age and chronic ethanol administration on quantitative neurohistology of ventrolateral striatum of the rat*

Variable	Density (N/mm^3)		
Age and treatment (rat no.)	Neuronal nuclei	Glial nuclei	Capillary fragments
Young control			
Y-2-C	154,208	51,132	75,724
Y-4-C	156,887	48,697	91,957
Y-6-C	151,773	59,492	94,716
Young EtOH			
Y-3-A	151,071	37,902	75,724
Y-7-A	119,065	46,019	91,956
Old control			
O-2-C	135,297	56,813	108,188
Old EtOH			
O-1-A	127,181	70,367	73,046
O-3-A	107,945	127,424	99,829

enough for statistical comparison, but there is a suggestion that the number of lipofuscin granules increased with age but not with alcohol treatment. Mitochondrial density in neuronal perikarya and neuropil was lowest in the old ethanol-treated rats, suggesting an age-ethanol interaction with regard to these organelles. The number of nerve endings per unit area was also determined in the neuropil of the lateral caudate-putamen. Again, the lowest values were observed in the oldest ethanol-treated group (Table 5).

We also studied mitochondrial and lipofuscin density in the larger pyramidal neurons of layer 3 in the motor cortex (Fig. 14). In all of the samples examined, no change was apparent in lipofuscin or mitochondrial size and density, either as a consequence of age or ethanol treatment (Table 5). Perhaps the sample number was too small (2–4 rats per group), or ultrastructural comparisons did not take into account the polar orientation of pigment granules in many pyramidal cells of the cortex. The accumulation of smooth and rough endoplasmic reticulum seemed to be less abundant in the old ethanol-treated animals than in the controls, but we did not attempt to verify this impression by quantitative procedures.

Quantitative neurohistologic techniques have revealed that long-term ethanol consumption, in the absence of malnutrition, produces neuronal loss in the central nervous system (44). There is also evidence that changes in aging rats may be characterized by a range of morphometric disturbances including neuronal loss, gliosis, lipofuscin accumulation (3,20), decreased mitochondria (30), and decrements in dendritic surface area (35). Our findings of neuronal loss (3), decreased mitochondrial density, and degeneration of nerve endings in the ventrolateral caudate-putamen (striatum) of the oldest ethanol-treated rats, compared with the ethanol-

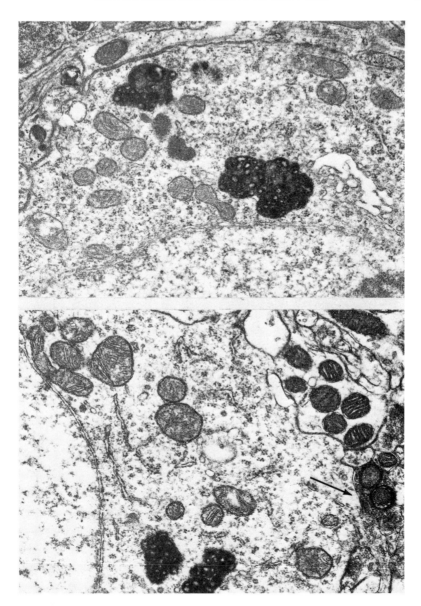

FIG. 10. (Top) Appearance of ultrastructure of ventrolateral striatum of 12-month-old control rat. ×25,200. **FIG. 11. (Bottom)** Twelve-month-old ethanol-treated rat (10% vol/vol for 6 months). Note enlarged mitochondria and degenerating nerve ending (*arrow*) in micrograph of ethanol-treated rat. ×25,200.

free controls, are in accord with these earlier findings. The fact that similar changes were not observed in the striatum of younger ethanol-treated rats or in the motor cortex at any age level following ethanol administration may indicate relative in-

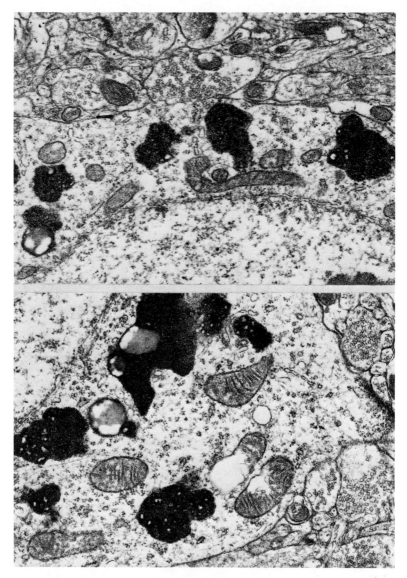

FIG. 12. (Top) Ultrastructural appearance of organelles in neurons of ventrolateral striatum of 34-month-old control rat. ×25,200. **FIG. 13. (Bottom)** Thirty-four-month-old rat on 10% (vol/vol) ethanol for 6 months. Note enlarged mitochondria and lipofuscin granules in micrograph of ethanol-treated rat. ×25,200.

sensitivity of these brain regions to ethanol. It is also apparent that one criterion of aging, universality, has not been established by using ethanol as an age-accelerating agent in this experiment.

TABLE 5. *Effects of age and chronic ethanol administration on quantitative distribution of organelles in hepatocytes, neurons, and neuropil of ventrolateral striatum and neurons of motor cortex in the rat*

Organelle concentration (N/mm^2)	Young		Old	
	Control	EtOH	Control	EtOH
Hepatocytes				
Mitochondria	28 ± 5	33 ± 4	32 ± 4	28 ± 3
Lipofuscin				
Nerve endings				
Ventrolateral striatum (neurons)				
Mitochondria	32 ± 7	38 ± 3	44 ± 8	24 ± 6
Lipofuscin	6.0 ± 0.4	5.8 ± 0.6	8.1 ± 1.2	8.5 ± 0.7
Nerve endings	26 ± 3	26 ± 2	27 ± 4	20 ± 3
Ventolateral striatum (neuropil)				
Mitochondria	50 ± 6	45 ± 8	52 ± 4	37 ± 3
Lipofuscin	26 ± 3	26 ± 2	27 ± 4	20 ± 3
Nerve endings				
Motor cortex (pyramidal neurons)				
Mitochondria	36 ± 3	33 ± 2	27 ± 3	31 ± 3
Lipofuscin	6.0 ± 0.4	3.7 ± 0.7	5.5 ± 0.8	4.3 ± 0.6
Nerve endings				

Values represent the mean ± SEM of results from 20 micrographs per region of 2 to 4 rats per group. Ages of rats at sacrifice were 12 months (young) and 34 months (old).

That lipofuscin pigment accumulates in many organs with aging is not disputed. If lipofuscin is a product of peroxidative damage and free-radical attack at the membrane level, it would not be surprising to find an increase in lipofuscin deposition in neurons in association with aging. Prolonged ethanol ingestion is also presumed to result in membrane damage (37,38). Yet, we found no evidence of increased lipofuscin deposition or any significant change in superoxide dismutase activity in our aged mice (34 months) after 6 months of ethanol ingestion. Consequently, questions of lipofuscin accumulation in relation to free-radical damage and the ensuing functional age-ethanol-related decrements remain unresolved.

CONCLUSION

This study used male C57BL/6J mice and male Sprague-Dawley rats of different ages to study the effects of long-term ethanol administration on brain and liver function and structure. Mice between the ages of 10 and 24 months and rats between ages 6 and 28 months were maintained on liquid diets containing 6 to 7% vol/vol of ethanol (36% of available calories) or pair-fed an equivalent diet in which sucrose was substituted isocalorically for ethanol (controls). The following results were noted:

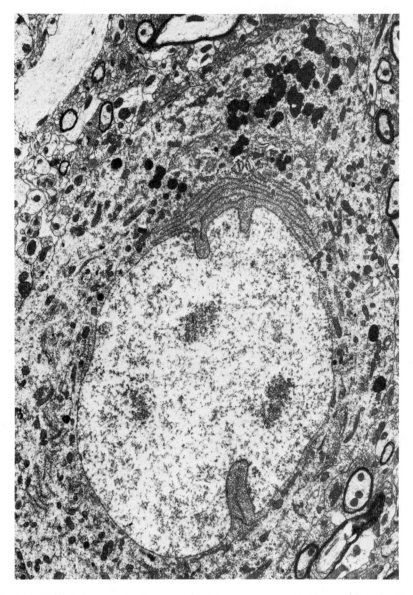

FIG. 14. Typical appearance of pyramidal cell in motor cortex of 12-month-old control rat. Note polar concentration of lipofuscin granules. ×5,670.

1. Exposure of ethanol-treated (4 months) and ethanol-free mice to a single dose of ethanol (2 mg/kg) revealed no significant age- or treatment-related differences in blood ethanol levels. Blood acetaldehyde levels were increased with age in both the ethanol-treated and ethanol-free groups of mice. Elevated acetaldehyde levels

in aged humans following alcohol ingestion could contribute to the sensitivity of older patients to ethanol.

2. There is an increase with age in mouse locomotor activity induced by ethanol withdrawal (6 to 11 days). Ethanol withdrawal-hyperexcitability may be a factor in the treatment of elderly alcohol abusers.

3. The administration of ethanol did not seem to affect hexobarbital narcosis. Fatty livers were observed in both young and old alcohol-treated rats, but ultra-structural and morphometric comparisons did not reveal any significant qualitative or quantitative differences in hepatocyte mitochondria. There was no apparent acceleration of aging in the liver according to any of the criteria used in this study.

4. There is a selective vulnerability of the aging nervous system to ethanol, as indicated by mitochondrial and nerve-ending damage and decreased cholinergic receptor binding in the basal ganglia of aged mice. There was also evidence of increased superoxide dismutase in some brain regions of the oldest ethanol-treated mice. Cell loss was enhanced by ethanol administration, but lipofuscin, regarded as a universal marker of aging in postmitotic cells like neurons, was not increased by ethanol at any age level. Taken together, these findings suggest that some regions of the brain are relatively more susceptible to ethanol damage than others. Further, the changes noted are more in the nature of a pathologic process rather than an indication of accelerated aging.

5. Finally, the experiments suggest that drugs that may be able to stimulate surviving cholinergic neurons may be useful in treating elderly alcoholics.

ACKNOWLEDGMENTS

The authors thank Lore Feldman, Carolyn Rolsten, Les Goekler, and Susan Sansom for their technical assistance.

REFERENCES

1. Abel, E. L. (1980): Procedural consideration in evaluating prenatal effects of alcohol in animals. *Neurobehavioral Toxicol.*, 2:167–174.
2. Bartus, R. T., Dean, R. L., Beer, B., and Lippa, A. S. (1982): The cholinergic hypothesis of geriatric memory dysfunction. *Science*, 217:408–417.
3. Brizzee, K. R., Samorajski, T., Smith, R. C., and Brizzee, D. L. (1981): The effect of age and chronic neuroleptic drug treatment on cell populations in the neostriatum of Fischer 344 rats. In: *Aging, Vol. 17: Brain Neurotransmitters and Receptors in Aging and Age-Related Disorders*, edited by S. J. Enna, T. Samorajski, and B. Beer, pp. 59–80. Raven Press, NY.
4. Carrico, R. J., and Deutsch, H. F. (1969): Isolation of human hepatocuprein and cerebrocuprein. Their identity with erythrocuprein. *J. Biol. Chem.*, 244:6087–6093.
5. Detering, N., Collins, Jr., R. M., Hawkins, R. L., Ozand, P. T., and Karahasan, A. (1980): Comparative effects of ethanol and malnutrition on the development of catecholamine neurons: Changes in neurotransmitter levels. *J. Neurochem.*, 34:1587–1593.
6. Drachman, D. A. (1977): Memory and cognitive function in man: Does the cholinergic system play a specific role? *Neurology*, 21:783–790.
7. Durkin, T. P., Hashem-Zedeh, H., Mandel, P., and Ebel, A. (1982): A comparative study of the acute effects of ethanol on the cholinergic system in hippocampus and striatum of inbred mouse strains. *J. Pharmacol. Exp. Ther.*, 220:203–208.

8. Freund, G. (1980): Cholinergic receptor loss in brains of aging mice. *Life Sci.*, 26:371–375.
9. Freund, G. (1982): Interactions of aging and chronic alcohol consumption on the central nervous system. In: *Alcoholism and Aging: Advances in Research*, edited by W. G. Wood and M. F. Elias, pp. 131–148. CRC Press, Boca Raton, FL.
10. Freund, G. (1982): The interaction of chronic alcohol consumption and aging in brain structure and function. *Alcoholism*, 6:13–21.
11. Fried, R., Ciesielski-Treska, J., Ledig, M., and Mandel, P. (1978): Superoxide dismutase activity in nerve cell culture. *Neurochem. Res.*, 3:635–639.
12. Gothóni, P., and Ahtee, L. (1980): Chronic ethanol administration decreases 5-HT and increases 5-HIAA concentration in rat brain. *Acta Pharmacol. Toxicol.*, 46:113–120.
13. Gottfries, C. G. (1981): Etiological and treatment considerations in SDAT. In: *Strategies for the Development of an Effective Treatment for Senile Dementia*, edited by T. Crook and S. Gershon, pp. 107–120. Mark Powley Associates, New Canaan, CT.
14. Harman, D. (1980): The aging process. *Proc. Natl. Acad. Sci. U.S.A.*, 78:7124–7128.
15. Hocman, G. (1980): Biochemistry of aging. *Int. J. Biochem.*, 12:515–522.
16. Hunt, W. A., and Dalton, T. K. (1981): Neurotransmitter-receptor binding in various brain regions in ethanol-dependent rats. *Pharmacol. Biochem. Behav.*, 14:733–739.
17. Korsten, M. A., Matsuzaki, S., Feinman, L., and Lieber, C. S. (1975): High blood acetaldehyde levels after ethanol administration. Differences between alcoholic and nonalcoholic subjects. *N. Engl. J. Med.*, 292:386–389.
18. Lancaster, F., Fenimore, D., and Samorajski, T. (1980): Effects of dihydroergotoxin (Hydergine) on peripheral blood alcohol levels. *Life Sci.*, 26:285–290.
19. Lancaster, F., Rolsten, C., and Samorajski, T. (1983): Effects of aging and chronic ethanol treatment on peripheral blood ethanol and acetaldehyde levels of mice. (*In preparation*).
20. Landfield, P. W., Braun, L. D., Pitler, T. A., Lindsey, J. D., and Lynch, G. (1981): Hippocampal aging in rats: A morphometric study of multiple variables in semithin sections. *Neurobiol. Aging*, 2:265–275.
21. Ledig, M., M'Paria, J-R., and Mandel, P. (1981): Superoxide dismutase activity in rat brain during acute and chronic alcohol intoxication. *Neurochem. Res.*, 6:385–390.
22. Lippa, A. S., Critchett, D. J., Bartus, R. T., Harrington, W., and Pelham, R. W. (1979): Electrophysiological and biochemical evidence for age-related alterations in hippocampal functioning. *Proc. Soc. Neurosci.*, 5:8.
23. McCord, J., and Fridovich, I. (1968): The reduction of cytochrome c by milk xanthine oxidase. *J. Biol. Chem.*, 243:5753–5760.
24. Muller, P., Britton, R. S., and Seeman, P. (1980): The effects of long-term ethanol on brain receptors for dopamine, acetylcholine, serotonin, and noradrenaline. *Eur. J. Pharmacol.*, 65:31–37.
25. Pelham, R. W., Marquis, J. K., Kugelmann, K., and Munsat, T. L. (1980): Prolonged ethanol consumption produces persistent alterations of cholinergic function in rat brain. *Alcoholism*, 4:282–287.
26. Reiss, U., and Gershon, D. (1976): Comparison of cytoplasmic superoxide dismutase in liver, heart and brain of aging rats and mice. *Biochem. Biophys. Res. Commun.*, 73:255–262.
27. Riley, J. N., and Walker, D. W. (1978): Morphological alterations in hippocampus after long-term alcohol consumption in mice. *Science*, 201:646–648.
28. Ritzmann, R. F., and Springer, A. (1980): Age-differences in brain sensitivity and tolerance to ethanol in mice. *Age*, 3:15–17.
29. Samorajski, T. (1977): Central neurotransmitter substances and aging: A review. *J. Am. Geriat. Soc.*, 25:337–348.
30. Samorajski, T., Friede, R. L., and Ordy, J. M. (1971): Age differences in the ultrastructure of axons in the pyramidal tract of the mouse. *J. Gerontol.*, 26:542–551.
31. Samorajski, T., Strong, J. R., and Sun, A. (1977): Dihydroergotoxin (Hydergine) and alcohol-induced variations in young and old mice. *J. Gerontol.*, 32:145–152.
32. Samorajski, T., Rolsten, C., and Pratte, K. (1978): Dihydroergotoxine (Hydergine) and ethanol-induced aging in C57BL/6J mice. *Pharmacology (Suppl. 1)*, 16:36–44.
33. Samorajski, T., Hicks, P. B., and Ordy, J. M. (1980): Metabolism of other neurotransmitters in degenerative syndromes associated with aging. In: *États Déficitaires Cérébraux Liés À L'Âge*, edited by R. Tissot, pp. 125–152. Georg et CIE S.A., Genève.
34. Samorajski, T., Strong, J. R., Volpendesta, D., Miller-Soule, D., and Hsu, L. (1982): The effects

of aging, ethanol, and dihydroergotoxin mesylate (Hydergine) alone and in combination on behavior, brain neurotransmitter, and receptor systems. In: *Alcoholism and Aging: Advances in Research*, edited by W. G. Wood, and M. F. Elias, pp. 115–129. CRC Press, Boca Raton, FL.

35. Scheibel, A. B. (1981): The gerohistology of the aging human forebrain: Some structuro-functional considerations. In: *Aging, Vol. 17: Brain Neurotransmitters and Receptors in Aging and Age-Related Disorders*, edited by S. J. Enna, T. Samorajski, and B. Beer, pp. 31–41. Raven Press, NY.

36. Strong, R., Hicks, P., Hsu, L., Bartus, R. T., and Enna, S. J. (1980): Age-related alterations in the rodent brain cholinergic system and behavior. *Neurobiol. Aging*, 1:59–63.

37. Sun, A. Y., Ordy, J. M., and Samorajski, T. (1975): Effects of alcohol on aging in the nervous system. In: *Neurobiology of Aging, Vol. 16*, edited by J. M. Ordy and K. R. Brizzee, pp. 505–520. Plenum Press, New York.

38. Sun, A. Y., and Sun, G. Y. (1979): Neurochemical aspects of the membrane hypothesis of aging. In: *CNS Aging and Its Neuropharmacology: Experimental and Clinical Aspects*, edited by W. Meier-Ruge, pp. 34–53. Karger, Basel.

39. Tabakoff, B., Munoz-Marcus, M., and Fields, J. Z. (1979): Chronic ethanol feeding produces an increase in muscarinic cholinergic receptors in mouse brain. *Life Sci.*, 25:2173–2180.

40. Tewari, S., Fleming, E. W., and Noble, E. P. (1975): Alterations in brain RNA metabolism following chronic ethanol ingestion. *J. Neurochem.*, 24:561–569.

41. Vanella, A., Geremia, E., D'Urso, G., Tiriolo, P., DiSilvestro, I., Grimaldi, R., and Pinturo, R. (1982): Superoxide dismutase activities in aging rat brain. *Gerontology*, 28:108–113.

42. Victor, M., Adams, R. D., and Collins, G. H. (1971): Pathological findings. In: *The Wernicke-Korsakoff Syndrome*, pp. 71–130. F.A. Davis, Philadelphia, PA.

43. Vijayan, V. K. (1977): Cholinergic enzymes in the cerebellum and the hippocampus of the senescent mouse. *Expl. Geront.*, 12:7–11.

44. Walker, D. W., Barnes, D. E., Zornetzer, S. F., Hunter, B. E., and Kubanis, P. (1980): Neuronal loss in hippocampus induced by prolonged ethanol consumption in rats. *Science*, 209:711–713.

45. Walker, D. W., Hunter, B. E., and Wickliffe, C. (1981): Neuroanatomical and functional deficits subsequent to chronic ethanol administration in animals. *Alcoholism*, 5:267–282.

46. von Wartburg, J. P. (1980): Acetaldehyde. In: *Psychopharmacology of Alcohol*, edited by M. Sandler, pp. 137–147. Raven Press, NY.

47. Yamamura, H., Kuhar, M. J., Greenberg, D., and Snyder, S. H. (1974): Muscarinic cholinergic receptor binding: Regional distribution in monkey brain. *Brain Res.*, 66:541–549.

Alcoholism in the Elderly, edited by
J. T. Hartford and T. Samorajski.
Raven Press, New York © 1984.

Neurotransmitter Function in Relation to Aging and Alcoholism

Gerhard Freund

*Veterans Administration Medical Center and Departments of Medicine and Neuroscience,
University of Florida College of Medicine, Gainesville, Florida 32602*

TYPES OF BRAIN LESIONS ASSOCIATED WITH AGING AND ALCOHOL ABUSE

Because both aging and alcohol abuse result in similar behavioral impairments, the question arose what, if any, relationships exist between these two processes. Two recent reviews of this subject have appeared (35,90).

Brain function, including sensory input, memory, associative processes of learning (cognitive function), and motor-verbal output, depends upon the functional integrity of neurons, their axons, and dendrites. Impaired function may result from a great variety of age-associated lesions ranging from gross morphological mass destruction (tumor, hemorrhage, infarction, normal pressure hydrocephalus) at one end of the spectrum to purely biochemical changes (hypothyroidism, generalized hypoxia) at the other end. In between these extremes may be the regional or generalized death of small groups of neurons as in the plaques of Alzheimer's disease—senile dementia. In other cases, individual, scattered neurons may die and disappear, as is inferred by a decreased number of cells in a given structure (12), although a loss of neurons with normal aging is questioned by some investigators (15,21,77). However, it is possible that neurons disappear without a change in cell numbers per area or in cell numbers per tissue volume if cell bodies and their surrounding neuropil dendrites are lost in equal proportions. Only a cell count of the entire structure would reveal such a loss (30). Local cell density could even increase if more neurons with large neuropils were lost than were neurons with small neuropils. In still other cases, the neuronal cell bodies appear intact morphologically and only the peripheral dendrites or axons and their associated synapses are affected (61,62,68). *In vivo*, the resulting atrophy in aging and alcohol abuse may now be recognized by computerized axial tomography (20,87). Finally, clinical dementia has been observed in patients when no morphological abnormalities were found, not even of the synapses, under the electron microscope (17). In these patients, it is reasonable to infer a purely biochemical lesion of synaptic transmitters, their enzymes, and their receptors. Similarly, "normal" aging in the absence of specific diseases such as atherosclerosis or Alzheimer's disease could also be manifest solely in biochemical changes in synapses.

SYNAPTIC FUNCTION

Synaptic Function and Clinical Behavior

Whatever the nature of an age- or alcohol-associated lesion that causes impaired brain function, it must ultimately result in absent or altered function of the synapses, their transmitters, and their receptors. The specific functions of the brain are carried out by neurons communicating with each other by releasing transmitters into the synaptic cleft and by presynaptic transmitters interacting with postsynaptic receptors of the message-receiving neuron. This is the common terminal and the rate-limiting pathway of brain function (30,66). Measures of synaptic transmitter turnover rates, their enzyme activities, and their receptors may therefore give important information not only about functional activity at a particular time but also about the maximal communication capacity of the system. A neuron that dies loses the afferent synapses on its own cell body and dendrites. Other neurons lose the synapses supplied by the efferent axon of the dead neuron. Because neurons cannot divide, the loss of neurons is permanent and irreplaceable. Therefore, reduction of the numbers of synaptic receptor molecules in a brain region indicates a decreased capacity to receive messages and probably a loss of entire synapses. Synaptic receptor numbers are a quantifiable chemical measure of synaptic functional capacity. The decline of receptor numbers may even precede a decrease in morphologically recognizable numbers of synapses. The degree of resultant impairment of behavioral function ranges from no demonstrable deficit or benign forgetfulness (48) to severe dementia. This will depend on the region, type, quantity, quality, rate of loss, and reserve capacity of the particular transmitter system involved (32). Finally, it is at the synaptic transmitter level of organization that pharmacological means may be employed to prevent or treat age- and alcohol-related brain dysfunctions.

Recovery of Synaptic Function from Injury

The CNS is static only in that neurons cannot divide and regenerate. However, brain function can recover, to some extent, for several reasons. First, there are excess spare cells, synapses, transmitters, and receptors; second, transmitter turnover and receptor number and affinity can be adaptively upregulated in those synapses that remain (70); third, formation of entirely new axonal processes with synapses by "sprouting" from undamaged neurons is possible.

When aging or alcohol abuse reduces brain tissue components, synaptic transmitter synthesis in the remaining components may initially increase. As the compensatory capacity is exceeded by further losses, the transmitter synthesis in a particular amount of tissue may decline below normal control values. Decreased presynaptic transmitter synthesis may lead to a compensatory increase in postsynaptic receptors and in enhanced affinity of the receptors for their respective transmitters or both. This "denervation supersensitivity" results in an enhanced postsynaptic response to a standard presynaptic stimulus, and the increased number of the receptors can be measured directly in the tissues.

The receptor molecules are synthesized in the neuronal cell body and transported by axoplasma flow to the synapses where they traverse the synaptic cleft to the postsynaptic cleft location. Therefore, if an axon is severed completely, the receptors accumulate proximal to the cut (84) and are lost in the synapses distant to the cut. If axotomy is proximal (close to the cell body) so that it causes retrograde degeneration of the cell, then the afferent synapses located on this cell body and their associated receptors are reduced. As the axon and its cell body recover, the receptors in the synapses return also (64). In summary, cell damage may cause loss of both proximal, afferent and distant, efferent synapses.

The severing of axons that supply a particular population of neurons results in loss of afferent input through the synapses derived from the axonal branches (deafferentation). Often this is followed by growth and branching of axons (sprouting) from other intact neurons that also supply the same partially deafferented cell. Usually the sprouting cells are anatomically and functionally different from the original neuron whose axon has been destroyed. But function may be restored if the sprouting neurons are from a contralateral, functionally equivalent region (67,89). This compensatory synaptic growth after neuronal death is less in old normal rats (16). Studies in man, however, suggest that the dendritic trees are greater in the clinically normal old brain than in young brain. In contrast, pathological senile dementia is associated with shrunken dendritic trees (13). One might speculate then that age- or alcohol-related death of neurons may be followed by some partial compensatory sprouting and the formation of new synapses. It is doubtful, however, that most of them are functionally equivalent to the original synapses they replace.

In summary, it is evident that the functional capacity of synaptic transmitters, enzymes, and receptors depends on a balance between the degree of destruction and the various compensatory responses. These responses include increased synthetic enzyme activities and receptor densities and affinities as well as regeneration by sprouting of new axonal processes. Both destruction and compensatory responses change with time and are in a dynamic equilibrium. When destruction is so extensive that the compensatory processes are insufficient, behavioral deficits will result. A small amount of additional anatomical or biochemical destruction may then cause a great degree of behavioral deficit (32). For these reasons, it is hardly surprising that morphological and biochemical correlations with the degree of behavioral impairment often are less than perfect, particularly if simple linear correlations are expected (32,35). As has been discussed elsewhere (32), no behavioral deficits at all may ensue, although there is a loss of functional units. Only after the reserve capacity is exhausted may a rapid, even exponential decline of function ensue. This course is compatible with clinical experience (44).

Neurochemical Methods for Assessing Synaptic Function

Historically, changes of synaptic function in response to various physiological and pathological stimuli were determined by measuring the concentrations of the putative transmitters in pieces of tissues. This appeared logical because the amount of transmitter released into the synpatic clefts is proportionate to the number of action potentials conducted by the axon. It soon became apparent that marked changes in the functional activities of synapses could occur with changes in transmitter turnover rate with little or no change in transmitter concentration. Thus the rate of transmitter production and accumulation could be measured in the presence of inhibitors of enzymes that catabolize the transmitters. The turnover could also be measured indirectly by assessing the activities of enzymes that either synthesize or catabolize transmitters.

Methodological difficulties have arisen from the lability of enzymes and their substrates, from the inability to determine in what cellular compartments substrates and enzymes are located and function, and from other problems. In studies using autopsy material from humans, these problems are compounded by variable time intervals between death and autopsy, the cause and mode of death, associated diseases and conditions (malnutrition, stress, institutionalization), medications affecting synaptic transmitters, circadian rhythm, and many physiological variables such as body temperature. Difficulties in interpreting results have arisen from the inability to prove causal relationships from associations between changes in transmitters and behavior. In addition, the magnitude of minute-to-minute fluctuations in transmitter function may be greater than differences associated with aging or alcohol abuse.

Transmitters interact with receptors as described in the foregoing section. Unlike the rapid fluctuations in transmitter concentrations and their enzymes, changes in receptors occur generally more slowly, and receptors are often less labile under various conditions. For this reason, and because the methods are relatively simple, the measurement of synaptic receptors has therefore been widely adopted.

In principle, receptors in a tissue slice or homogenate are exposed to a radioactively labeled transmitter or a drug that binds like a transmitter (agonist or antagonist drug). After an incubation period, the tissue, or its homogenate, is washed to remove the unbound transmitter or drug. The remaining bound amount of radioactivity is a measure of the number of receptor molecules and of nonspecific binding to sites other than receptors (58). These methods can be applied to animals injected *in vivo* or to brain homogenates or slices *in vitro* where radioactivity can be autoradiographically visualized. Nonspecific binding (to sites other than receptors) is then determined and subtracted from total binding. Nonspecific binding of radioactivity is determined in the presence of large amounts of nonradioactive transmitters (or drugs), which block almost all the specific binding sites because of very high affinity to the receptor and very little affinity to the nonspecific binding sites on proteins and lipids. Affinity, the strength of transmitter-receptor interaction, is determined in the presence of increasing amounts of unlabeled transmitters that displace the radioactive transmitter from the receptor. The smaller the amount of radioactive transmitter that is displaced from its receptor by a particular amount of unlabeled transmitter, the greater is the affinity of the receptor for its transmitter.

Recently, the investigation of synaptic receptors has become much more complex with the realization that a single, particular type of transmitter can interact with several different kinds of receptors (72). These different subpopulations of receptors may regulate different kinds of functions or, like isoenzymes, may differ in structure but serve the same function. For example, one kind of benzodiazepine receptor may regulate the seizure threshold, and another receptor may regulate the level of anxiety (46). This may explain why the single type of benzodiazepine drug has several different kinds of functions, including anxiolytic, muscle relaxant, and anticonvulsive (76). In other cases, these different receptors, which interact with the same transmitter, may serve the same function but may be distributed in different proportions in different brain regions or structures. Every time receptors are found to be heterogeneous, the question arises whether they are distinctly different types, or the same type of molecule interconvertible to different stereoconfigurational states. Because the functions of different receptor types or configurations may be different, it becomes critically important to distinguish the effects of aging and alcohol abuse not only on total receptor populations but also on its different subpopulations, some of which may be affected more than others.

Linearized binding or saturation curves obtained by adding increasing amounts of the radioactive labeled ligand (transmitter or drug) to brain tissue homogenates are called Scatchard plots. Alternatively, the addition of increasing concentrations of unlabeled ligand to homogenates with constant concentrations of a radioactive labeled ligand results in similar displacement curves. The presence of an S-shaped plot instead of a straight line is often the first indication that multiple binding sites of differing degrees of affinity *may* exist or that the degree of affinity may be altered, depending on the *in vitro* conditions. In the case of benzodiazepine (BZ) receptors, different drugs may react differentially with the different types of receptors (57,73,88). For example, type I BZ receptor mediates anxiolytic actions, has a high affinity for both BZ and triazolopyridazines (TPZ), and is not coupled to gamma-aminobutyric acid (GABA) receptors or to chloride ionophores. Type II mediates anticonvulsive and spasmolytic actions, has little affinity for TPZ, and is coupled to GABA and chloride ionophores or to both (46). The actual separation by electrophoresis of different BZ receptor molecules suggests different molecular structures rather than mere steric interconversion (70). Some receptors may be physiologically active only in a low- or a high-affinity state. Finally, the receptors for two different kinds of transmitter may interact with each other as do BZ and GABA receptors in the regulation of a chloride channel (59).

Because of space limitations, only one more example, the muscarinic acetylcholine receptor, will be given to illustrate, in principle, the importance of the heterogeneity of receptors for aging and alcohol research. Heterogeneity of these receptors was first suspected because the binding curves of the high-affinity antagonist drugs, such as quinuclidinyl benzilate (QNB), were uniform but the curves of low-affinity (not of high-affinity) agonist drugs suggested the presence of three types of receptors—low-, high-, and a minor super-high-affinity population (8,43). It was subsequently shown by autoradiography (83) and binding curves (9,23,47) that the proportions of these receptors with different affinities are different in various brain structures and regions. For example, high-affinity receptor sites were present in particularly high concentrations in lamina IV of the cerebral cortex, *nucleus tractus diagonalis*, and some thalamic nuclei of the rat brain (83). The usual question then arose whether the receptors with different degrees of affinity were interconvertible stereoconfigurations of the same molecule or whether they were completely different molecules. Interconvertibility of the conformational states of a single molecule was suggested because (a) disulfide bond reducing agents like cystine diminished binding and (b) reversible reduction and reoxidation diminished and restored high affinity. The importance of thiol groups in this process was suggested by experiments with *N*-ethylmaleimide and similar agents (3,4,41). Again, drugs with selective affinity for only one subtype of receptor can be used for the separation (40).

What is the functional significance of these subtypes with different affinities? The low-affinity site is thought to be coupled to the muscarinic receptor, i.e., the physiologically active form important for neurotransmission. In contrast, the high-affinity form may be a functionally inactive "reserve" precursor or degradation (8) form. [See McKinney and Coyle (55) for further discussion.] Although these findings have not been applied to research in aging and alcohol abuse, their implications are clear. For instance, if only the low-affinity binding sites were the sites relevant for cognitive and memory function, this fraction could decline with aging or alcohol abuse even if the total number of binding sites did not change significantly. The conversion of inactive (high-affinity) to active (low-affinity) state could be impaired in aging and alcohol abuse.

Some receptors are located not only in the postsynaptic membrane but also in the presynaptic membrane. There they serve to regulate the rate of release of transmitter by negative feedback mechanisms (autoregulation). For instance, the subtype α_1 adrenergic receptor is located postsynaptically and the α_2 presynaptically (42). Some portion of the low-affinity muscarinic receptor in CNS also may be located presynaptically (1,75). The effect of changes in membranes surrounding the receptors on their binding properties has barely begun to be explored (51). For example, the addition of phosphatidylserine to brain homogenates enhances specific muscarinic binding (2). The effects of aging and alcohol abuse on receptor function could be mediated by such membrane effects.

As the complexity of transmitter-receptor interactions unfolds, so does the complexity of potential receptor changes induced by aging and alcohol abuse.

Possible Relationships Between Synaptic Function in Aging and Alcohol Abuse

Impaired behavioral performance can be conceptualized as interference with the chain of events that leads from electrical and molecular events to overt behavior.

The many consecutive and parallel steps, regions, and systems involved in processing sensory input, storage, retrieval, associative processes, and motor output offer many possibilities where age- or alcohol-related processes could interfere with normal function. Probably several, rather than single, systems or steps are involved. It is conceivable that aging and alcohol abuse share or overlap to some extent in these molecular-behavioral chains of events. At one end of the spectrum, totally different molecular changes might result in the same kind of impaired behavior. This is called "independent decrement hypothesis" in behavioral studies (65). The same clinical picture of dementia can be caused by a great variety of mechanisms ranging from circumscribed local lesions to lead poisoning. At the other end of the spectrum is the possibility that both chronological aging and alcohol abuse cause impaired memory by a shared molecular mechanism ("premature" or "accelerated" aging hypothesis). For instance, both processes could enhance free radical formation and propagation to which cholinergic synapses in the hippocampus may be especially sensitive (as they are to hypoxia). This could result in membrane lipid changes that, in turn, might prevent the conversion of the muscarinic receptor from the high-affinity to the coupled, low-affinity state. The participation of hippocampus in normal memory processes would be impaired. This could happen in the absence of any morphologically visible change. Between these two extreme examples, there are innumerable possibilities.

The real problem is probably not whether or not aging and alcohol abuse interact with each other, but rather how, to what extent, at what levels of biological organization, and under what environmental and genetic conditions do they interact (32). Overt behavior is only at the end of a very complex chain of biological events. The same molecular process could operate in aging and alcohol abuse. But the behavioral outcome could differ because this same molecular process may be more active in a different brain structure or region in aging as compared with alcohol abuse.

One school of thought attributes alcohol-associated brain impairment entirely to vitamin deficiency (80) except in cases of hepatic encephalopathy. If that were the case, there would be no molecular relationship between aging- and alcohol-associated deficits because aging is clearly not caused by vitamin deficiency nor can the consequences of aging be prevented with vitamins. The data and arguments against this hypothesis have been presented elsewhere (27,32,33).

At the molecular and synaptic levels of biological organization, ethanol has many effects that could modify the various processes involved in normal and in pathological aging. At one end of the spectrum is a purely physical effect by intercalation of ethanol molecules between the lipid chains of membranes, which increases the disorder or fluidity of membranes in general and around important functional proteins. The membrane effects could also enhance the formation and propagation of free radicals. At the other end of the spectrum are chemical effects that result from the metabolism of ethanol and acetaldehyde and include changes in redox state, inductions of liver enzymes, and changes in lipoproteins. However, all of these phenomena are of short duration, measured in hours or days. They are often followed by compensatory changes that reestablish homeostasis. For instance, increased membrane fluidization by ethanol over a period of several days induces changes in membrane composition that reestablish the original state of fluidity while ethanol is present (38). It is completely unknown how such temporary changes could be transformed into permanent, largely irreversible alterations of synapses.

A first step toward understanding the molecular changes in synapses induced by aging and alcohol abuse is to compare synaptic function of different systems in normal young and old brains and in alcohol-exposed young and old brains. Similarities in changes of synaptic function in old brains and in ethanol-exposed brains suggest, but do not prove, related mechanisms. Once similarities have been found, the second step from correlative data to proof of causality would be an active manipulation (prevention or acceleration) of age- and ethanol-induced synaptic changes and their behavioral correlates. Such manipulations could be pharmacological; for example, administering precursors of transmitters or inhibiting destruction or enhancing formation of transmitters. Other methods could be genetic selection of strains resistant or susceptible to certain effects of aging or ethanol on synaptic receptors and brain function. Environmental procedures could include impoverishment, enrichment, nutrition, behavioral training, brain stimulation, lesions, and many others. There may be, of course, findings that are different in aging and ethanol abuse either because the mechanisms differ or because their changes are not relevant to the common behavioral deficits. The subsequent review of some of the studies will show that very little of what could be studied actually has been investigated.

In the subsequent sections, alterations in transmitter enzymes and receptors with aging and prolonged alcohol consumption are reviewed. The exposure to alcohol in single doses or for 1 to 3 weeks in small doses is unlikely to be relevant to long-term changes. Furthermore, synaptic changes observed during a 24-hr withdrawal period from alcohol are important for the elucidation of physical dependence but not of prolonged alcohol exposure. These studies are not included here. The many methodological and theoretical considerations involved in experiments with ethanol have been reviewed elsewhere (26,28,29,53).

SYNAPTIC TRANSMITTER-RECEPTOR FUNCTION IN LEARNING AND MEMORY

To understand how pathological conditions like alcohol abuse interfere with synaptic and behavioral functions, it is necessary to understand the normal functions. Much of our current knowledge is derived from studies in which different types of transmitters were stimulated or inhibited regionally or generally by drugs, and the resultant effects on behavior were observed (54,92).

The acetylcholinergic system is perhaps the most extensively explored because clinical observations had long ago recognized the amnestic effects of the central cholinergic-inhibiting drug scopolamine. The effect of this drug on short-term memory is similar to the effects of aging (22). Recently, the degeneration of the cholinergic projections from the nucleus basalis of Meynert to the cerebral cortex is thought to be of prime importance in the etiology of the senile dementia of Alzheimer's disease (86). A detailed review of this subject is beyond the scope of this chapter. The reader is referred to several excellent reviews of this topic (6,7,18,19,24,25,49). There is experimental evidence that almost all transmitter types besides the cholinergic are involved in normal cognitive functions and their pathological impairments, although their relative importance and their mechansims may vary. For example, adrenergic synapses may be important for the state of arousal (attention) and anxiolytic (BZ) or analgetic (endorphin) synapses for the degree of motivation to learn pain-motivated behaviors.

RECEPTOR SYSTEMS IN AGING AND ALCOHOLISM

Studies in Animals

There are no animal models for those diseases, such as Alzheimer's or vascular diseases, that cause dementia in aged humans. Therefore, all changes in animal behavior and synaptic function associated with aging are comparable to "normal" aging that is not associated with specific, clearly defined diseases. Chronic alcohol consumption as 35 to 40% of total calories by animals more nearly resembles alcohol abuse by humans. In rodents, after the acute effects of alcohol have subsided, this causes impaired performance of a wide variety of different memory and learning paradigms. The impairment is dose-dependent, not induced by accompanying malnutrition, specific in that it is not induced by sedatives other than alcohol, and is irreversible with the passage of time (36,81,82). The ethanol- and age-induced behavioral impairments in rodents are qualitatively identical but occur at an earlier age in the alcohol-exposed animals (36). In that sense, alcohol may "accelerate" the age-induced deterioration of learning. However, this descriptive concept based only on time relationships may be too simplistic to explain any of the age-ethanol interactions (32).

Can changes of transmitter-receptors in aged and chronically ethanol-treated animals explain the deficits in behavior? Table 1 summarizes the results of recent studies with cholinergic markers. Subpopulations of receptors, such as low-affinity acetylcholinergic receptors, have not been reported. Patterns quite different from those listed in the Table 1 could emerge if this were done. The absolute numbers of receptors reported in different studies may not be directly comparable because some investigators use whole brain tissue homogenates, 1,000-g supernatants, or 50,000-g crude mitochondrial pellets after various numbers of centrifugations before and after freezing. Some investigators express receptor numbers in reference to fresh tissue weights or protein determined in any one of the aforementioned centrifugal fractions. Some investigators compare maximal binding determined directly under specified conditions, whereas others use values calculated from Scatchard plots. For instance, some (60) do not indicate whether the homogenates had been centrifuged to remove endogenous ligands. All of these variables could affect the final results.

TABLE 1. *Cholinergic changes with aging and alcohol consumption in animals*

Methods	Species	Region	Age (months)	Ethanol Mode of admin.	Duration of exposure	Duration of withdrawal (weeks)	Density (%)	Affinity (%)	CAT (%)	Comments	Ref.
QNB	Mouse, C-57Bl	Whole brain	(a) 5–18 (b) 26 and 30	0	0	0	(a) NC (b) ↓ 10 and 20	NC NC	0 0	↓ Exponential	30
QNB	Mouse, C-57Bl	(a) Cortex (b) Striatum (c) Hippocampus (d) Stem (e) Cerebellum	4 and 29	0	0	0	(a) ↓ 20 (b) ↓ 28 (c) ↓ 10 (d) ↓ 18 (e) ↓ 5	NC ↑ 35 NC NC NC	0 0 0 0 0	NC at 15–25 m NS	50
QNB	Mouse, C-57Bl	(a) Cortex (b) Striatum (c) Hippocampus	6 and 30	0	0	0	(a) ↓ 34 (b) ↓ 30 (c) ↓ 27	NC NC NC	NC ↓ 20 NC	NC 6–12 m	74
	Rat, S-Dawley	(a) Cortex (b) Striatum (c) Hippocampus	10 and 26	0	0	0	(a) ↓ 20 (b) ↓ 25 (c) NC	NC ↑ 18 NC	↓ 54 ↓ 13 NC	NC 10–18 m	74
QNB	Rat, L-Evans	(a) Striatum (b) Cerebellum	4 and 22	0	0	0	(a) ↓ 28 (b) ↓ 25	NC NC	↓ 38 ↓ 36	Cortex, hippocampus Hypothalamus, amygdala; NC	56
QNB	Rat, Holtzman	(a) Striatum (b) Mammillary body	Adult	Liquid diet ad lib	(a) 2 w (b) 4 m (a) 2 w (b) 4 m	2 4 2 4	(a) NC (b) ↑ 117 (a) NC (b) ↑ 12	NC NC NC NC	NC ↓ 53 NC ↓ 58	Cortex, hippocampus NC	60

CAT, choline acetyltransferase; QNB, quinuclidinyl benzilate; m, months; 0, not reported; NC, no change; ↑ ↓, by % of base line; cortex, cerebral cortex; NS, not statistically significant; w, weeks.

The impression that emerges from inspecting the data in Table 1 is that aging causes a decrease of cholinergic receptor numbers in most regions under most conditions only in really old, not in "middle-aged" animals. This decline of receptor density occurs when brain acetylcholine synthesis decreases by 40% in 10-month-old mice and by 60% in 30-month-old mice (37). The data on the effects of ethanol are still sparse. But the consumption of ethanol for 4 months appears to cause a decrease in presynaptic choline acetyltransferase (CAT) activity and a compensatory ("denervation hypersensitivity") increase in the postsynaptic receptor numbers restricted to the striatum and mammillary body (60). More prolonged ethanol consumption possibly would lead to changes that are similar to those found in old animals. The changes are similar to those in aging rats (25).

B-adrenergic receptor binding as measured with ^{3}H-dihydroalprenolol (DHA) decreases with aging on the order of 25% in various regions in rodents and in humans (25). In only one reported study has ethanol in liquid diet been administered to rats for 2 months (5). The rats (of unspecified age, sex, and strain) were pair-fed with diets isocaloric in sucrose. Whole brain homogenates were prepared while the rats consumed ethanol and 1, 2, and 3 days after discontinuation of ethanol. A progressive increase on days 2 and 3 of 30% and 46% total DHA binding was reported. This was attributed to a hyperadrenergic state of ethanol withdrawal reaction after physical dependence. Effects persisting longer after withdrawal were not investigated.

Dopaminergic (spiroperidol or haloperidol) binding with aging (63) generally is decreased on the order of 30 to 50% either as a result of decreased receptor density or affinity. Pelham et al. (60) report a 29% decrease of specific haloperidol binding in striatum after the consumption of liquid diet containing ethanol for 13 months. The affinity was reduced by only 10%. It is not stated how soon after withdrawal from ethanol these measurements were made and, therefore, to what extent these findings could result from acute ethanol intoxication or postwithdrawal illnesses.

GABA and BZ receptor functions are partially linked to each other and to a chloride channel (59). These synapses are widely distributed in the brain and probably serve several different functions, depending upon regions, subtypes, and linkages. It is well established that certain, currently unknown, endogenous ligands occupy the same receptors as do BZ drugs and thereby relieve anxiety induced by a variety of environmental conflict and fear-inducing situations (76).

Not only is there substantial evidence that BZ-mimicking endogenous transmitters are released in response to fear-inducing situations, but also there are rat strains genetically predisposed to a greater reaction to fear-inducing stimuli. These rats have fewer BZ receptors than do the fear-resistant strains (69). "Emotionality," whether related to genetic factors or aging, clearly affects arousal, motivational, and other aspects of performance in tests of memory and learning (54). It has also been proposed that the loss of BZ receptors with chronic alcohol intoxication may further enhance the perception of fear and thereby perpetuate the consumption of the sedative alcohol. Thus, a self-perpetuating circle could be initiated that involves both emotional and neurochemical factors that promote alcohol abuse (31). This, of course, is different from the suggestion that the manifestations of ethanol withdrawal illnesses could also be factors that perpetuate ethanol consumption by negative reinforcement (45). These two and other possible contributory causes of alcohol abuse are not mutually exclusive. Because relatively small amounts of BZ drugs block the effects of ethanol-withdrawal signs, including seizures, it has been proposed that there is a close interaction between the purely physical effects of ethanol in membranes and the BZ receptors in mediating at least some effects of ethanol (31).

The enzyme glutamic acid decarboxylase (GAD) produces GABA from its precursor glutamic acid. There is no significant change with aging in rat and mouse hippocampus and striatum. In cerebral cortex, there is a decrease of 50% in brains of rats between ages 10 and 26 months and no change in mouse brains (25). The age- and alcohol-related changes are summarized in Table 2.

Studies in Humans

There are few studies concerned with age- or alcohol-associated changes of synpatic function in human brains free of specific brain diseases ("normal aging"). Most of the literature is concerned with the effects of specific brain diseases on synaptic function (7,91) and is not reviewed here. It is currently unknown whether alcohol abuse protects against or predisposes to Alzheimer's senile dementia or to cerebral vascular sclerosis. Several laboratories have reported that normal aging does not affect presynaptic CAT enzyme activity but that in Alzheimer's dementia, it is decreased and the muscarinic cholinergic receptors are normal (18). However, these receptor densities are "normal" only when compared with age-matched, presumably nondiseased brains. Because of the decreased cholinergic input, these receptors should be upregulated. The fact that they are not may indicate pathological involvement and inability of the synapses to respond appropriately. The cholinergic receptor density may be called "normal" when it is really inappropriately low, considering the decreased synaptic input.

Normal aging has been reported to result in a 25% decrease of cholinergic (QNB) binding in the frontal and temporal cortex and no change in CAT between the ages of 70 to 90 years (11,85). B-adrenergic binding was decreased by 50% in the cerebellum but not in cerebral cortex from the ages of 62 to 80 years. There was no change from ages 40 to 60 (52).

Only two reports in the literature examine the effects of alcohol abuse on receptor binding in postmortem brain samples (78,79). In one series of 17 male alcoholics, aged 39 to 68, all patients consumed hard liquor daily until the time of hospital admission in undetermined stages of alcohol intoxification or withdrawal illnesses (78). Most patients had severe liver disease resulting in hepatic failure (9) or hepatic encephalopathy (6). The "supernatant fractions of patient brain extracts" did not change receptor binding in fresh rat brain membranes. However, it is not possible to know what the content of such drugs was in patients' blood (because of the drugs' lipid solubility and binding to carrier proteins) or to what extent the effects

TABLE 2. Benzodiazepine and GABA changes with aging and alcohol consumption in animals

Methods	Species	Region	Age (months)	Ethanol Mode of admin.	Duration of exposure (months)	Duration of withdrawal (months)	Results Density (%)	Affinity (%)	GAD (%)	Comments	Ref.
FNP	Mouse, C57Bl	Whole brain	11	Liquid diet	7	1	↓ 12	↓	0		31
FNP	Mouse, C57Bl	(a) Cortex (b) Striatum	12	Liquid diet	8	1	(a) ↓ 14 (b) NC	NC NC	0 0	Addition of GABA ↑ 36% in both groups	34
FNP	Mouse	(a) Cortex (b) Striatum (c) Hippocampus (d) Stem (e) Cerebellum	4 and 29	0	0	0	(a) ↓ 12 (b) ↓ 9 (c) ↓ 13 (d) ↓ 15 (e) ↓ 15	NC ↑ 35 NC NC NC	0 0 0 0 0		50
FNP	Rat, Füllin	Cortex	2 and 14	0	0	0	NC	NC	0		39
MUS	Rat, Wistar	Cortex, stem, cerebellum	3, 12, and 24	0	0	0	NC	NC	0		52
—	Rat, S-Dawley	(a) Cortex (b) Hippocampus (c) Striatum	10, 18, and 26	0	0	0	0	0	(a) ↓ 40, 50 (b) NC (c) NC		25
—	Mouse, C57Bl	(a) Cortex (b) Hippocampus (c) Striatum	6, 12, and 30	0	0	0	0	0	(a) NC (b) NC (c) NC		60

GAD, glutamic acid decarboxylase; FNP, flunitrazepam—BZ receptors; ↑ ↓, by % of base line; 0, not reported; NC, no change; MUS, muscimol—GABA receptors.

of such drugs on receptors persist after the drugs themselves have disappeared from tissues. No brain histology data were reported to determine the presence or absence of brain diseases that are unrelated to alcohol abuse. The control patients were older than the alcoholics (mean age, 53 versus 60 years; age ranges, up to 68 versus 82). The terminal mode of death in the alcoholics was generally acute, whereas the control subjects died mostly from chronic wasting diseases such as cancers. The results were calculated as binding per milligram of fresh tissue or protein with no determination of brain water or edema.

Given these caveats, the findings in one region, cerebral cortical slices through the superior frontal gyrus, were as follows: There was no significant difference in mean receptor density expressed in femtomoles per milligram of tissue, wet weight, and affinity of BZ [flunitrazepam (FNP)], and muscarinic cholinergic (QNB) binding. B-adrenergic (DHA) receptors were decreased by 15% ($p<0.03$), and GABA (muscimol) receptors were increased in alcoholics by 23% with no change in affinity. There was no difference between the subgroups with and without hepatic failure or undefined "anoxic changes of brain tissue" or 12 patients receiving six different CNS active drugs including BZ. The lack of effect of drugs is particularly surprising in view of previous demonstrations of downregulation of receptor binding in response to drug treatments (14,71). Overall, this very limited study is a beginning to define the effects of chronic alcohol abuse on receptors.

Another postmortem investigation was published in preliminary abstract form (79). Six alcoholics and matched nonalcoholic patients were studied. There were no differences in presynaptic enzyme activities of CAT, tyrosine hydroxylase, and monoamineoxidase. QNB receptor density was decreased in caudate and frontal cortex. Dopamine (spiroperidol) receptor number and affinity were unchanged. Affinity (not density) of dihydromorphine receptors was decreased in all brain areas studied. The authors concluded that "the data suggests that alcohol abuse results in rather specific changes in brain receptors." This author agrees and concludes that the currently available postmortem data are much too limited to meaningfully compare the patterns induced by normal aging and alcohol abuse.

SUMMARY AND CONCLUSIONS

Behavioral-cognitive function declines with aging and chronic exposure to alcohol. The morphological basis for this functional decline ranges from gross lesions (diffuse or focal) to the loss of scattered isolated cells, their processes, or both. The end result, the terminal common pathway of all these lesions, is the loss of synaptic function. The maximal capacity of synaptic function that remains determines the ability of neurons to communicate with each other and ultimately the limits of behavior. The qualitative (regions, transmitter type) and quantitative (rate) extent of synaptic losses depends on a balance between destructive and compensatory processes. The latter consists of sprouting of new neuronal processes with their synapses from surviving neurons, enhanced presynaptic enzyme activities, and postsynaptic upregulation of receptors and possibly coupling processes beyond (10).

Some behavioral consequences of aging and alcohol abuse could be the result solely of molecular changes in synapses without any morphologically visible changes. This possibility could be but never has been explored.

There are similarities of some of the behavioral changes in alcohol abuse and in aging not associated with specific brain lesions. The question arises whether this similarity is merely the end result of biologically totally different processes. Many entirely unrelated diseases can cause dementia and destroy brain cells. Alternatively, a molecular process such as free radical formation might be common to both aging and alcohol abuse. Such a shared molecular mechanism need not necessarily result in identical morphological, electrophysiological, or behavioral changes because the expression of the molecular mechanism could be modified at a higher level of organization. For example, ethanol could differentially alter blood flow to various brain regions so that flow patterns differ from those in aging. Different cell types could be sensitized by alcohol to the effects of free radicals only in specific brain structures not greatly affected by aging. Certain ischemic regional patterns in aging brains could inhibit or enhance the effects of free radicals in specific regions. Many genetic and environmental factors could potentially alter the same basic molecular mechanism so that the behavioral responses are modified to some extent.

The currently available data from man and animals are much too sketchy to determine what, if any, patterns of synaptic dysfunctions are present or shared by normal aging and alcohol abuse. It is also not known to what extent behavioral impairment results from purely biochemical lesions of the synapses in the absence of morphologically visible pathological changes. Interactions between aging and alcohol abuse could occur at any level of biological organization from the molecular to the behavioral. Some similarities of behavioral changes in aging and alcohol abuse suggest that alcohol may advance the clock of aging. If that were the case, research in both aging and alcohol could greatly benefit.

ACKNOWLEDGMENT

Dr. Freund's research is supported by the Medical Research Service of the Veterans Administration.

REFERENCES

1. Aguilar, J. S., Criado, M., and DeRobertis, E. (1979): Pre- and postsynaptic localization of central muscarinic receptors. *Eur. J. Pharmacol.*, 57:227–230.
2. Aronstam, R. S., Abood, L. G., and Baumgold, J. (1977): Role of phospholipids in muscarinic binding by neural membranes. *Biochem. Pharmacol.*, 26:1689–1695.
3. Aronstam, R. S., Abood, L. G., and Hoss, W. (1978): Influence of sulfhydryl reagents and heavy metals on the functional state of the muscarinic acetylcholine receptor in rat brain. *Mol. Pharmacol.*, 14:575–586.
4. Aronstam, R. S., Hoss, W., and Abood, L. G. (1977): Conversion between configurational states of the muscarinic receptor in rat brain. *Eur. J. Pharmacol.*, 46:279–282.
5. Banerjee, S. P., Sharma, V. K., and Khanna, J. M. (1978): Alterations in β-adrenergic receptor binding during ethanol withdrawal. *Nature (Lond.)*, 276:407–409.
6. Bartus, R. T. (1980): Cholinergic drug effects on memory and cognition in animals. In: *Aging in*

the 1980's: Psychological Issues, edited by L. W. Poon, pp. 163–180. American Psychological Association, Washington, D.C.

7. Bartus, R. T., Dean, R. L., III, Beer, B., and Lippa, A. S. (1982): The cholinergic hypothesis of geriatric memory dysfunction. *Science*, 217:408–417.

8. 'Birdsall, N. J. M., Burgen, A. S. V., and Hulme, E. C. (1978): The binding of agonists to brain muscarinic receptors. *Mol. Pharmacol.*, 14:723–736.

9. Birdsall, N. J. M., Hulme, E. C., and Burgen, A. (1980): The character of the muscarinic receptors in different regions of the rat brain. *Proc. R. Soc. Lond. [Biol.]*, 207:1–12.

10. Bonnet, K. A. (1979): Adaptive alterations in receptor mediated processes and their implications for some mental disorders. *Adv. Exp. Med. Biol.*, 116:247–259.

11. Bowen, D. M., Spillane, J. A., Curzon, G., Meier-Ruge, W., White, P., Goodhardt, M. J., Iwangoff, P., and Davison, A. N. (1979): Accelerated ageing or selective neuronal loss as an important cause of dementia? *Lancet*, 1:11–14.

12. Brody, H. (1978): Cell counts in cerebral cortex and brainstem. In: *Aging, Vol. 7: Alzheimer's Disease: Senile Dementia and Related Disorders*, edited by R. Katzman, R. D. Terry, and K. L. Bick, pp. 345–351. Raven Press, NY.

13. Buell, S. J., and Coleman, P. D. (1979): Dendritic growth in the aged human brain and failure of growth in senile dementia. *Science*, 206:854–856.

14. Chiu, T. H., and Rosenberg, H. C. (1978): Reduced diazepam binding following chronic benzodiazepine treatment. *Life Sci.*, 23:1153–1158.

15. Coleman, P. D., and Goldman, G. (1981): Neuron counts in locus coeruleus of aging rat. In: *Aging, Vol. 17: Brain Neurotransmitters and Receptors in Aging and Age-Related Disorders*, edited by S. J. Enna, T. Samorajski, and B. Beer, pp. 23–30. Raven Press, NY.

16. Cotman, C. W., and Scheff, S. W. (1979): Compensatory synapse growth in aged animals after neuronal death. *Mech. Ageing Dev.*, 9:103–117.

17. Cragg, B. G. (1975): The density of synapses and neurons in normal, mentally defective and ageing human brains. *Brain*, 98:81–90.

18. Davies, P. (1978): Studies on the neurochemistry of central cholinergic systems in Alzheimer's disease. In: *Aging, Vol. 7: Alzheimer's Disease: Senile Dementia and Related Disorders*, edited by R. Katzman, R. D. Terry, and K. L. Bick, pp. 453–459. Raven Press, NY.

19. Davis, K. L., and Yamamura, H. I. (1978): Minireview: cholinergic underactivity in human memory disorders. *Life Sci.*, 23:1729–1734.

20. de Leon, M. J., Ferris, S. H., George, A. E., Reisberg, B., Kricheff, I. I., and Gershon, S. (1980): Computed tomography evaluations of brain-behavior relationships in senile dementia of the Alzheimer's type. *Neurobiology of Aging*, 1:69–79.

21. Diamond, M. C., and Connor, J. R., Jr. (1981): A search for the potential of the aging brain. In: *Aging, Vol. 17: Brain Neurotransmitters and Receptors in Aging and Age-Related Disorders*, edited by S. J. Enna, T. Samorajski, and B. Beer, pp. 43–58. Raven Press, NY.

22. Drachman, D. A., and Leavitt, J. (1974): Human memory and the cholinergic system: A relationship to agingπ. *Arch. Neurol.*, 30:113–121.

23. Ellis, J., and Hoss, W. (1980): Analysis of regional variations in the affinities of muscarinic agonists in the rat brain. *Brain Res.*, 193:189–198.

24. Enna, S. J., Samorajski, T., and Beer, B., editors (1981): *Brain Neurotransmitters and Receptors in Aging and Age-Related Disorders*. Raven Press, NY.

25. Enna, S. J., and Strong, R. (1981): Age-related alterations in central nervous system neurotransmitter receptor binding. In: *Aging, Vol. 17: Brain Neurotransmitters and Receptors in Aging and Age-Related Disorders*, edited by S. J. Enna, T. Samorajski, and B. Beer, pp. 133–142. Raven Press, NY.

26. Eriksson, K., Sinclair, J. D., and Kiianmaa, K. (1980): *Animal Models in Alcohol Research*. Academic Press, NY.

27. Freund, G. (1973): Chronic central nervous system toxicity of alcohol. *Annu. Rev. Pharmacol.*, 13:217–227.

28. Freund, G. (1979): Physical dependence on ethanol: Conceptual considerations. *Drug Alcohol Depend.*, 4:173–178.

29. Freund, G. (1980): Physical dependence on ethanol: Methodological considerations. *Adv. Exp. Med. Biol.*, 126:211–229.

30. Freund, G. (1980): Cholinergic receptor loss in brains of aging mice. *Life Sci.*, 26:371–375.

31. Freund, G. (1980): Benzodiazepine receptor loss in brains of mice after chronic alcohol consumption. *Life Sci.*, 27:987–992.
32. Freund, G. (1982): Interactions of aging and chronic alcohol consumption on the central nervous system. In: *Alcoholism and Aging: Advances in Research*, edited by W. G. Wood and M. F. Elias, pp. 131–148. CRC Press, Boca Raton, FL.
33. Freund, G. (1982): The interaction of chronic alcohol consumption and aging on brain structure and function. *Alcoholism (NY)*, 6:13–21.
34. Freund, G. (1982): Decreased benzodiazepine receptors in cerebral cortex of mice after prolonged ethanol consumption. *Alcoholism (NY)*, 6:141.
35. Freund, G., and Butters, N. (1982): Alcohol and aging: challenges for the future. Editorial, Symposium: Neurobiological Interactions Between Aging and Alcohol Abuse. *Alcoholism (NY)*, 6:1–2.
36. Freund, G., and Walker, D. W. (1971): Impairment of avoidance learning by prolonged ethanol consumption in mice. *J. Pharmacol. Exp. Ther.*, 179:284–292.
37. Gibson, G. E., Peterson, C., and Jenden, D. J. (1981): Brain acetylcholine synthesis declines with senescence. *Science*, 213:674–676.
38. Goldstein, D. B., and Chin, J. H. (1981): Disordering effect of ethanol at different depths in the bilayer of mouse brain membranes. *Alcoholism (NY)*, 5:256–258.
39. Haefely, W., Bandle, E. F., Burkhard, W. P., da Prada, M., Keller, H. H., Kettler, R., Mohler, H., and Richards, J. G. (1980): Pharmacology of central neurotransmitters in advanced age. In: *États Déficitaires Cérébraux Liés À l'Age*, pp. 329–353. Librarie de l'Université, Georg, Geneva.
40. Hammer, R., Berrie, C. P., Birdsall, N. J. M., Burgen, A. S. V., and Hulme, E. C. (1980): Pirenzepine distinguishes between different subclasses of muscarinic receptors. *Nature (Lond.)*, 283:90–92.
41. Hedlund, B., and Bartfai, T. (1979): The importance of thiol- and disulfide groups in agonist and antagonist binding to the muscarinic receptor. *Mol. Pharmacol.*, 15:531–544.
42. Hoffman, B. B., and Lefkowitz, R. J. (1981): Alpha-adrenergic receptor subtypes. *N. Engl. J. Med.*, 302:1390–1396.
43. Hulme, E. C., Birdsall, N. J. M., Burgen, A. S. V., and Mehta, P. (1978): The binding of antagonists to brain muscarinic receptors. *Mol. Pharmacol.*, 14:737–750.
44. Jarvik, L. F. (1978): Genetic factors and chromosomal aberrations in Alzheimer's disease, senile dementia, and related disorders. In: *Aging, Vol. 7: Alzheimer's Disease: Senile Dementia and Related Disorders*, edited by R. Katzman, R. D. Terry, and K. L. Bick, pp. 273–277. Raven Press, NY.
45. Kissin, B. (1979): Biological investigations in alcohol research. *J. Stud. Alcohol [Suppl.]*, 40:146–181.
46. Klepner, C. A., Lippa, A. S., Benson, D. I., Sano, M. C., and Beer, B. (1979): Resolution of two biochemically and pharmacologically distinct benzodiazepine receptors. *Pharmacol. Biochem. Behav.*, 11:457–462.
47. Kloog, Y., Egozi, Y., and Sokolovsky, M. (1979): Characterization of muscarinic acetylcholine receptors from mouse brain: Evidence for regional heterogeneity and isomerization. *Mol. Pharmacol.*, 15:545–558.
48. Kral, V. A. (1978): Benign sensescent forgetfulness. In: *Aging, Vol. 7: Alzheimer's Disease: Senile Dementia and Related Disorders*, edited by R. Katzman, R. D. Terry, and K. L. Bick, pp. 47–51. Raven Press, NY.
49. Kubanis, P., and Zornetzer, S. F. (1981): Age-related behavioral and neurobiological changes: A review with an emphasis on memory. *Behav. Neural Biol.*, 31:115–172.
50. Kubanis, P., Zornetzer, S. F., and Freund, G. (1982): Memory and postsynaptic cholinergic receptors in aging mice. *Pharmacol. Biochem. Behav.*, 17:313–322.
51. Loh, H. H., and Law, P. Y. (1980): The role of membrane lipids in receptor mechanisms. *Annu. Rev. Pharmacol. Toxicol.*, 20:201–234.
52. Maggi, A., Schmidt, M. J., Ghetti, B., and Enna, S. J. (1979): Effect of aging on neurotransmitter receptor binding in rat and human brain. *Life Sci.*, 24:367–374.
53. Majchrowicz, E., and Noble, E. P. (1979): *Biochemistry and Pharmacology of Ethanol.* Plenum Press, NY.
54. McGaugh, J. L. (1973): Drug facilitation of learning and memory. *Annu. Rev. Pharmacol.*, 13:229–241.

55. McKinney, M., and Coyle, J. T. (1982): Regulation of neocortical muscarinic receptors: effects of drug treatment and lesions. *J. Neurosci.*, 2:97–105.
56. Morin, A. M., and Wasterlain, C. G. (1980): Aging and rat brain muscarinic receptors as measured by quinuclidinyl benzilate binding. *Neurochem. Res.*, 5:301–308.
57. Nielsen, M., and Braestrup, C. (1980): Ethyl β-carboline-3-carboxylate shows differential benzodiazepine receptor interaction. *Nature*, 286:606–607.
58. O'Brien, R. D. (1979): The receptors: A comprehensive treatise. In: *General Principles and Procedures*, p. 345. Plenum Press, NY.
59. Paul, S. M., Marangos, P. J., and Skolnick, P. (1981): The benzodiazepine—GABA—chloride ionophore receptor complex: Common site of minor tranquilizer action. *Biol. Psychiatry*, 16:213–229.
60. Pelham, R. W., Marquis, J. K., Kugelmann, K., and Munsat, T. L. (1980): Prolonged ethanol consumption produces persistent alterations of cholinergic function in rat brain. *Alcoholism*, 4:282–287.
61. Pentney, R. (1982): Age and ethanol-associated changes in cerebellar Purkinje cells. In: *Alcoholism and Aging: Advances in Research*, edited by W. G. Wood and M. F. Elias, pp. 149–169. CRC Press, Boca Raton, FL.
62. Riley, J. N., and Walker, D. W. (1978): Morphological alterations in hippocampus after long-term alcohol consumption in mice. *Science*, 201:646–648.
63. Roth, G. S. (1981): Steroid and dopaminergic receptors in the aged brain. In: *Aging Vol. 17: Brain Neurotransmitters and Receptors in Aging and Age-Related Disorders*, edited by S. J. Enna, T. Samorajski, and B. Beer, pp. 163–169. Raven Press, NY.
64. Rotter, A., Birdsall, N. J. M., Burgen, A. S. V., Field, P. M., and Raisman, G. (1977): Axotomy causes loss of muscarinic receptors and loss of synaptic contacts in the hypoglossal nucleus. *Nature (Lond.)*, 266:734–735.
65. Ryan, C. (1982): Alcoholism and premature aging: A neuropsychological perspective. *Alcoholism (NY)*, 6:22–30.
66. Samorajski, T. (1981): Normal and pathologic aging of the brain. In: *Aging, Vol. 17: Brain Neurotransmitters and Receptors in Aging and Age-Related Disorders*, edited by S. J. Enna, T. Samorajski, and B. Beer, pp. 1–12. Raven Press, NY.
67. Scheff, S. W., and Cotman, C. W. (1977): Recovery of spontaneous alternation following lesions of the entorhinal cortex in adult rats: Possible correlation to axon sprouting. *Behav. Biol.*, 21:286–293.
68. Scheibel, A. B. (1978): Structural aspects of the aging brain: Spine systems and the dendritic arbor. In: *Aging, Vol. 7: Alzheimer's Disease: Senile Dementia and Related Disorders*, edited by R. Katzman, R. D. Terry, and K. L. Bick, pp. 353–373. Raven Press, NY.
69. Shephard, R. A., Nielsen, E. B., and Broadhurst, P. L. (1982): Sex and strain differences in benzodiazepine receptor binding in Roman rat strains. *Eur. J. Pharmacol.*, 77:327–330.
70. Sieghart, W., and Karobath, M. (1980): Molecular heterogeneity of benzodiazepine receptors. *Nature*, 286:285–287.
71. Synder, S. H. (1979): Receptors, neurotransmitters and drug responses. *N. Engl. J. Med.*, 300:465–472.
72. Synder, S. H., and Goodman, R. R. (1980): Multiple neurotransmitter receptors. *J. Neurochem.*, 35:5–15.
73. Squires, R. F., Benson, D. I., Braestrup, C., Coupet, J., Klepner, C. A., Myers, V., and Beer, B. (1979): Some properties of brain specific benzodiazepine receptors: New evidence for multiple receptors. *Pharmacol. Biochem. Behav.*, 10:825–830.
74. Strong, R., Hicks, P., Hsu, L., Bartus, R. T., and Enna, S. J. (1980): Age-related alterations in the rodent brain cholinergic system and behavior. *Neurobiol. Aging*, 1:59–63.
75. Szerb, J. C. (1978): The characterization of presynaptic muscarinic receptors in central cholinergic neurons. In: *Cholinergic Mechanisms and Psychopharmacology*, edited by D. J. Jenden, pp. 49–60. Plenum Press, NY.
76. Tallman, J. F., Paul, S. M., Skolnick, P., and Gallager, D. W. (1980): Receptors for the age of anxiety: Pharmacology of the benzodiazepines. *Science*, 207:274–281.
77. Terry, R. D. (1978): Discussion in: *Aging, Vol. 7: Alzheimer's Disease: Senile Dementia and Related Disorders*, edited by R. Katzman, R. D. Terry, and K. L. Bick, pp. 396–399. Raven Press, NY.

78. Tran, V. T., Snyder, S. H., Major, L. F., and Hawley, R. J. (1981): GABA receptors are increased in brains of alcoholics. *Ann. Neurol.*, 9:289–292.

79. Valverius, P., Borg, S., Fields, J., Hoffman, P. L., Knobloch, M., Lee, J., Moses, F., Munoz-Marcus, M., Perry, B. D., Prichard, D. U., Stibler, H., and Tabakoff, B. (1982): Brain neurotransmitter receptors in alcoholics—a postmortem study. *Alcoholism (NY)*, 6:137.

80. Victor, M., and Banker, B. Q. (1978): Alcohol and dementia. In: *Aging, Vol. 7: Alzheimer's Disease: Senile Dementia and Related Disorders*, edited by R. Katzman, R. D. Terry, and K. L. Bick, pp. 149–170. Raven Press, NY.

81. Walker, D. W., Barnes, D. E., Zornetzer, S. F., Hunter, B. E., and Kubanis, P. (1980): Neuronal loss in hippocampus induced by prolonged ethanol consumption in rats. *Science*, 209:711–713.

82. Walker, D. W., Hunter, B. E., and Abraham, W. C. (1981): Neuroanatomical and functional deficits subsequent to chronic ethanol administration in animals. *Alcoholism (NY)*, 5:267–282.

83. Wamsley, J. K., Zarbin, M. A., Birdsall, N. J. M., and Kuhar, M. J. (1980): Muscarinic cholinergic receptors: Autoradiographic localization of high and low affinity agonist binding sites. *Brain Res.*, 200:1–12.

84. Wamsley, J. K., Zarbin, M. A., and Kuhar, M. J. (1981): Muscarinic cholinergic receptors flow in the sciatic nerve. *Brain Res.*, 217:155–161.

85. White, P., Hiley, C. R., Goodhardt, M. J., Carrasco, L. H., Keet, J. P., Williams, I. E. I., and Bowen, D. M. (1977): Neocortical cholinergic neurons in elderly people. *Lancet*, 1:668–671.

86. Whitehouse, P. J., Price, D. L., Struble, R. G., Clark, A. W., Coyle, J. T., and DeLong, M. R. (1982): Alzheimer's disease and senile dementia: Loss of neurons in the basal forebrain. *Science*, 215:1237–1239.

87. Wilkinson, A. D. (1982): Examination of alcoholics by computed tomography (CT) scans: A critical review. *Alcoholism (NY)*, 6:31–45.

88. Williams, E. F., Rice, K. C., Paul, S. M., and Skolnick, P. (1980): Heterogeneity of benzodiazepine receptors in the central nervous system demonstrated with kenazepine, an alkylating benzodiazepine. *J. Neurochem.*, 35:591–597.

89. Wilson, R. C., Levy, W. B., and Steward, O. (1979): Functional effects of lesion-induced plasticity: Long term potentiation in normal and lesion-induced temporodentate connections. *Brain Res.*, 176:65–78.

90. Wood, W. G., and Elias, M. F., editors (1982): *Alcoholism and Aging: Advances in Research.* CRC Press, Boca Raton, FL.

91. Yamamura, H. I. (1981): Neurotransmitter receptor alterations in age-related disorders. In: *Aging, Vol. 17: Brain Neurotransmitters and Receptors in Aging and Age-Related Disorders*, edited by S. J. Enna, T. Samorajski, and B. Beer, pp. 143–147. Raven Press, NY.

92. Zornetzer, S. F. (1978): Neurotransmitter modulation and memory: A new neuropharmacological phrenology? In: *Psychopharmacology: A Generation of Progress*, edited by M. A. Lipton, A. DiMascio, and K. F. Killam, pp. 637–649. Raven Press, NY.

Alcoholism in the Elderly, edited by
J. T. Hartford and T. Samorajski.
Raven Press, New York © 1984.

Changes in Biogenic Amines and Their Metabolites with Aging and Alcoholism

Richard E. Wilcox

*Alcohol and Drug Abuse Research Program, Department of Pharmacology and
Toxicology, College of Pharmacy, University of Texas, Austin, Texas 78712*

The aging process and the chronic ingestion of large quantities of ethanol may well have profound actions on a large number of neurotransmitter-neuromodulator systems within the brain (119,153), including those with peptidergic mediation whose messenger is yet to be characterized. In all likelihood, significant changes in the balances among the neurotransmitters of the brain result from the effects of alcoholism and aging (11,12,29). The focus of this review is on putative aging-alcohol interactions on dopaminergic, noradrenergic, and serotonergic functions within regions of the brain. Thus, although ethanol abuse and aging each take their toll on cholinergic and gamma-aminobutyric acid (GABA)ergic functions, (9,22,39, 67,133,177,186,187,191,199) the catecholamines and serotonin represent neuro-transmitters whose morphology and regulation have been particularly well characterized in relation to alcohol administration and aging (135,136). Unfortunately, the adequacy of the characterization of the brain dopamine (DA), norepinephrine (NE), and serotonin systems in relation to aging and ethanol is only relative. Only recently have a number of studies begun to emerge in which functional parameters of each transmitter system have been assessed (178), and only some of these studies have reported brain regional effects of either aging or alcohol. Perhaps just as significant is that only a very few of the recent state-of-the-art technical studies also included adequate nutritional controls so that the distinct actions of chronic alcohol or aging versus partial starvation, debilitation, or frank disease become discernible.

From such a dearth of material, it is only possible to speculate concerning the true effects of alcoholism throughout the life-span, yet the speculations are exciting (200,204). In man, chronic alcoholism appears to reproduce many of the changes in striatal dopamine function produced with advanced age. Similarly, long-term ethanol abuse produces changes in regional NE, which also mirror the deficits that are brought about with sufficient longevity. An interesting divergence between the results of prolonged alcoholism and senescence seems to occur in relation to seroto-nin. The effects of normal aging are relatively modest decreases in serotonin, in contrast with severe insults to the catecholamine systems, but chronic alcoholism is associated with severe deficits in brain serotonin that are comparable to those observed with NE. The actual magnitude of the changes in transmitter levels during the normal life-span and long-term alcohol abuse may or may not be indicative of meaningful functional derangements in the brain (70). It is, nevertheless, striking that the changes observed in the older alcoholic are so similar to the changes observed in animal models of aging versus chronic ethanol effects. That these changes in brain transmitters in aging ethanol addicts may actually have functional significance is suggested by the recent observation of transient symptoms of Parkinson's disease in seven alcoholics (aged 53–70) during alcohol withdrawal or chronic severe intoxication (18). We provide a brief overview of aging-ethanol relationships in each brain system, and then we briefly discuss selected aspects of the anatomy and regulation of DA, NE, and serotonin systems of the brain, which make them intriguing models for the study of aging-ethanol interactions. Subsequently, we summarize the effects of aging versus ethanol on each system and conclude our discussion with some suggestions about the direction of future studies in the area.

DOPAMINE: THE NIGROSTRIATAL SYSTEM

Ethanol-Aging Interactions on Brain Dopamine

Carlen and co-workers (18) reported transient symptoms of Parkinson's disease in seven alcoholics (aged 53–70) during either alcohol withdrawal or chronic severe intoxication. The median duration of ethanol abuse in these individuals was 20 years (range = 10–42 years) and was not related to liver disease. All patients showed recovery or improvement of the motor disorder with a shift to more temperate habits. The dopaminergic deficits and imbalances between DA and other (e.g., cholinergic and GABAergic) mediators that occur in parkinsonism (104,105,110,112) also occur during normal aging (6,106). Thus, alcoholism appears to be able to produce a pattern of disruption of striatal DA activity via a DA blocker-like effect, which resembles the insults produced by Parkinson's disease or by aging (158,172). It is interesting in this regard that there is a widely held view that parkinsonism represents an accelerated aging of the nigrostriatal DA system (6,156). In another recent study of alcoholics, Carlsson and colleagues (19) noted that the levels of striatal DA were depressed to less than 50% in the caudate nucleus of the 70-year-old control values, whereas hypothalamic dopamine was depressed by nearly 100% in 50-year-old alcoholics. Hippocampal values for the dopamine metabolite homovanillic acid (HVA) were found also to be depressed by 47% in the hippocampus of the alcoholics. These changes in brain DA are particularly striking relative to the profound deficits in DA function, which normally occur with aging (189), and when considering that the alcoholics were 20 years younger than the controls.

Anatomy and Regulation

Studies suggesting an integral involvement of the nigrostriatal DA system in the pathogenesis of Parkinson's disease (48,64,72), in the motor deficits of Huntington's chorea (50), and in the tardive dyskinesia side effects of antischizophrenic pharmacotherapy (48) have helped to make the nigrostriatal DA system one of the best understood in the brain (12,96,97,114). This DA pathway is also one of the most profoundly affected by the normal aging process (7,81,86,189).

The dorsal compact zone of the substantia nigra is the major origin of the DA projection to the caudate nucleus and putamen (together, striatum) of the basal ganglia. This projection, accounting for 80% of the brain's DA, is highly organized topographically (44,121). Impulse flow in nigrostriatal DA neurons results in an increase in DA synthesis and turnover and in the accumulation of DA metabolites in the striatum. Thus, increased DA turnover seems to reflect an increase in the activity of the rate-limiting enzyme in DA (and NE) synthesis, tyrosine hydroxylase (TH). But, paradoxically, if impulse flow is reduced in nigrostriatal neurons, the neurons also respond by increasing DA synthesis. The mechanism for the enhanced DA synthesis with increased or decreased nigrostriatal impulse flow is a focus of highly active research efforts (68,128,147,152,190,194). The response of nigrostriatal neurons to the cessation of impulse flow is not as predictable from changes in synthesis as is the response of noradrenergic neurons, and it is important to remember this difference in evaluating the effects of ethanol.

The Aging Nigrostriatal Dopamine System

Striatal DA levels decline in adult man at a rate of about 1% per year (2,20,146), whereas DA declines in rodent neostriatum somewhat more slowly—20% by 28 months [(45,47,49) but see (131)]. An important concern is whether different DA pools (85a,165) are differentially affected by aging (185). TH activity shows similar modest declines (15–25%) at least in mice (45,71,190). Similarly, there occurs only modest (20%) decrements in striatal DA uptake with age in some studies (45,79), whereas others (81) report no change. As might be expected, activities of both monoamine oxidase (MAO) and catechol-O-methyl transferase (COMT), in contrast, show increases with age (149,175).

Basal activity for striatal DA-sensitive adenylate cyclase is not consistently altered during aging, whereas decreases in DA-stimulated cyclic adenosine monophosphate (AMP) accumulation have been observed in aged organisms of several species (51,52, 101–103,137,138,159). These findings reinforce the idea presented above that the dynamic function of a neural system provides a better index of its integrity than do presumed steady-state assessments (e.g., turnover versus levels). Most significantly, deficits in DA-stimulated adenylate cyclase appear to occur between 3 and 12 months of age in the rodent (159), with no further declines in the later life-span, and the deficits are substantial 30 to 50% decreases. DA receptor binding is reduced in aging in the striata of several species (52,80,82,101,140,163,184). These decreases are profound (50%), with the major change being a decreased receptor density with an occasional report of reduced affinity [see Roth (151) for discussion].

Age-related changes in the ability of nigrostriatal DA neurons to compensate for acute (10) or chronic drug treatment have also begun to be evaluated in several

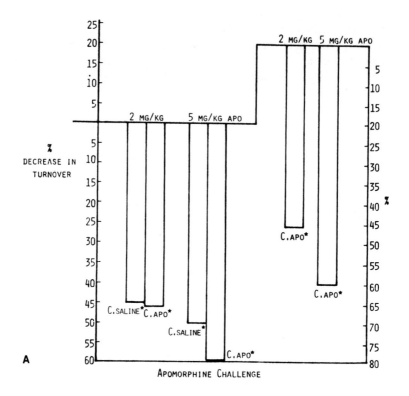

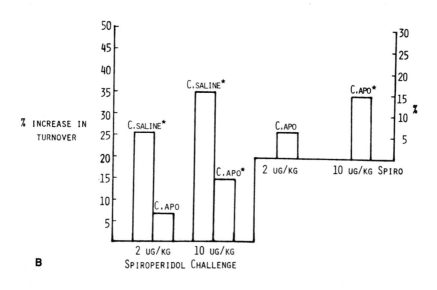

FIG. 1.

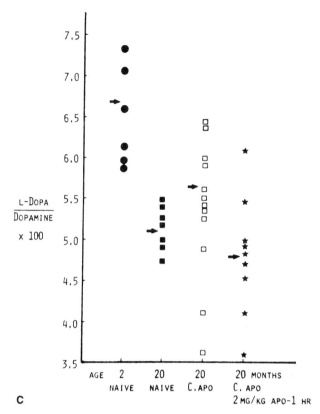

C

FIG. 1. Nigrostriatal plasticity during aging. Changes in striatal DA turnover after chronic DA agonist administration to young vs old mice. *In vivo* accumulation of DOPA vs DA was determined after decarboxylase inhibition using HPLC (reverse phase with electrochemical detection) after chronic treatment of male CD-1 mice with apomorphine (APO) (30 mg/kg, intraperitoneal) or saline. Control values were 6.6 ± 0.3 ng DOPA per mg protein per 30 min vs 101.3 ± 4.1 ng DA per mg protein per 30 min after 100 mg/kg NSD1015. **A.** Amorphine inhibition of DA turnover after chronic apomorphine. Data from 2-month-old mice are expressed as % change in DOPA/ DA 60 min after acute challenge with APO or saline. *$p < 0.05$ vs control of $N \geqslant 10$ per group. **B.** Spiroperidol stimulation of DA turnover after chronic apomorphine. Data from 2-month-old mice are expressed as % change in DOPA/DA 60 min after acute challenge with spiroperidol (Spiro) or saline. *$p < 0.05$ vs control of $N \geqslant 10$ per group. **C.** DA turnover in aged mice. Data from 2-month-old and 20-month-old mice are expressed as L-DOPA/DA × 100 60 min after APO or saline (Naive). *Arrows* indicate means. Data from Vaugh and Wilcox (190).

recent papers. Long-term neuroleptic administration (6–12 months) (24,25, 26,132,150,192) results in changes that are generally consistent with the results of other chronic studies with DA blockers (21,124,198) in showing supersensitive receptors after drug administration is terminated. However, a recent report by Randall et al. (142) suggests that old (24–26 months) mice did not show striatal supersensitization responses (via striatal ^{3}H-spiroperidol binding or apomorphine-induced stereotypy) after 3 weeks of haloperidol treatment. In contrast, Hefti et al.

(71) reported no change in striatal DA turnover in mice after 18 months of dihydroxyphenylalanine (L-DOPA) administration (5 g/kg/day), and Randall et al. (142) found striatal desensitization to chronic bromocriptine (a DA agonist) to occur throughout the life-span. In another report (189) it was observed that aged (20 months) mice were still capable of responding to 2 weeks of apomorphine (APO) treatment with an increase in *in vivo* DOPA accumulation (after decarboxylase inhibition). The animals also responded to chronic APO followed by acute *in vivo* APO challenge with the expected reduction in DOPA accumulation and to chronic APO followed by acute *in vivo* spiroperidol challenge with the expected increases in DOPA accumulation. However, the magnitude of the changes in the old animals in response to chronic APO treatment was reduced when compared with the changes shown by 2-month-old chronic APO-treated controls (Fig. 1). Taken together, these results suggest that the plasticity of the nigrostriatal DA system changes with aging in a somewhat selective manner (being preserved with some DA agonists for certain parameters). The effects of chronic ethanol administration on these neural compensatory mechanisms could well be quite profound. This point is highlighted by the recent observation (156) that in a rodent model of Parkinson's disease, young rats with incomplete lesions of the nigrostriatal system show transient motor impairment with subsequent recovery (Fig. 2A) only to have the symptoms reappear as the animals age (Fig. 2B). This is strikingly reminiscent of the emergence of parkinsonian symptoms in aging alcoholics.

Effects of Ethanol on Brain Dopamine

In the striatum, some reports indicate that acute ethanol administration enhances both DA synthesis and metabolism [(43) but see (36)], whereas chronic administration of alcohol is associated with tolerance to the ethanol effect on TH activity (183). These ethanol-induced effects are, unfortunately, not common to all brain regions (Tables 1 and 2) (16,17,43,188) nor to all studies of striatum (116). A threefold caveat concerning the apparent conflicts in the literature may be appropriate at this point. First, the duration of chronic ethanol treatment and the elapsed time following cessation of treatment can strongly affect both the magnitude and the direction of the observed neurochemical responses of the organism, since neurons adapt to the presence of drug and then readapt (with rebound?) in the absence of drug. Second, maintaining the health and nutritional status of the animal during long-term ethanol treatment and comparing the results from ethanol-treated subjects with appropriate control data are key requirements that are still too often overlooked in studies of chronic alcoholism (33–35,41,59,118). Third, as was mentioned earlier, topographically innervated subdivisions of brain regions probably are not homogenous in their neurochemistry, so they should not be expected to be homogenous in their response to drugs. Thus, "minor" differences between investigators in dissection protocols might result in two laboratories consistently sampling two different portions of a given brain region.

Acute ethanol administration increases striatal DOPA formation and levels of dihydroxyphenylacetic acid (DOPAC), whereas complete tolerance to the stimulant

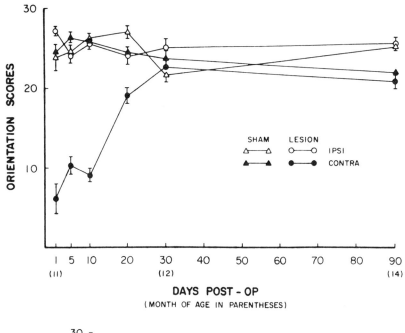

DAYS POST - OP
(MONTH OF AGE IN PARENTHESES)

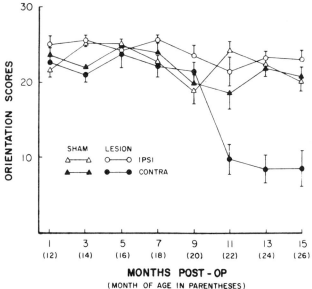

MONTHS POST - OP
(MONTH OF AGE IN PARENTHESES)

FIG. 2. Reemergence of behavioral deficits in "recovered" nigrostriatal-lesioned rats as a function of aging. Male Long-Evans rats, 11 months old at time of surgery, received unilateral electrolytic lesions of the medial forebrain bundle in the lateral hypothalamic area. Behavioral tests were carried out as described in ref. 156. Data from Schallert (156).

TABLE 1. *Effects of ethanol (EtOH) on brain regional biogenic amines*

	Cortex	Striatum	Accumbens	Hippocampus	Olfactory tubercle	Amygdala	Hypothalamus	Nigra	Cerebellum	Brainstem
Levels										
DA	↑ (171)	↑ (116)	—	—	—	—	—	—	↑ (171)	↑ (171)
NE	↑ (171), ↓ (126)	↑ (171)	—	—	—	—	↓ (126)	—	↑ (171)	↑ (171), ↓ (126)
5-HT	↑ (126), NC (60,171)	NC (171)	—	↑ (126)	—	—	—	—	NC (171)	NC (171)
Turnover										
DA	NC (43)	↑ (43), ↓ (116), NC (43,143, 147,176)	—	—	↓ (16)	—	—	NC (43)	—	—
NE	↑ (60, 126), NC (171)	—	—	—	—	—	—	—	—	—
5-HT	NC (171)	—	—	—	—	—	—	—	NC (171)	↑ or NC (60), NC (171)
Receptors										
DA	NC (75)	↑ or NC (5,90,141), ↓ (73), ↑ (144), NC (125)	↓ (125)	—	—	—	—	—	—	—
NE	↑ (87), NC (75)	—	NC (75)	NC (75)	—	—	NC (75)	—	↑ (23), NC (75)	—
5-HT	NC (75)	NC (75)	—	NC (75)	—	—	—	—	—	—

↑, increase; ↓, decrease; NC, no change.
Numbers refer to references at end of chapter.

TABLE 2A. *Effects of ethanol (EtOH) on biogenic amine functions: dopamine synthesis*

Study	Action	Comments
Fadda et al. (43) (SD[a] rat) 3.2 g/kg EtOH	DOPA: Caudate-acute ↑ Substantia nigro-acute NC Frontal cortex-acute NC Caudate-chronic NC Substantia nigra-chronic NC	
Umezu et al. (188) (SD rat)	Catechol olfactory tubercle ↓	³H-Catechol from labeled tyrosine
Mena and Herrera (116) (Wistar rat)	DOPA striatum NC DA striatum ↑	
Detering et al. (33) (rats)	DA levels striatum ↓	Pups-prenatal EtOH
Strombom et al. (176) (NMRI mice, female)	DOPA: EtOH enhanced APO-induced Striatum ↓ Limbic system ↓ Hemispheres ↓	EtOH did not change DOPA accumulation by itself
Tabakoff & Hoffman (183)	Chronic EtOH produces tolerance to stimulation of DOPA accumulation after neuroleptics	
Bustos et al. (16) (SD rats)	EtOH: DA synthesis ↓ (olfactory tubercle) EtOH: NC DA release (olfactory tubercle)	From ¹⁴C-Tyrosine
Soliman et al. (171) (SD rats)	DA levels ↑ cerebellum, cortex, pons	3 hr after 2 g/kg EtOH
Murphy et al. (126) (Wistar rats)	EtOH-preferring pons- midbrain DA ↓	Selectively bred

↑, increase; ↓, decrease; NC, no change.
[a]Sprague-Dawley.

effect on DOPA formation developed after 60 days of alcohol treatment (43). One day after ethanol withdrawal, striatal DA and DOPAC levels were unchanged in the chronically treated rats, but acute ethanol challenge to withdrawing chronic ethanol-treated animals was followed by a decrease in DA and an increase in DOPAC in striatum, frontal cortex, and substantia nigra. Fadda et al. (43) suggested that both acute and chronic administration of ethanol releases DA but that in the acute condition, DA depletion is prevented by increased synthesis. Such studies highlight the need for evaluating changes in both DOPA versus DA and in DA versus its major metabolites (3,4-DOPAC, HVA, and 3-methoxytyramine) in attempts to evaluate changes in DA function associated with chronic ethanol ingestion.

TABLE 2B. *Effects of EtOH on biogenic amine functions:*
dopamine metabolism

Study	Action	Comments
Barbaccia et al. (5)	DOPAC: DBA2J NC acute NC withdrawal C57 13L 16J acute ↑ NC withdrawal Swiss albino acute ↑ NC withdrawal	
Fadda et al. (43) (SD[a] rat)	DOPAC: Caudate-acute ↑ Substantia nigra-acute NC Frontal cortex NC	
Weiner et al. (197) (monkey)	Caudate: DOPAC NC HVA NC DOPAL[b] NC DOPET[c] NC	Push-pull perfusion
Reggiani et al. (144) (SD rats)	Acute EtOH: DOPAC ↑ (striatum)	

↑, increase; ↓, decrease; NC, no change.
[a]Sprague-Dawley.
[b]3,4,-dihydroxyphenylacetaldehyde.
[c]3,4-dihydroxyphenylethanol.

It is conceivable that the tolerance to the ethanol action on striatal DA synthesis observed after chronic administration (plus acute ethanol challenge) may reflect an adaptation of DA autoreceptors on terminals of nigrostriatal neurons (53). Partial support for this view is obtained from the report by Strombom et al. (176) in which doses of apomorphine small enough to selectively stimulate DA autoreceptors (and so inhibit DA synthesis and, perhaps, release) were found to produce a dose-dependent supression of low-dose ethanol-induced locomotor stimulation and of striatal DOPA accumulation. If ethanol in low doses is capable of acting effectively on DA autoreceptors, then a major portion of ethanol's chronic effects on striatal DA synthesis might be mediated at presynaptic sites. An autoreceptor action of ethanol might also help to explain why in limbic system sites, which have a less well-documented contribution of autoreceptors to DA regulation (4a), the effects of chronic ethanol ingestion are different. For example, acute ethanol administration leaves DA synthesis and metabolism unaffected in frontal cortex, whereas decreases in DA and DOPAC are still observed after chronic ethanol administration followed by acute ethanol challenge (43).

Using slices from rat olfactory tubercle, Bustos et al. (16) noted that acute *in vitro* ethanol challenges inhibited DA synthesis from labeled tyrosine. It is difficult to determine if these results contradict the statement above—that acute ethanol does

TABLE 2C. *Effects of EtOH on biogenic amine functions: dopamine receptors*

Study	Action	Comments
Hunt & Dalton (75) (4 days EtOH; SD[a] rat)	DA binding: Caudate-APO NC	0.5 nm ^{3}H-APO ± 300 nm APO
	Caudate-ADTN[b] NC	8 nm ^{3}H-ADTN ± 5 m nm ADTN
	Caudate-haloperidol NC	3 nm ^{3}H-Haloperidol ± 100 mcm DA
Barbaccia et al. (5) (3 weeks low dose EtOH; mice)	Caudate-Swiss albino ↑ Caudate-C57 BL/6J ↑ Caudate-DBA2J NC	0.3 nm ^{3}H-Spiroperidol ± 10^{-4}m DA
Rabin & Molinoff (141) (*in vitro* EtOH; mouse)	Caudate-binding NC	^{3}H-Spiroperidol 80–650 pm ± 2 mcm d-Butaclamol
	Caudate-adenylate cyclase ↑	
Muller et al. (125) (Wistar rats)	Caudate NC	^{3}H-Haloperidol 3 nm ± 100 nm
	Mesolimbic ↓	d-Butaclamol
Hruska & Silbergeld (73) (*in vitro* rats)	Caudate-binding ↓	^{3}H-Spiroperidol 5-200 nm ± 1mcm . d-Butaclamol
Lai et al. (89) (SD rats)	Caudate-binding Acute NC	3 g/kg (by mouth); ^{3}H-Spiroperidol "various concentrations" ± 1 mcm d-Butaclamol
	Chronic	6 g/kg/day (by mouth), 14 days
Reggiani et al. (144) (SD rats)	Chronic EtOH ↑ striatal binding	^{3}H-Spiroperidol K_d ↑

↑, increase; ↓, decrease; NC, no change.
[a]Sprague-Dawley.
[b]2-amino-6,7 dihydroxy-1,2,3,4-tetrahydronaphthalene.

not alter DA synthesis in limbic areas—since differences in brain region, assay method, and nature of ethanol challenge all differed between studies.

The acute actions of alcohol have been reported to result in decreased DA receptor binding in nucleus accumbens (73). In contrast, the determination of the effects of chronic ethanol on brain DA function in limbic and other regions are less easy to characterize. In part, the difficulty arises because of differing definitions of the term "chronic" among laboratories. Also, the way that DA receptors are defined, e.g., what type of radioligand is used in binding assays, can play a significant role in the outcome of experiments. Both of these sources of confusion are highlighted by the recent literature. Several reports have noted that the binding of the DA antagonist, spiroperidol, is enhanced in the striatum after chronic ethanol treatment

TABLE 2D. *Effects of EtOH on biogenic amine functions: dopamine behavior*

Study	Action	Comments
Lai et al. (89)	Acute-APO stereotypy ↑	3 g/g (by mouth)
(SD[a] rats)	Acute-locomotor NC	—
	Chronic-APO stereotypy ↑	6 g/kg/day (by mouth); 14 days
	Chronic-locomotor NC	—
Strombom et al. (176)	APO ↓ EtOH-stimulation of	—
(NMRI mice, female)	locomotor activity	

↑, increase; ↓ decrease; NC, no change.
[a]Sprague-Dawley.

(5,144). However, other laboratories report no change in striatal DA binding [(5) in DBA2J mice; (75,125)]. In the Muller et al. (125) and Hunt and Dalton (75) reports, striatal assays were carried out with ^{3}H-haloperidol rather than ^{3}H-spiroperidol. Although both ligands are certainly appropriate for labeling "DA receptors" (161), both ligands also label alpha-adrenergic and 5-hydroxytryptamine (5-HT) receptors (88), the latter even more strongly labeled by spiroperidol than by haloperidol. Thus, the positive results in the Reggiani et al. (144) and Barbaccia et al. (5) studies might, for example, be due to ethanol-induced changes in serotonergic function (supported by 125 via changes in 5-HT binding; see below).

In many ways the Hunt and Dalton (75) report is a prototype of a careful brain regional analysis of the effects of chronic ethanol on a number of neurotransmitter systems. However, 4 days of intensive ethanol intubations, although certainly producing severe ethanol withdrawal signs (76), may not be inducing the same pattern of compensatory changes as longer periods of exposure to alcohol. Rather than being critical of the "4-day" dosing model (which offers compelling parallels to an alcoholic "binge"), the divergent results of binding studies should emphasize the need to evaluate thoroughly a variety of durations of exposure to alcohol.

NOREPINEPHRINE: THE LOCUS CERULEUS PROJECTIONS

Ethanol-Aging Interactions on Brain Norepinephrine

A cogent recent study of changes in brain NE in middle-aged alcoholics was carried out by a group of Swedish investigators (19). In the hypothalamus, 50-year-old alcoholics were found to have NE levels that were 66% of that of 70-year-old controls. Hippocampal NE levels were observed to be reduced by 30% in comparison with the 70-year-old control group. NE levels in the cingulate gyrus were depressed by more than 50% in aging alcoholics, whereas in the caudate nucleus, a 35% reduction in the catecholamine was noted. Taken together with the data on the reductions of brain-regional DA in older ethanol abusers, these results suggest that the middle-aged alcoholic is an octogenarian in terms of brain catecholamines.

TABLE 2E. *Effects of EtOH on biogenic amine functions: norepinephrine synthesis*

Study	Action	Comments
Borg et al. (13a)	MOPEG:[a] Acute alcoholics ↑ Acute nonalcoholics ↑	CSF
Hawley et al. (69)	NE alcoholic withdrawal ↑	CSF
Umezu et al. (188) (SD[b] rat)	Catechol hippocampus NC	^{3}H-Catechol from ^{3}H-Tyrosine
Mena & Herrera (116) (Wistar rat)	NE levels ↑ in diencephalon	
Detering et al. (33) (rat)	NE levels ↓ whole brain	Pups-prenatal EtOH
Detering et al. (34) (rat)	NE levels ↓ hypothalamus	Pups-prenatal EtOH
	NE disappearance ↓ hypothalamus	FLA-63; pups, prenatal, or postnatal EtOH
Detering et al. (35) (rat)	TH ↑ DBH[c] ↑ prenatal DBH ↓ postnatal DDC[d] ↑ MAO ↓ COMT ↓	Pups
Baizer et al. (4) (mice)	EtOH (hypothalamus):	
	TH ↑ 25 min in short sleep TH ↑ 125 min in long sleep	Recover righting at 25 min Recover righting at 125 min
Soliman et al. (171) (SD rats)	NE levels ↑ caudate, cerebellum, cortex, midbrain, pons	1–3 hr after 2 g/kg EtOH
Murphy et al. (126) (Wistar rats)	EtOH-nonpreferring: Cortex ↓ NE Hypothalamus ↓ NE Midbrain ↓ NE Midbrain ↓ NE EtOH-preferring Midbrain ↓ NE	Selectively bred

↑, increase; ↓, decrease; NC, no change.
[a]5-methoxy-γ-hydroxy-phenylglycol.
[b]Sprague-Dawley.
[c]Dopamine β-hydroxylase.
[d]DOPA decarboxylase.

Anatomy and Regulation

The locus ceruleus (LC) is the largest NE-containing nucleus in mammalian brain, with almost 50% of all brain NE (129). It projects extensively throughout much of the brainstem and forebrain, including the entire isocortex. Generally, the LC projections are not as topographically organized as those of the nigrostriatal

TABLE 2F. *Effects of EtOH on biogenic amine functions: norepinephrine receptors*

Study	Action	Comments

Hunt & Dalton (75)
(4 days EtOH)
	Alpha-NE binding:
	  Cortex NC
	  Hypothalamus NC
	  Cerebellum NC
	  Hippocampus NC
	  Accumbens NC
		0.37nm ^{3}H-
		  Dihydroergokryptine $\pm$
		  100 mcm $(-)-$NE

	Beta-NE binding:
	  Cortex NC
	  Hypothalamus NC
	  Cerebellum NC
	  Hippocampus NC
	  Accumbens NC
		1.8nm ^{3}H-Dihydroalprenolol
		  $\pm$ 10 mcm
		d, 1-Propranolol

Kuriyama et al. (87) (3–10 days EtOH)	Beta-NE binding Cortex ↑	
Smith et al. (170) (SD[a] rat; 4 days EtOH)	Cortex-adenylate cyclase ↑	
Weitbrecht & Cramer (195a) (Wistar rat; acute EtOH)	Cyclic AMP ↓ Cyclic GMP ↓	CSF CSF

Church & Feller (23) (mice)	Cyclic AMP:
	  C57BL/6By ↓
	    cerebellum
	  (after EtOH challenge)
	  BALB/CByJ
		Shorter sleep times

Rangaraj & Kalant (142a) (Wistar rat)	EtOH + NE ↓ Na^+-K^+ATPase whole brain	

↑, increase; ↓, decrease; NC, no change.
[a]Sprague-Dawley.

system, and projections of the LC are widespread to include (from dorsal NE bundle) thalamus, amygdala, septum, habenular nuclei, olfactory bulb, anterior olfactory nucleus, piriform cortex, hippocampus, neocortex (from other LC projections), hypothalamus, cerebellum, brainstem, and spinal cord. Regulation of LC NE neurons is controlled in a manner similar to that observed in peripheral postganglionic sympathetic neurons. Thus, electrical stimulation of LC neurons or acute stress (3) increases TH activity, enhances NE turnover and the accumulation of 3-methoxy, 4-hydroxyphenyl-ethyleneglycol (MHPG) in cortex. Decreases in impulse flow in the same neurons reduce NE turnover with little effect on NE levels (27). Thus, in contrast to the increases in DA synthesis, which result from increases or decreases in impulse flow, changes in NE synthesis rates in LC neurons appear to be a better predictor of impulse flow in central NE neurons.

The Aging Locus Ceruleus Norepinephrine System

Brain concentrations of NE decline with age in brainstem and hypothalamus of rhesus monkey (155). This finding correlates well with an observed decrease in

TABLE 2G. *Effects of EtOH on biogenic amine functions: norepinephrine behavior*

Study	Action	Comments
Kiianmaa (85)	EtOH intake ↑ EtOH-hypothermia ↓	6-OHDA[a] ↓ NE + DA
Sharkawi (164)	Loss of righting ↑ to EtOH by FLA-63[b]	FLA-63 ↓ disappearance of EtOH from brain, etc.
Kiianmaa and Attila (84) (Alko alcohol rats)	EtOH intake NC EtOH sleep time ↑	Neonate
Strombom et al. (176) (NMRI mice, female) Blum et al. (13) (Swiss Webster mice)	Clonidine ↓ EtOH- stimulated α-MPT[c] ↑ EtOH withdrawal	Locomotor activity
	α-MPT ↑ EtOH narcosis	α-MPT alone and after imipramine pretreatment

↑, increase; ↓, decrease; NC, no change.
[a]6-Hydroxydopamine.
[b]*bis*-(1-methyl-4-homopiperazinyl-thiocarbonyl) disulfide.
[c]α-methyl-*p*-tyrosine.

hindbrain NE in aged man (148). Indeed, in the case of at least some of the LC projections, striking parallels are found with the profound effects of age on nigro-striatal DA. However, a lack of age-related changes has been reported for NE in cerebellum, hypothalamus, and brainstem of mice in a report in which age-associated decreases in DA were found (45). A recent experiment by Estes and Simpkins (42) may help to resolve some of the apparent discrepancies relating to the effects of age on the hypothalamus (Table 3) (45,90,131,155) and, by extrapolation, perhaps provide general insights for resolving discrepancies in studies of other brain regions. Estes and Simpkins (42) assayed DA and NE concentrations in discrete hypothalamic regions. Both catecholamines were found to decline with age in portions of the medial basal hypothalamus, whereas NE concentrations were only slightly decreased in the preoptic area. Since different pathways project to these two hypothalamic regions, the data of Estes and Simpkins are consistent with potentially differential age effects on the two systems. Similarly, the absence of an age effect in a given brain region does not necessarily rule out highly significant changes in more circumscribed subregions.

Consistent with the above, NE turnover has generally been reported to decline with age in brainstem, cerebellum, and hypothalamus (45,74,134,167). Both TH and DA beta-hydroxylase activities show age effects, with the former increasing slightly while the latter decreases (145). MAO and COMT activities generally increase with age; for example, MAO-B activity is enhanced within hippocampus, brainstem, and amygdala (50).

In man, cerebellar beta-NE receptor binding declines significantly with age (99), and similar effects also occur in rats (65,99). Similar reductions in beta-NE binding in rat brainstem have also been reported (99). Decreases in beta- and alpha-NE binding in cerebral cortex have also been noted (120), although the literature is not

TABLE 2H. *Effects of EtOH on biogenic amine functions: serotonin synthesis*

Study	Action	Comments
Branchey et al. (14) (human)	↓ 5-HTP	Alcoholics and controls
(rats)	↓ 5-HT whole brain	6 weeks EtOH vs balanced diet
	↓ 5-HIAA baboon	
Gothoni & Ahtec (60) (Wistar rats)	↓ 5-HT; NC 5-HIAA hemispheres minus cortex	Chronic, intoxicated
	↓ 5-HT, NC 5-HIAA pons & medulla	Withdrawn
	NC 5-HT, ↑ 5-HIAA cortex	
	NC 5-HT, ↑ 5-HIAA hemispheres minus cortex	
	NC 5-HT, ↑ 5-HIAA pons & medulla	
	NC 5-HT, ↑ 5-HIAA cortex	EtOH may ↓ 5-HIAA removal from brain via probenecid
Fukumori et al. (55) (Wistar rats)	EtOH: NC 5-HT ↑ 5-HIAA (whole brain)	Disulfiram
	Disulfiram: ↑ 5-HT ↓ 5-HIAA	
	EtOH + disulfiram: ↑ 5-HT ↓ 5-HIAA	
Fukumori et al. (54) (Wistar rats)	Disulfiram: ↑ 5-HT ↑ 5-HIAA (whole brain)	↓ Transport of 5-HIAA brain tissue
Murphy et al. (126) (Wistar rats)	EtOH-nonpreferring: Cortex 5-HT ↑ Thalamus 5-HT ↑ Cortex 5-HIAA ↑	Selectively bred
Soliman et al. (171) (SD[a] rats)	Acute EtOH: 5-HT 5-HIAA Caudate NC NC Cerebellum NC NC Cortex NC NC Midbrain NC NC Pons NC NC	

↑, increase; ↓, decrease; NC, no change.
[a]Sprague-Dawley.

entirely consistent in this regard (99). Decreased sensitivity of NE-stimulated aden-ylate cyclase activity in hippocampus (193), cortex (8,102,138), cerebellum (157,193), and hypothalamus (102,138) has also been reported, but the literature is by no means consistent (Table 3).

Similar to results on changes in age-related plasticity after chronic DA blockers, reserpine (a vesicular reuptake inhibitor and, hence, depleter of catecholamines and 5-HT) administration to old rats was not associated with the compensatory increases

TABLE 2I. *Effects of EtOH on biogenic amine functions: serotonin receptors*

Study	Action	Comments
Hunt and Dalton (75) (4 days EtOH)	Serotonin binding: Caudate NC Hippocampus NC Cortex NC	4nm ³H-Serotonin ± 10 mcm Serotonin
Muller et al. (125) (11–15 days EtOH)	Caudate ↑ Hippocampus ↓	3nm ³H-Serotonin ± 100 nm Serotonin

↑, increase; ↓, decrease; NC, no change.

TABLE 2J. *Effects of EtOH on biogenic amine functions: serotonin behavior*

Study	Action	Comments
Frankel et al. (51) (Wistar rat)	PCPA[a] ↑ tolerance loss	Motor impairment
Yojay et al. (203) (Swiss As/W mice)	PCPA ↓ EtOH narcosis	Imipramine pretreatment
Le et al. (93) (Wistar rat)	5,7-Dihydroxytryptamine ↓ tolerance to EtOH Motor impairment Hypothermia	
Geller et al. (58) (SD[b] rats)	5-HTP ↓ EtOH drinking	

↑, increase; ↓, decrease; NC, no change.
[a]p-chlorophenylalanine.
[b]Sprague-Dawley.

in beta-NE receptor density in the cerebellum and cortex observed in young rats (66). In the same report, desmethylimipramine (a NE uptake inhibitor) treatment (reminiscent of bromocriptine) was found to maintain its ability to induce a beta-NE subsensitivity. Thus, a selective (to antagonists) reduction in the plasticity of brain catecholamine neurons with age may be a somewhat general phenomenon.

Effects of Ethanol on Brain Norepinephrine

NE synthesis (as a function of TH activity) is increased in the hypothalamus of long-sleep and short-sleep mice at the times when each strain of animal is recovering the righting reflex (4). Similarly, other recent studies of NE levels [which, as critically discussed in McGeer et al. (107), do not provide a particularly useful estimate of NE function] have, nevertheless, generally supported the conclusions of earlier work (76,133a) (Table 2) that acute ethanol challenge decreases NE turnover whereas NE turnover appears enhanced with chronic NE administration.

TABLE 3. *Effects of aging on brain regional biogenic amines*

	Cortex	Striatum	Accumbens	Hippocampus	Septum	Amygdala	Hypothalamus	Nigra	Cerebellum	Brainstem
Levels										
DA	—	↓ (2,20,46, 90,146)	—	—	—	—	↑ or ↓ (regionally) (42)	↓ (2), NC (131)	—	—
NE	—	—	—	↓ (2)	—	—	↑ (154), ↑ or ↓ (regionally) (42), ↓ (89,131), NC (45) ↓ (154,167)	NC (131)	NC(45)	↓ (148,149,154)
5-HT	—	—	—	↓ (113)	—	—	—	—	—	↓ (113)
Turnover										
DA	—	↓ (45), NC (32,71, 131,163)	—	↓ (32)	—	—	↓ (45, 131), NC or ↓ (74)	—	—	↓ (45)
NE	—	—	—	—	—	—	↓ (45,131), NC or ↓ (74)	—	↓ (45)	↓ (45)
5-HT	—	—	—	—	—	—	↑ (167) (Pargyline)	—	—	—
Reuptake										
DA	↓ (61)	—	—	—	—	—	↓ (61)	—	—	—
NE	NC (61)	—	—	—	—	—	NC (61)	—	—	—
5-HT	NC (61)	—	—	—	—	—	NC (61)	—	—	—
Synthetic enzymes										
DA	—	↓ (28,108,109, 111,145)	↓ (145)	—	—	—	—	—	—	—
NE	—	—	—	—	—	—	↓ (145)	—	—	—
5-HT	—	—	—	↓ (113)	NC (113)	—	—	—	—	↓ (113), NC (145)
Receptors										
DA	↓ (102)	↓ (63,82,83, 94,101,120, 137,162, 184,193), ↓ or NC (138)	↓ (162)	↓ (193), NC (138)	—	—	↓ (102, 138)	↓ (62,83, 137,162, 193)	—	—
NE	↓ (8,120), NC (99)	—	—	—	—	—	—	—	↓ (65,99, 157,193)	↓ (99)
5-HT	↓ (166)	—	—	—	—	—	—	—	—	—

↑, increase; ↓, decrease; NC, no change.
Numbers refer to references at end of chapter.

In this context, the results of the Baizer et al. (4) long-sleep/short-sleep study suggest that useful information about the functional significance of ethanol-induced changes in NE turnover might be obtained by measurements made at several times after ethanol challenge (e.g., before and after depression of the righting reflex) in a number of strains.

An interesting approach to the study of putative ethanol-catecholamine interactions has been provided by Carlsson's group (176). Small doses of a DA agonist (apomorphine) and a NE agonist (clonidine) appropriate for selective stimulation of autoreceptors supressed the locomotor stimulation induced by low doses of ethanol in mice. Moreover, these low doses of ethanol (which did not alter DOPA accumulation after decarboxylase inhibition) did affect the inhibition in striatum produced by the catecholamine agonists. Ethanol enhanced the reduction in DOPA accumulation by APO but slightly inhibited the reduction in DOPA associated with clonidine injection. Thus, the consistency of the behavioral and turnover data with regard to DA provides an exciting link between ethanol stimulation and autoreceptors. The lack of consistency with regard to NE suggests that the ethanol-clonidine interaction on behavior may be secondary to an effect on some other system.

Recent receptor studies of the actions of chronic ethanol on NE have typically reported increased postsynaptic receptor activity using radioligand binding or adenylate cyclase assays as probes [(23) in BALB/CByJ mice; (87,170)]. However, a recent study of NE binding after chronic ethanol by Hunt and Dalton (75) showed no change in markers of alpha- and beta-NE binding. It is good to recall, however, that the 4-day duration of repeated ethanol dosing in the latter report was not comparable to that of other studies.

SEROTONIN: THE RAPHE NUCLEI PROJECTIONS

Ethanol-Aging Interactions on Brain Serotonin

A series of brains from middle-aged alcoholics investigated for changes in serotonin indicated that the most profound changes in content of the transmitter occurred in the hypothalamus, with decreases of 91% observed relative to aged controls (19). The ratio of 5-HT to 5-hydroxyindole-3-acetic acid (5-HIAA) was 32% in hypothalamus, which was the lowest ratio of transmitter to metabolite found within the serotonin system in any of the brain regions examined. Hippocampal levels of serotonin were reduced by 53% in older alcoholics (mean age, 53 years) whereas 5-HIAA values were less depressed (5-HT/5-HIAA, 80%). Serotonin levels in the cingulate gyrus were found reduced to 57% of the values found in controls, whereas 5-HIAA levels were only depressed by 9%. Caudate nucleus levels of serotonin were reduced by 70% while 5-HT/5-HIAA was found to be 32%.

Anatomy and Regulation

In marked contrast to most of the catecholaminergic cell groups, serotonergic (5-HT) neurons are mainly distributed within specific cytoarchitectonic entities (the raphe nuclei) often with other types of neurons (31,130). The nucleus dorsalis raphe is the largest of the three serotonin cell groups of the midbrain and seems to contain predominantly 5-HT neurons. Taken together, the raphe nucleu project to striatum, hippocampus, habenula, thalamus, hypothalamus, amygdala, anterior olfactory nucleus, olfactory bulb, and cortex. The widespread distribution of the raphe projections is reminiscent of the LC projections and similarly implies a highly collateralized axonal system from each serotonin neuron (44). Serotonin is synthesized by 5-hydroxylation of L-tryptophan with subsequent decarboxylation of 5-hydroxytryptophan (5-HTP) by aromatic L-amino acid decarboxylase (DOPA decarboxylase). Manipulation of 5-HT function by administration of L-tryptophan is complicated by the fact that only a small fraction of a given dose of the amino acid is metabolized to 5-HT and by the observation that high concentrations of tryptophan metabolites (such as kynurenine) or tryptophan itself may inhibit conversion of tryptophan to serotonin (57). The use of 5-HTP also presents a potential problem because it requires only aromatic L-amino acid decarboxylase for conversion to 5-HT. This enzyme is not restricted to 5-HT neurons (it catalyzes the conversion of L-DOPA to DA in dopaminergic, noradrenergic, and adrenergic neurons as well), and it is present in large excess so that its activity would have to be inhibited almost completely for 5-HT synthesis to be decreased substantially (56,139). Blockade of dopaminergic and noradrenergic receptors causes a compensatory enhancement of neurotransmitter turnover (107). One might then reasonably expect that blockade of central 5-HT receptors would similarly increase serotonin turnover. This turns out not to be the case for most 5-HT blockers [methysergide, cyproheptadine, lysergic acid-diethylamide, and mianserin (56,174)]. Only methiothepin (which also blocks catecholamine receptors) enhances 5-HT turnover (56). Therefore, the effects of ethanol on biogenic amine function must be interpreted with full cognizance of the disparate mechanisms regulating transmitter release within each brain system.

The Aging Raphe Serotonin Systems

In contrast to the profound effects of aging on brain catecholamine systems, the serotonergic pathways appear to be much less susceptible to changes over the lifespan. Thus, 5-HT levels decline in hippocampus and brainstem (113) but not in septum (113) or in hypothalamus (155,167). The clearance of 5-HIAA in hypothalamus does appear to decrease with age, resulting in smaller decreases in 5-HIAA after MAO inhibition (167). Whether this relates to the observed increases in cerebrospinal fluid (CSF) 5-HIAA in human subjects over 70 years old (61) or to age-related increases in MAO (149) remains to be demonstrated. Serotonin uptake is unaltered in the striatum with age (79). TH activity has been found to decrease in rat hippocampus and brainstem but not septum (113) whereas 5-HT binding in human cortex similarly declines (166) in aging.

Effects of Ethanol on Brain Serotonin

Early (36) and more recent (171) reports are consistent in suggesting that acute ethanol challenge has only minimal effects on 5-HT levels or turnover. In contrast, brain serotonin function as estimated by plasma precursor (5-HTP) levels has been reported to be decreased in alcoholics (14). In chronically intoxicated rats, 5-HT levels were found to be decreased in cerebral hemispheres minus cortex and in pons/medulla while 5-HIAA was unaltered (60). However, these same authors observed that under the same conditions, cortical serotonin exhibited no change whereas increases in 5-HIAA were observed. In the same study, regional assays were repeated in rats withdrawn from alcohol. In all regions, 5-HT was unaltered while 5-HIAA increased. Similarly, selectively bred ethanol-nonpreferring rats exhibited, in the absence of drug treatment, increased 5-HT in cortex and thalamus and increased 5-HIAA in cortex when compared with controls (126), although significant changes from control were not apparent in the ethanol-preferring animals. Thus, chronic ethanol may be associated with decreased serotonin turnover during the later stages of intoxication and in early withdrawal. However, this conclusion must be tentative since earlier studies of turnover have tended to report either no change (51) or increases (87). However, both of these studies utilized pargyline (to inhibit MAO). Pargyline may not completely prevent the disappearance of 5-HT from the brain [some O-sulphate may be formed (57)] and may alter serotonin synthesis (98) so that the results of the early and more recent studies may not be strictly comparable. Nevertheless, Curzon (30) has recently concluded that pargyline, decarboxylase inhibition, probenecid, and radiolabeled tryptophan methods all give comparable estimates of 5-HT synthesis rates. Thus, it is important for studies of the effects of ethanol on brain 5-HT turnover using MAO versus decarboxylase inhibition procedures to be carried out to resolve this discrepancy in the 5-HT ethanol literature.

Radioactive 5-HT binding has been reported to be enhanced after chronic ethanol in striatum (recall studies of changes in ^{3}H-spiroperidol binding) but to be decreased in the hippocampus (125). However, Hunt and Dalton (75) reported no change in ^{3}H-5-HT binding in striatum, hippocampus, or cerebral cortex after 4-day ethanol intubations. Besides a difference in length of ethanol treatment (2 weeks versus 4 days), there is a second potentially significant difference between the two conflicting studies. Although both laboratories used virtually the same concentration of ^{3}H-serotonin (at or below the K_d), the blank concentrations, which actually define specific binding (15,161,196), differed by 100-fold between the two reports. It is likely, therefore, that the binding labeled "specific" in the Hunt and Dalton (75) experiment included a significant portion of nonspecific (i.e., nonserotonergic) binding as well.

CONCLUSIONS

Behavioral studies have suggested that potential significant interactions may exist between the effects of alcoholism and aging (153). As we have discussed, both aging and ethanol are known to exert profound actions on brain catecholamine functions and on the activity of other chemical mediators as well (1,40,83,100, 180,181). Furthermore, ethanol and the process of aging each appear to exert a variety of somewhat selective actions on the chemical transmission within different brain regions.

Future studies of aging-ethanol interactions must focus on maintaining adequate nutritional-health status of the subjects for the data to have relevance for the specific interaction of the drug abuse-aging process. Also, studies of chronic ethanol should standardize dose and duration of drug, bearing in mind the truly long-term nature (20 years) of the ethanol abuse facing the clinician. Such studies must begin to shift emphasis toward brain regional or subregional characterization of functional parameters of transmitters (synthesis, turnover, release, etc.) and away from whole brain analyses of transmitter levels. Neurotransmitter balances may be more profoundly affected by alcohol-aging interactions than are aspects of the function of a single transmitter. These should be evaluated carefully and the functional significance of disruptions in chemical mediator relationships explored by showing that pharmacological manipulations of brain transmitters that correct a deficit or restore a balance have some ameliorative action toward the ravages of chronic alcohol use in aging man.

The current paucity of neurochemical data on ethanol-aging relationships reflects the difficulty of the task and the fact that the requisite background studies of the actions of ethanol or aging on brain regional neurotransmitter parameters have only recently begun to approach a critical mass. The challenge of the moment is to assess the current core of studies of the effects on aging versus alcohol on all neuromodulators in such a way that a productive course is charted for the future. The pleasant task of this review has been to help portend the road ahead. The delightful task of the reader will be to travel that road by carrying out the needed future studies of alcohol-aging effects. In so doing, the way will be paved for elimination of a disease and for procurement of richer lives for those now addicted to ethanol.

ACKNOWLEDGMENTS

This work was supported in part by a grant from the National Institutes of Mental Health (MH333442) to William H. Riffee and R. E. Wilcox. The author is grateful to Dr. T. Samorajski for encouragement and to Dr. S. W. Leslie and Dr. C. K. Erickson for many helpful suggestions. Special thanks are provided to Kaye Chung and Laura Sundquist for typing of the manuscript.

REFERENCES

1. Amaducci, L., Davison, A. N., and Amtuono, P., editors (1980): *Aging, Vol. 13: Aging of the Brain and Dementia.* Raven Press, NY.
2. Adolfsson, R., Gotlfrier, C. G., Roos, B. E., and Winblad, B. (1979): Postmortem distribution of dopamine and homovanillic acid in human brain, variations related to age and a review of the literature. *J. Neural Transm.*, 45:81–105.
3. Antelman, S. M., and Caggiula, R. (1980): Norepinephrine-dopamine interactions and behavior. *Science*, 195:646–653.

4. Baizer, L., Masserano, J. M., and Weiner, N. (1981): Ethanol-induced changes in tyrosine hydroxylase activity in brains of mice selectively bred for differences in sensitivity to ethanol. *Pharmacol. Biochem. Behav.*, 15:945–949.

4a. Bannon, M. J., Michaud, R. L., and Roth, R. H. (1981): Mesocortical dopamine neurons. Lack of autoreceptors modulating dopamine synthesis. *Mol. Pharmacol.*, 19:270–275.

5. Barbaccia, M. L., Reggiani, A., Spano, P. F., and Trabucchi, M. (1981): Ethanol-induced changes of dopaminergic function in three strains of mice characterized by a different population of opiate receptors. *Psychopharmacology*, 74:260–262.

6. Barbeau, A. (1979): Newer therapeutic approaches in Parkinson's disease. In: *Advances in Neurology*, Vol. 24, edited by L. J. Poirier, T. L. Sourkes, and P. J. Bedard, pp. 433–450. Raven Press, NY.

7. Barbeau, A. (1980): Biochemical aging in Parkinson's disease. In: *Aging*, Vol. 13, Aging of the Brain and Dementia, edited by L. Amaducci, A. N. Davidson, and P. Antuono, pp. 275–287. Raven Press, NY.

8. Berg, A., and Zimmerman, I. D. (1975): Effects of electrical stimulation and norepinephrine on cyclic-AMP levels in the cerebral cortex of the aging rat. *Mech. Ageing Dev.*, 4:377–383.

9. Bernasconi, R., Maitre, L., Martin, P., and Raschdorf, F. (1982): The use of inhibitors of GABA-transaminase for the determination of GABA turnover in mouse brain regions: an evaluation of aminooxyacetic acid and gabaculine. *J. Neurochem.*, 38:57–66.

10. Bhattacharyya. A. K., and Pradham, S. N. (1980): Comparative effects of dopamine agonists in young and old rats. *Fed. Proc.*, 39:508.

11. Bianchine, J. R. (1980): Drug for Parkinson's disease. In: *The Pharmacological Basis of Therapeutics*, edited by A. G. Gilman, L. S. Goodman, and A. Gilman, pp. 475–494. Macmillan, NY.

12. Blecher, M., and Bar, R. S. (1981): *Receptors and Human Disease.* Williams and Wilkins, Baltimore.

13. Blum, K., and Wallace, J. E. (1974): Effects of catecholamine synthesis inhibition of ethanol-induced withdrawal symptoms in mice. *Br. J. Pharmac.*, 51:109–111.

13a. Borg. S., and Kvande, H. (1981): Central norepinephrine metabolism during alcohol intoxication in addicts and healthy volunteers. *Science*, 213:1135–1137.

14. Branchey, L., Shaw, S., and Lieber, C. S. (1981): Ethanol impairs tryptophan transport into the brain and depresses serotonin. *Life Sci.*, 29:2751–2755.

15. Burt, D. R. (1980): Basic receptor methods. II. Problems of interpretation in binding studies. *Receptor Binding Techniques: Society for Neuroscience 1980 Short Course Syllabus. Society for Neuroscience*, Bethesda, MD, pp. 53–70.

16. Bustos, G., Liberona, J. L., and Gysling, K. (1981): Regulation of transmitter synthesis and release in mesolimbic dopaminergic nerve terminals. *Biochem. Pharmacol.*, 30:2157–2164.

17. Bustos, G., and Roth, R. H. (1976): Effect of acute ethanol treatment on transmitter synthesis and metabolism in central dopaminergic neurons. *J. Pharm. Pharmacol.*, 28:580–582.

18. Carlen, P. I., Lee, M. A., and Jacob, M. (1981): Parkinsonism provoked by alcoholism. *Ann. Neurol.*, 9:84–86.

19. Carlsson, A., Adolfsson, R., Aquilonius, S. M., Gottfries, C. G., Oreland, L., Svennerholm, L., and Winblad, B. (1980): Biogenic amines in human brain in normal aging, senile dementia, and chronic alcoholism. In: *Ergot Compounds and Brain Function. A Neuroendocrine and Neuropsychiatric Aspects*, edited by M. Goldstein, pp. 295–304. Raven Press, NY.

20. Carlsson, A., and Winblad, B. (1976): The influence of age and time interval between death and autopsy on dopamine and 3 methoxytyramine levels in human basal ganglia. *J. Neural Trans.*, 83:271–276.

21. Cattabeni, F., Racagni, G., Spano, P. F., and Costa, E., editors (1980): Long-Term Effects of Neuroleptics. *Advances in Biochemical Psychopharmacology*, Vol. 24. Raven Press, NY.

22. Caudill, W. L., Houck, G. P., and Wightman, R. M. (1982): Determination of gamma-aminobutyric acid by liquid chromatography with electrochemical detection. *J. Chromatogr.*, 227:331–339.

23. Church, A. C., and Feller, D. (1979): The influence of mouse genotype on the changes in brain cyclic nucleotide levels induced by acute alcohol administration. *Pharmacol. Biochem. Behav.*, 10:335–338.

24. Clow, A., Theodorou, A., Jenner, P., and Marsdin, C. D. (1980): Changes in rat striatal dopamine

turnover and receptor activity during one year neuroleptic administration. *Eur. J. Pharmacol.*, 63:135–144.

25. Clow, A., Theodorou, A., Jenner, P., and Maraden, C. D. (1980): Cerebral dopamine function in rats following withdrawal from one year of continuous neuroleptic administration. *Eur. J. Pharmacol.*, 63:145–157.

26. Clow, A., Theodorou, A., Jenner, P., Maradin, C. D. (1980): A comparison of striatal and mesolimbic dopamine function in the rat during 6 month trifluoperazine administration. *Psychopharmacology*, 69:227–233.

27. Cooper, J. R., Bloom, F. E., and Roth, R. H. (1982): *The Biochemical Basis of Neuropharmacology*. Oxford, NY.

28. Cote, L. J., and Kremzner, L. T. (1974): Changes in neurotransmitter systems with increasing age in human brain. In: *Trans. Am. Soc. Neurochem.*, 5th Annual Meeting, New Orleans, La. p. 83.

29. Cote, L. (1981): Basal ganglia, the extrapyramidal motor system, and diseases of transmitter metabolism. In: *Principles of Neural Science*, edited by E. R. Kandel and J. H. Schwartz, pp. 347–357. Elsevier, NY.

30. Curzon, G. (1981): The turnover of 5-hydroxytryptamine. In: *Central Neurotransmitter Turnover*, edited by C. J. Pycock and P. V. Taberner, pp. 59–81. University Park Press, Baltimore, MD.

31. Dahlstrom, A., and Fuxe, K. (1964): Evidence for the existence of monoamine-containing neurons in the central nervous system. *Acta Physiol. Scand.*, 62, Suppl. 232.

32. Demarest, K. T., Riegle, G. D., and Moore, K. E. (1980): Characteristics of dopaminergic neurons in the aged male rat. *Neuroendocrinology*, 31:222–227.

33. Detering, N., Collins, Jr., R. M., Hawkins, R. L., Ozand, P. T., and Karahasan, A. (1980): Comparative effects of ethanol and malnutrition on the development of catecholamine neurons: changes in neurotransmitter levels. *J. Neurochem.*, 34:1587–1593.

34. Detering, N., Collins, Jr., R. M., Hawkins, R. L., Ozand, P. T., and Karahasan, A. (1980): A comparative effect of ethanol and malnutrition on the development of catecholamine neurons: changes in norepinephrine turnover. *J. Neurochem.*, 34:1788–1791.

35. Detering, N., Edward, E., Ozand, P., and Karahasan, A. (1980c): Comparative effects of ethanol and malnutrition on the development of catecholamine neurons: changes in specific activities of enzymes. *J. Neurochem.*, 34:297–304.

36. Deitrich, R. A. (1976): Biochemical aspects of alcoholism. *Psychoneuroendocrinology*, 1:325–346.

37. Dray, A. (1980): The physiology and pharmacology of mammalian basal ganglia. *Prog. Neurobiol.*, 14:223–335.

38. Enna, S. J., and Snyder, S. H. (1975): Properties of gamma-aminobutyric acid (GABA) receptor binding in rat brain synaptic membrane fractions. *Brain Res.*, 100:81–97.

39. Enna, S. J., and Snyder, S. H. (1977): Influence of ions, enzymes and detergents on gamma-aminobutyric acid receptor binding in synaptic membranes of rat brain. *Molec. Pharmacol.*, 13:442–453.

40. Enna, S. J., Samorajski, T., and Beer, B., editors (1981): *Aging, Vol. 17: Brain Neurotransmitters and Receptors in Aging and Age-Related Disorders*. Raven Press, NY.

41. Erickson, C. K. (1976): Regional distribution of ethanol in rat brain. *Life Sci.*, 19:1439–1446.

42. Estes, K. S., and Simpkins, J. W. (1980): Age-related alterations in catecholamine concentrations in discrete preoptic area and hypothalamic regions in the male rat. *Brain Res.*, 194:556–560.

43. Fadda, F., Argiolas, A., Melis, M. R., Serra, G., and Gessa, G. L. (1980): Differential effect of acute and chronic ethanol on dopamine metabolism in frontal cortex, caudate nucleus and substantia nigra. *Life Sci.*, 37:979–986.

44. Fallon, J. H., and Moore, R. Y. (1978): Catecholamine innervation of the basal forebrain. IV. Topography of the dopamine projection to the basal forebrain and neostriatum. *J. Comp. Neurol.*, 180:545–580.

45. Finch, C. E. (1973): Catecholamine metabolism in the brains of aging male mice. *Brain Res.*, 52:261–276.

46. Finch, C. E. (1976): The regulation of physiological changes during mammalian aging. *Q. Rev. Biol.*, 51:49–83.

47. Finch, C. E. (1978): Age related changes in brain catecholamines: a synopsis of findings in C57BL/6J mice and other rodent models. In: *Advances in Experimental Medicine and Biology, Vol. 113.*

Parkinson's Disease-II. edited by C. E. Finch, D. E. Potter, and A. D. Denny, pp. 15–39. Plenum Press, NY.
48. Finch, C. E., Randall, P. K., and Marshall, J. F. (1981): Aging and basal gangliar functions. *Ann. Rev. Geront. Geriatr.*, 2:49–87.
49. Finch, C. E. (1977): Neuroendocrine and autonomic aspects of aging. *Handbook of the Biology of Aging*. Van Nostrand Reinhold, New York.
50. Finch, C. E. (1980): The relationships of aging changes in the basal ganglia to manifestations of Huntington's chorea. *Ann. Neurol.*, 7:406–411.
51. Frankel, D., Khanna, J. M., Kalant, H., and Leblanc, A. E. (1978): Effect of p-chlorophenyla-lanine on the loss and maintenance of tolerance to ethanol. *Psychopharmacology*, 56:139–143.
52. Freund, G. (1984): Neurotransmitter function in relation to aging and alcoholism. In: *Alcoholism in the Elderly*, edited by T. Samorajski, pp. 65–84. Raven Press, New York.
53. Frye, G. D., and Breese, G. R. (1981): An evaluation of the locomotor stimulating action of ethanol in rats and mice. *Psychopharmacology*, 75:372–379.
54. Fukumori, R., Minegishi, A., Satoh, T., Kitagawa, H., and Yanaura, S. (1979): Effect of di-sulfiram on turnover of 5-hydroxytryptamine in rat brain. *Life Sci.*, 25:123–130.
55. Fukumori, R., Minegishi, A., Satoh, T., Kitagawa, H., and Yanaura, S. (1980): Changes in the serotonin and 5-hydroxyindoleacetic acid contents in rat brain after ethanol and disulfiram treat-ments. *Eur. J. Pharmacol.*, 61:199–202.
56. Fuller, R. W. (1980): Pharmacology of central serotonin neurons. *Annu. Rev. Pharmacol. Toxicol.*, 20:111–127.
57. Gal, E. M., Young, R. B., and Sherman, A. D. (1978): Tryptophan loading: consequent effects on the synthesis of kynurenine and 5-hydroxyindoles in rat brain. *J. Neurochem.*, 31:237–244.
58. Geller, L., Hartmann, R. J., and Messiha, F. S. (1981): Blockade of 5-HTP reduction of ethanol drinking with the decarboxylase inhibitor, R04-4602. *Pharmacol. Biochem. Behav.*, 15:871–874.
59. Goldman, M. E., Miller, S. S., Shorey, R. L., and Erickson, C. K. (980): Ethanol dependence produced in rats by nutritionally complete diets. *Pharmacol. Biochem. Behav.*, 12:503–507.
60. Gothoni, P., and Ahtee, L. (1980): Chronic ethanol administration decreases 5-HT and increases 5-HIAA concentration in rat brain. *Acta Pharmacol. Toxicol.*, 46:113–120.
61. Gottfries, C. G., Gottfries, I., Johansson, B., Olsson, R., Persson, T., Roos, B. E., and Sjostrom, R. (1971): Acid monoamine metabolites in human cerebrospinal fluid and their relations to age and sex. *Neuropharmacology*, 10:665–672.
62. Govoni, S., Loddo, P., Spano, P. F., and Trabucchi, M. (1977): Dopamine receptor sensitivity in brain and retina of rats during aging. *Brain Research*, 138:565–570.
63. Govoni, S., Memo, M., Saiani, L., Spano, P. F., and Trabucchi, M. (1980): Impairment of brain neurotransmitter receptors in aged rats. *Mech. Ageing Dev.*, 12:39–46.
64. Govoni, S., Olgiati, V. R., Trabucchi, M., Garau, L., Stefanini, E., and Spano, P. F. (1978): (3H)-Haloperidol and (3H)-spiroperidol receptor binding after striatal injection of kainic acid. *Neurosci. Lett.*, 8:207–210.
65. Greenberg, L. H., and Wiss, B. (1978): Beta-adrenergic receptors in aged rat brain: Reduced number and capacity of pineal gland to develop supersensitivity. *Science*, 201:61–63.
66. Greenberg, L. H., and Weiss, B. (1979): Ability of aged rats to alter β-adrenergic receptors of brain in response to repeated administration of reserpine and desmethylimipramine. *J. Pharmacol. Exp. Ther.*, 211:209–316.
67. Hakkinen, H. M., and Kulonen, E. (1979): Ethanol intoxication and the activities of glutamote decarboxylase and γ-aminobutyrate aminotransferase in rat brain. *J. Neurochem.*, 33:943–946.
68. Haubrich, D. R., and Pflueger, A. B. (1982): The autoreceptor control of dopamine synthesis. An *in vitro* and *in vivo* comparison of dopamine agonists. *Mol. Pharmacol.*, 21:114–120.
69. Hawley, R. J., Major, L. F., Schulman, E. A., and Lake, C. R. (1981): CSF levels of norepi-nephrine during alcohol withdrawal. *Arch. Neurol.*, 38:289–292.
70. Haycock, J. W., White, W. F., McGaugh, J. L., and Cotman, C. W. (1977): Enhanced stimulus-secretion coupling from brains of aged mice. *Exp. Neurol.*, 57:873–882.
71. Hefti, F., Milamed, E., Bhawn, J., and Wurtman, R. J. (1981): Long-term administration of L-dopa does not damage dopaminergic neurons in the mouse. *Neurology* (NY), 31:1194–1195.
72. Hornykiewicz, O. (1976): The neurochemistry of Parkinson's disease: Effect of l-dopa therapy. *J. Pharmacol. Exp. Ther.*, 195:453–464.
73. Hruska, R. E., and Silbergeld, E. K. (1980): Inhibition of (3H)-spiroperidol binding by *in vitro* addition of ethanol. *J. Neurochem.*, 35:750–752.

74. Huang, H. H., Simphins, J. W., and Meites, J. (1977): Hypothalmic norepinephrine (NE) and dopamine (DA) turnover and relation to LH, FSH, and prolacting release in old female rats. *Endocrinology [Suppl.]*, 100:331.

75. Hunt, W. A., and Dalton, T. K. (1981): Neurotransmitter-receptor binding in various brain regions in ethanol-dependent rats. *Pharmacol. Biochem. Behav.*, 14:733–739.

76. Hunt, W. A., and Majchrowicz, E. (1974): Alterations in the turnover of brain norepinephrine and dopamine in alcohol-dependent rats. *J. Neurochem.*, 23:549–552.

77. Jacoby, J. H., Shabshelowitz, H., Fernstrom, J. D., and Wurtman, R. (1975): The mechanisms by which methiothepin, a putative serotonin receptor antagonist, increases brain 5-hydroxyindole levels. *J. Pharmacol. Exp. Ther.*, 195:257–264.

78. Jacoby, J. H., Poulakos, J. J., and Bryce, G. F. (1978): On the central anti-serotoninergic actions of cyproheptadine and methysergide. *Neuropharmacology*, 17:299–306.

79. Jones, V. J., and Finch, C. E. (1975): Senescent and dopamine uptake by subcellular fractions of C57BL/6J male mouse brain. *Brain Res.*, 91:197–215.

80. Jonsson, G., and Ponzio, F. (1979): A rapid and simple method for the determination of picogram levels of serotonin in brain tissue using liquid chromatography with electrochemical detection. *J. Neurochem.*, 32:129–132.

81. Joseph, J. A., Berger, R. E., Engel, B. T., and Roth, G. S. (1981): Age-related changes in the nigrostriatum: a behavioral and biochemical analysis. *J. Gerontol.*, 33:643–649.

82. Joseph, J. A., Filburn, C. R., and Roth, G. S. (1978): Development of dopamine receptor denervation supersensitivity in the neostriatum of the senescent rat. *Life Sci.*, 29:575–584.

83. Katzman, R., Terry, R. D., and Bick, K. L., editors (1978): *Aging, Vol. 7: Alzheimer's Disease: Senile Dementia and Related Disorders*. Raven Press, NY.

84. Kiianmaa, K., and Attila, L. M. J. (1979): Alcohol intake, ethanol-induced narcosis and intoxication in rats following neonatal 6-hydroxydopamine or 5,7-dihydroxytryptamine treatment. *Naunyn-Schmiedeberg's Arch. Pharmacol.*, 308:165–170.

85. Kiianmaa, K. (1980): Alcohol intake and ethanol intoxication in the rat: effect of a 6-OHDA-induced lesion of the ascending noradrenaline pathways. *Eur. J. Pharmacol.*, 64:9–19.

85a. Korf, J. (1981): The turnover of neurotransmitters in the brain: an introduction. In: *Central Neurotransmitter Turnover*, edited by C. J. Pycock and P. V. Taberner, pp. 1–20. University Park Press, Baltimore.

86. Kubanis, P., and Zornetzer, S. F. (1971): Review age-related behavioral and neurobiological changes: a review with an emphasis on memory. *Behav. Neur. Biol.*, 31:115–172.

87. Kuriyama, K., Muramatsu, M., Aiso, M., and Ueno, E. (1971): Alteration in beta-adrenergic receptor binding in brain, lung and heart during morphine and alcohol dependence and withdrawal. *Neuropharmacology*, 20:659–666.

88. Laduron, P. (1981): Dopamine receptor: from an *in vivo* concept towards a molecular characterization. In: *Towards Understanding Receptors*, edited by J. W. Lamble. *Current Reviews in Biomedicine*, 1:105–111. Elsevier/North Holland, Amsterdam.

89. Lai, H., Kazi, S., Carino, M. A., and Horita, A. (1982): Chronic haloperidol treatment potentiates apomorphine- and ethanol-induced hypothermia in the rat. *Life Sci.*, 30:821–826.

90. Lanfield, P. W., Baskin, R. K., and Pitler, T. A. (1981): Brain aging correlates: retardation by hormonal-pharmacological treatments. *Science*, 214:581–584.

91. Langer, S. Z. (1981): Presynaptic regulation of the release of catecholamines. *Pharmacol. Rev.*, 32:337–362.

92. Larsen, T. A., and Calne, D. B. (1982): Recent advances in the study of Parkinson's disease. *Trends Neurosci.*, Jan., 10–12.

93. Le, A. D., Khanna, J. M., Kalant, H., and LeBlanc, A. E. (1980): Effect of 5,7-dihydroxytryptamine on the development of tolerance to ethanol. *Psychopharmacology*, 67:143–146.

94. Levin, P., Janda, J. K., Joseph, J. A., Ingram, D. K., and Roth, G. S. (1981): Dietary restriction retards age-associated loss of rat striatal dopaminergic receptor. *Science*, 214:30.

95. Leysen, J. E., Gommeren, W., and Laduron, P. M. (1978): Spipirone: a ligand of choice for neuroleptic receptors. 1. Kinetics and characteristics of in vitro binding. *Biochem. Pharmacol.*, 27:307–316.

96. Lindvall, O., and Bjorklund, A. (1974): The organization of the ascending CA neuron-systems in the rat brains as revealed by the glyoxylic acid fluorescence method. *Acta Physiol. Scand. [Suppl.]*, 412:1–48.

97. Lloyd, K. G. (1978): Neurotransmitter interactions related to central dopamine neurons. In: *Essays in Neurochemistry and Neuropharmacology*, Vol. 3, pp. 131–207. John Wiley, NY.
98. Maggi, A., U'Prichard, D. C., and Enna, S. J. (1980): Differential effects of antidepressant treatment on brain monoaminergic receptors. *Eur. J. Pharmacol.*, 61:91–98.
99. Maggi, A., Schmidt, M. J., Ghetti, B., and Enna, S. J. (1979): Effect on aging on neurotransmitter receptor binding in rat and human brain. *Life Sci.*, 24:367–374.
100. Majchrowicz, E., and Noble, E. P., editors (1979): *Biochemistry and Pharmacology of Ethanol*. Plenum Press, NY.
101. Makman, N. H., Ahn, H. S., Thal, L., Dvorkin, B., Horowitz, S. G., Harpless, N., and Rosenfield, N. (1978): Decreased brain biogenic amine-stimulated adenylate cyclase and spiroperidol binding sites with aging. *Fed. Proc.*, 37:548.
102. Makman, N. H., Ahn, H. S., Thal, L. J., Sharpless, N. S., Dvorkin, B., Horowitz, S. G., and Rosenfield, M. (1979): Aging and monoamine receptors in brain. *Fed. Proc.*, 38:1922–1926.
103. Makman, M. H., Ahn, H. S., Thal, L. J., Sharpless, N. S., Dvorkin, B., Horowitz, S. G., and Rosenfield, M. (1980): Evidence for selective loss of brain dopamine and histamine-stimulated adenylate cyclase activities in rabbits with aging. *Brain Res.*, 192:177–183.
104. Marsh, G. R., and Thompson, L. W. (1977): Psychophysiology of aging. In: *Handbook for the Psychology of Aging*, edited by J. E. Birren and K. W. Schaie, pp. 219–248. Van Nostrand Reinhold, NY.
105. Marshall, J. F., and Berrois, N. (1979): Movement disorders of aged rats: Reversal by dopamine receptor stimulation. *Science*, 206:477–479.
106. McGeer, E. G. (1981): Neurotransmitter systems in aging and senile dementia. *Prog. Neuro-psychopharmacol.*, 5:435–445.
107. McGeer, P. L., Eccles, J. C., and McGeer, E. G. (1978): *Molecular Neurobiology of the Mammalian Brain*. Plenum Press, NY.
108. McGeer, E. G., Fibiger, H. C., McGeer, P. L., and Wickson, V. (1971): Aging and brain enzymes. *Exp. Gerontol.*, 6:391–396.
109. McGeer, E. G., and McGeer, P. L. (1976): Neurotransmitter metabolism in the aging brain. In: *Neurobiology of Aging*, Vol. 3, edited by R. D. Terry and S. Gershon, pp. 389–403. Raven Press, NY.
110. McGeer, P. L., McGeer, E. G., and Suzuki, J. S. (1977): Aging and extrapyramidal function. *Arch. Neurol.*, 34:33–35.
111. McGeer, E. G., and McGeer, P. L. (1975): Age changes in human for some enzymes associated with metabolism of catecholamines. GABA, and acetylcholine. In: *Neurobiology of Aging*, edited by J. M. Ordy and K. R. Brizzee, pp. 287–305. Plenum Press, NY.
112. McGeer, E. G., and McGeer, P. L. (1980): Aging and neurotransmitter systems. In: *Neuroendocrine and Neuropsychiatric Aspects of Aging*, edited by M. Goldstein, pp. 305–314. Raven Press, NY.
113. Meek, J. L., Bertilsson, L., Cheney, D. L., Zsilla, G., and Costa, E. (1977): Aging-induced changes in ACh and 5-HT content of discrete brain nuclei. *J. Gerontol.*, 32:129–131.
114. Meier-Ruge, W., Iwangoff, P., Reichlmeir, K., and Sandoz, P. (1980): Neurochemical findings in the aging brain. In: *Ergot Compounds and Brain Function: Neuroendocrine and Neuropsychiatric Aspects*, edited by M. Goldstein, et al. Raven Press, NY.
115. Memo, M., Lucchi, L., Spano, P. E., and Trabucchi, M. (1980): Aging process affects a single class of dopamine receptors. *Brain Res.*, 202:488–492.
116. Mena, M. A., and Herrera, E. (1980): Monoamine metabolism in rat brain regions following long term alcohol treatment. *J. Neural. Trans.*, 47:227–236.
117. Miller, A. E., Shaar, C. J., and Riegle, G. D. (1976): Aging effects on hypothalmic dopamine and norepinephrine content in the male rat. *Exp. Aging Res.*, 2:475–480.
118. Miller, S. S., Goldman, M. E., Erickson, C. K., and Shorey, R. L. (1980): Induction of physical dependence and tolerance to ethanol in rats fed a new nutritionally complete and balanced liquid diet. *Psychopharmacology*, 68:55–59.
119. Mishara, B. L., and Kastenbaum, R. (1980): *Alcohol and Old Age*. Grune and Stratton, NY.
120. Misra, C. H., Shelat, H. G., and Smith, R. C. (1980): Effect of age in adrenergic and dopaminergic receptor binding in rat brain. *Life. Sci.*, 27:521–526.
121. Moore, R. Y., and Bloom, F. E. (1978): Central CA neuron systems: Anatomy and physiology of the DA systems. *Annu. Rev. Neurosci.*, 1:129–169.

122. Moore, R. Y., and Bloom, F. E. (1979): Central catecholamine neuron systems: anatomy and physiology of the norepinephrine and epinephrine systems. *Annu. Rev. Neurosci.*, 2:113–168.

123. Moore, R. Y., Halaris, A. E., and Jones, B. E. (1978): Serotonin neurons of the midbrain raphe: ascending projections. *J. Comp. Neurol.*, 180:417–438.

124. Muller, P., and Seeman, P. (1978): Dopaminergic supersensitivity after neuroleptics: time-course and specificity. *Psychopharmacology*, 60:1–11.

125. Muller, P., Britton, R. S., and Seeman, P. (1980): The effects of long-term ethanol on brain receptors for dopamine, acetylcholine, serotonin and noradrenaline. *Eur. J. Pharmacol.*, 65:31–37.

126. Murphy, J. M., McBride, W. J., Lumeny, L., and Li, T.-K. (1982): Regional brain levels of monoamines in alcohol-preferring and -nonpreferring lines of rats. *Pharmacol. Biochem. Behav.*, 16:145–149.

127. Naber, D., Wirz-Justice, A., Kafka, M. S., and Wehr, T. A. (1980): Dopamine receptor binding in rat striatum: ultradian rhythm and its modification by chronic imipramine. *Psychopharmacology*, 68:1–5.

128. Nakano, S., Hara, C., and Ogawa, N. (1980): Circadian rhythm of apomorphine-induced stereotypy in rats. *Pharmacol. Biochem. Behav.*, 12:459–461.

129. Nestoros, J. N. (1980): Ethanol specifically potentiates GABA-mediated neurotransmission in feline cerebral cortex. *Science*, 209:708–710.

130. Nieuwenhuys, R., Voogd, J., and van Huijzen, Chr. (1978): *The Human Central Nervous System. A Synopsis and Atlas.* Springer-Verlag, NY.

131. Osterburg, H. H., Donahue, H. G., Severson, J. A., and Finch, C. E. (1981): Catecholamine levels and turnover during aging in brain regions of male C57BL/6J mice. *Brain Res.*, 224:337–352.

132. Owen, J., Cross, A. J., Waddington, J. L., Poulter, M., Gamble, S. J., and Crow, T. J. Dopamine mediated behavior and 3H-spiperone binding to striatal membranes in rats after nine months haloperidol administration. *Life Sci.*, 26:55–59.

133. Perry, T. L., Kish, S. J., Buchanan, J., and Hansen, S. (1979): Gamma-aminobutyric acid deficiency in brain of schizophrenic patients. *Lancet*, 1:237–239.

133a. Pohorecky, L. A. (1974): Effects of ethanol on central and peripheral noradrenergic neurons. *J. Pharmacol. Exp. Ther.*, 189:380–391.

134. Ponzio, F., Brunello, N., and Algeri, S. (1978): Catecholamine synthesis in brain of aging rats. *J. Neurochem.*, 30:1617–1620.

135. Pradhan, S. N. (1980): Central neurotransmitters and aging. *Life Sci.*, 26:1643–1656.

136. Pradhan, S. N., Aulakh, C. S., and Bhatta-Charyya, A. K. (1980): Behavioral and neurochemical alterations with aging in rats. *Fed. Proc.*, 39:508.

137. Puri, S. K., and Volicer, L. (1977): Effects of aging on cyclic AMP levels and adenylate cyclase and phosphodiesterase activities in the rat corpus striatum. *Mech. Ageing Dev.*, 6:53–58.

138. Puri, S. K., and Volicer, L. (1981): Age-related changes of cyclic nucleotide levels in rat brain regions. *Mech. Ageing Dev.*, 15:239–242.

139. Pycock, C. J., and Taberner, P. V. (1981): *Central Neurotransmitter Turnover.* University Park Press, Baltimore, MD.

140. Randall, P. K. (1980): Functional aging of the nigro-striatal system. *Peptide.* Vol. 1. Suppl. 1, pp. 177–184.

141. Rabin, R. A., and Molinoff, P. B. (1981): Activation of adenylate cyclase by ethanol in mouse striatal tissue. *J. Pharmacol. Exp. Ther.*, 216:129–134.

142. Randall, P. K., Severson, J. A., and Finch, C. E. (1981): Aging and the regulation of striatal dopaminergic mechanisms in mice. *J. Pharmacol. Exp. Ther.*, 219:690–700.

142a. Rangaraj, N., and Kalant, H. (1979): Interaction of ethanol and catecholamines on rat brain $(Na^+ + K^+)$-ATPase. *Can. J. Physio. Pharmacol.*, 57:1098–1106.

143. Reggiani, A., Barbaccia, M. L., Spano, P. F., and Trabucchi, M. (1980a): Acute and chronic ethanol administration on specific (3H)-GABA binding in different rat brain areas. *Psychopharmacology*, 67:261–264.

144. Reggiani, A., Barbaccia, M. L., Spano, P. F., and Trabucchi, M. (1980b): Dopamine metabolism and receptor function after acute and chronic ethanol. *J. Neurochem.*, 35:34–37.

145. Reis, D. J., Ross, R. A., and Joh, T. H. (1977): Changes in the activity and amounts of enzymes

synthesizing catecholamines and acetylcholine in brain, adrenal medulla, and sympathetic ganglia of aged rat and mouse. *Brain Res.*, 136:465–474.

146. Riederer, P., and St. Wuketich. (1976): Time course of nigrostriatal degeneration in Parkinson's disease. *J. Neural Trans.*, 38:277–301.

147. Riffee, W. H., Wilcox, R. E., Vaughn, D. M., and Smith, R. V. (1982): Dopamine receptor sensitivity after chronic dopamine agonists. Striatal (3H)-spiroperidol binding in mice after chronic administration of high doses of apomorphine, N-*n*-propylnorapomorphine and dextroamphetamine. *Psychopharmacology*, 77:146–149.

148. Robinson, D. S. (1975): Changes on MAO and monoamines with human development and aging. *Fed. Proc.*, 34:103–107.

149. Robinson, D. S., Davis, J. N., Nies, A., Colburn, R. W., Davis, J. M., Bourne, H. R., Bunney, W. E., Shaw, D. M., and Coppen, A. J. (1972): Aging monoamines and monoamine-oxidase levels. *Lancet*, 1:290–291.

150. Roffman, M., Condasco, F., and King, A. (1980): Apomorphine-induced stereotypy in mature and senescent rats following cessation of chronic haloperidol treatment. *Comm. Psychopharmacol.*, 4:283–286.

151. Roth, G. S. (1981): Steroid and dopaminergic receptors in the aged brain. In: *Aging, Vol. 17: Brain Neurotransmitters and Receptors in Aging and Age-Related Disorders*, pp. 163–171. Raven Press, NY.

152. Roth, R. H. (1979): Dopamine autoreceptors: pharmacology, function and comparison with post-synaptic dopamine receptors. *Comm. Psychopharmacol.*, 3:429–445.

153. Ryan, C. (1982): Alcoholism and premature aging: a neuropsychological perspective. *Alcoholism*, 6:22–30.

154. Samorajski, T., and Rolsten, C. (1973): Age and regional differences in the chemical composition of brains of mice, monkeys and humans. In: *Progress in Brain Research, Vol. 40: Neurobiological Aspects of Maturation and Aging*, edited by D. H. Ford, pp. 253–265. Elsevier, Amsterdam.

155. Samorajski, T., Rolsten, C., and Ordy, J. M. (1971): Changes in behavior, brain, and neuroendocrine chemistry with age and stress in C57BL/10 male mice. *J. Gerontol.*, 26:168–175.

156. Schallert, T. (1982): Sensorimotor impairment and recovery of function in brain damaged rats: reappearance of symptoms during old age. *J. Comp. Physiol. Psychol.* (in *press*).

157. Schmidt, M. J., and Thornberry, J. F. (1978): Cyclic AMP and cyclic GMP accumulation in vitro in brain regions of young, old, and aged rats. *Brain. Res.*, 139:159–177.

158. Schmidt, M. J. (1980): The pharmacotherapy of Parkinson's disease. In: *Neuropharmacology of Central Nervous System and Behavioral Disorders*, edited by G. C. Palmer, pp. 149–171. Academic Press, NY..

159. Schmidt, M. J. (1981): The cyclic nucleotide system in the brain during aging. In: *Aging, Vol. 17: Brain Neurotransmitters and Receptors in Aging and Age-Related Disorders*, pp. 171–195. Raven Press, New York.

160. Schochen, D. D., and Roth, G. S. (1977): Reduced beta-adrenergic receptor concentrations in ageing man. *Nature (Lond.)*, 267:856–858.

161. Seeman, P. (1980): Brain dopamine receptors. *Pharmacol. Rev.*, 32:230–313.

162. Severson, J. A., and Finch, C. E. (1980a): Age changes in human basal ganglion dopamine receptors. *Fed. Proc.*, 39:508.

163. Severson, J. A., and Finch, C. E. (1980b): Reduced dopaminergic binding during aging in the rodent striatum. *Brain Res.*, 192:147–162.

164. Sharkawi, M. (1980): Pharmacological and metabolic interactions between ethanol and the dopamine-beta-hydroxylase inhibitor FLA 63 in mice. *Neuropharmacology*, 19:277–280.

165. Sharman, D. F. (1981): The turnover of catecholamines. In: *Central Neurotransmitter Turnover*, edited by C. J. Pycock and P. V. Taberner, pp. 20–59. University Park Press, Baltimore, MD.

166. Shih, J. C., and Young, H. (1978): The alteration of serotonin binding sites in aged human brain. *Life Sci.*, 23:1441–1448.

167. Simpkins, J. W., Mueller, G. P., Huang, H. H., and Meiter, J. (1977): Evidence for depressed catecholamine and inhanced serotonin metabolism in aging male rats: possible relation to gonadotropin secretion. *Endocrinology*, 100:1672–1678.

168. Singer, G., and Kelly, J. (1972): Cholinergic and adrenergic interaction in the hypothalamic control of drinking and eating behavior. *Physio. Behav.*, 8:885–890.

169. Sjöquist, B. (1975): Mass fragmentographic determination of 4-hydroxy-3-methoxyphenylglycol

(HMPG) in urine, cerebrospinal fluid, plasma and tissues using a deuterium-labelled internal standard. *J. Chromatog.*, 105:309–316.

170. Smith, T. L., Jacobyansky, A., Shen, A., Pathman, D., and Thurman, R. G. (1981): Adaptation of cyclic AMP generating system in rat cerebral cortical slices during chronic ethanol treatment and withdrawal. *Neuropharmacology*, 20:67–72.

171. Soliman, K. F. A., Walker, C. A., and Ross, F. H. (1981): Effects of acute ethanol administration on brain biogenic amines. *Chronopharmacology and Chronotherapeutics*, pp. 109–114. Florida A&M University Foundation, Tallahassee, Fla.

172. Sourkes, T. L. (1981): Parkinson's disease and other disorders of the basal ganglia. In: *Basic Neurochemistry (3rd ed.)*, edited by G. J. Siegel, R. W. Albers, B. W. Agranoff, and R. Katzman, pp. 719–733. Little, Brown and Co., Boston, MA.

173. Starke, K., Taube, H. B., and Borowski, E. (1977): Presynaptic receptor systems in catecholaminergic transmission. *Biochem. Pharmacol.*, 26:259–268.

174. Starke, K. (1981): Presynaptic receptors. *Annu. Rev. Pharmacol. Toxicol.*, 21:7–30.

175. Stramentinole, G., Gualano, M., Catto, E., and Algeri, S. (1977): Tissue levels of S–adenosylmethionine in aging rats. *J. Gerontol.*, 32:392–394.

176. Strombom, U., Svensson, T. H., and Carlsson, A. (1977): Antagonism of ethanol's central stimulation in mice by small doses of catecholamine-receptor agonists. *Psychopharmacology*, 51:293–299.

177. Supavilai, P., and Karobath, M. (1980): Ethanol and other CNS depressants decrease GABA synthesis in mouse cerebral cortex and cerebellum *in vivo*. *Life Sci.*, 27:1035–1040.

178. Svensson, T. H., and Waldeck, B. (1973): Significance of acetaldehyde in ethanol-induced effects on catecholamine metabolism and motor activity in the mouse. *Psychopharmacologia*, 31:229–238.

179. Symposium (1980): *Receptor Binding Techniques*. Society for Neuroscience short course syllabus. Society for Neuroscience, Bethesda.

180. Symposium (1981): Neurobiological correlates of intoxication and physical dependence upon ethanol. (Majchrowicz, E., and Hunt, W. A.). *Fed. Proc.*, 40:2048.

181. Symposium (1982): Neurobiological interactions between aging and alcohol abuse. (Freund, G., and Butters, N.). *Alcoholism*, 6:1.

182. Tallarida, R. J., and Murray, R. B. (1981): *Manual of Pharmacologic Calculations with Computer Programs*, Springer-Verlag, NY.

183. Tabakoff, B., and Hoffman, P. L. (1978): Alterations in receptors controlling dopamine synthesis after chronic ethanol ingestion. *J. Neurochem.*, 31:1223–1229.

184. Thal, L. J., Horowitz, S. G., Dvorkin, B., and Makman, M. H. (1980): Evidence for loss of brain (3H)-spiroperidol and (3H) ADTN binding sites in rabbit brain with aging. *Brain Res.*, 192:185–194.

185. Thompson, J. M., Whitaker, J. R., and Joseph, J. A. (1981): (3H) dopamine accumulation and release from striatal slices in young, mature, and senescent rats. *Brain Res.*, 224:436–440.

186. Ticku, M. J. (1980): The effects of acute and chronic ethanol administration and its withdrawal on gamma-aminobutyric acid receptor binding in rat brain. *Br. J. Pharmacol.*, 70:403–410.

187. Ticku, M. K., and Burch, T. (1980): Alterations in γ-aminobutyric acid receptor sensitivity following acute and chronic ethanol treatments. *J. Neurochem.*, 34:417–423.

188. Umezu, K., Bustos, G., and Roth, R. H. (1980): Regional inhibitory effects of ethanol on monoamine synthesis regulation within the brain. *Biochem. Pharmacol.*, 29:2477–2483.

189. Vaughn, D. M., and Wilcox, R. E. (1983): Plasticity of the nigrostriatal dopamine system during aging. Changes in dopamine turnover and apomorphine-induced stereotypic activity after chronic spiroperidol or apomorphine. *J. Pharmacol. Exp. Ther. (submitted)*.

190. Vaughn, D. M., and Wilcox, R. E. (1982b): Plasticity of the nigrostriatal dopamine system after chronic dopamine agonist treatment. Changes in striatal dopamine turnover suggest possible autoreceptor subsensitivity. *Eur. J. Pharmacol., (submitted)*.

191. Volicer, L. (1980): GABA levels and receptor binding after acute and chronic ethanol administration. *Brain Res. Bull. [Suppl.]*, 2:809–813.

192. Waddington, J. L., and Gamble, S. J. (1980): Neuroleptic treatment for a substantial proportion of adult life: Behavioral sequelae of 9 months haloperidol administration. *Eur. J. Pharmacol.*, 67:363–369.

193. Walker, J. B., and Walker, J. P. (1973): Properties of adenylate cyclase from senescent rat brain. *Brain Res.*, 54:391–396.

194. Waggoner, W. G., Mc.Dermed, J., and Leighton, H. J. (1980): Presynaptic regulation of tyrosine hydroxylase activity in rat striatal synaptosomes by dopamine analogs. *Mol. Pharmacol.*, 18:91–99.

195. Wagner, L. A. (1975): Subcellular storage of biogenic amines. *Life Sci.*, 17:1755–1762.

195a. Weibrecht, W., and Cramer, H. (1980): Depression of cyclic AMP and cyclic GMP in the cerebrospinal fluid of rats after acute administration of ethanol. *Brain Res.*, 200:478–480.

196. Weiland, G. A., and Molinoff, P. B. (1981): Quantitative analysis of drug-receptor interactions. I. determination of kinetic and equilibrium properties. *Life Sci.*, 29:313–330.

197. Weiner, H., Myers, R. D., Simpson, C. W., and Thurman, J. A. (1980): The effects of alcohol on dopamine metabolism in the caudate nucleus of an unanesthetized monkey. *Alcoholism*, 4:427–429.

198. Wilcox, R. E., Smith, R. V., Anderson, J. A., and Riffee, W. H. (1979): Apomorphine-induced stereotypic cage climbing in mice as a model for studying changes in dopamine receptor sensitivity. *Pharmacol. Biochem. Behav.*, 12:29–33.

199. Williams, M., and Risley, E. A. (1979): Characterization of the binding of (3H)-muscimol, a potent gamma-aminobutyric acid agonist to rat brain synaptosomal membranes using a filtration assay. *J. Neurochem.*, 32:713–718.

200. Wood, W. G., Elias, M. F., editors (1981): *Alcoholism and Aging: Current Advances in Research.* CRC Press, Boca Raton, FL.

201. Yamamura, H. I., Enna, S. J., and Kuhar, M. J., editors (1978): *Neurotransmitter Receptor Binding.* Raven Press, NY.

202. Yamamura, H. I., and Enna, S. J., editors (1981): *Neurotransmitter Receptors. Part 2. Biogenic Amines. Receptors and Recognition. Series B. Vol. 10.* Chapman and Hall, NY.

203. Yojay, L., Yojay, R., and Munoz. (1981): Influence of imipramine on the narcosis induced by ethanol in mice. *Prog. Med. Sci.*, 9:334–375.

204. Zimberg, S. (1978): Diagnosis and treatment of the elderly alcoholic. *Alcoholism*, 2:27–41.

Alcoholism in the Elderly, edited by
J. T. Hartford and T. Samorajski.
Raven Press, New York © 1984.

Age and Development of Tolerance to and Physical Dependence on Alcohol

Ronald F. Ritzmann and Christine L. Melchior

Alcohol and Drug Abuse Research and Training Program, Department of Physiology and Biophysics, University of Illinois at the Medical Center, Chicago, Illinois 60680

Ethanol is probably one of the oldest and most commonly used psychoactive drugs. It is also becoming apparent that it is one of the most widely abused drugs in history. (The National Council on Alcoholism has reported that alcoholism is the second most frequent disease in the United States.) Unlike many other drugs of abuse, ethanol appeals to individuals over a wide range of age groups. Until recently, little emphasis has been given to the possible differential effects of ethanol on individuals in different stages of ontological development, particularly the later stages of this development. However, the recent projected increases in the elderly proportion of the population that comprises our society has created a need to evaluate the effect of a number of pharmacological agents, including ethanol, on older age groups.

Considering that many of the effects of ethanol are mediated by the central nervous system (CNS) and that many aspects of CNS functional components are subject to age-related changes, one would expect some changes in the effects of the drug during the aging process. In support of this premise, it has been reported that although the overall intake of ethanol in elderly individuals is less than in the population as a whole (5,11), the number of ethanol-related disorders among the elderly is greater than that observed in the total population (92). These observations indicate that there may be changes in acute sensitivity, development of physical dependence, and development of tolerance to ethanol in elderly individuals. Although any or all of these changes are clearly possible, it is the change in the development of tolerance and of physical dependence that is of particular interest, both because these factors may regulate the intake of the drug over a period of time and because changes in the ability to develop or maintain tolerance may be indicative of changes in CNS adaptability. Several theories of aging have suggested that there is a decrease in CNS adaptability at later ages, this being particularly evident in the inability to formulate new memories. Since some forms of tolerance have been proposed to be similar to memory, as discussed later in this chapter, one might anticipate similar losses in the ability to develop tolerance as have been reported for memory processes. In addition, correlating age-induced changes in various neurochemical systems with changes in the response to the drug may lead to a clear understanding of the role these systems have in mediating the action of ethanol.

DEFINITION OF TOLERANCE AND PHYSICAL DEPENDENCE

Repeated administration of ethanol leads to the development of tolerance and physical dependence. Tolerance is defined as a diminished response to the drug on successive exposures. Physical dependence (89) can be demonstrated by two components; first, withdrawal symptoms once use of the drug is discontinued and, second, drug-seeking behavior. Whereas classic theories of chronic drug usage have considered tolerance and physical dependence as a singular phenomenon, more recent observations suggest that this may be an oversimplification of the relationship (55,87). In brief, manipulation of a number of factors can alter the development of tolerance without affecting physical dependence (104). Although the concept involving either aspect of physical dependence appears straightforward, tolerance now appears to be a multifaceted phenomenon. Traditionally, tolerance has been divided into two components: (a) dispositional tolerance, which includes uptake, distribution, metabolism, and elimination of the drug and (b) functional tolerance, which is demonstrated by either a decreased response to a given drug level at the drug's site of action, or the necessity of increasing the amount of the drug present to achieve a given response. Since functional tolerance is, by definition, linked to some response, and since it has been known for some time that the rate at which tolerance develops is dependent upon the response measured, it has been suggested that different types of tolerance may be mediated by different mechanisms.

Tolerance represents a physiological adaptation to the presence of ethanol. It has been considered analogous to learning, which is also an adaptive physiological response to stimuli. However, a more direct role for learning in the expression of tolerance has also been suggested. Under appropriate circumstances, an organism may learn a particular response that diminishes the effect of a given dose of ethanol, which thus may be interpreted as tolerance. Although the type (or types) of learning (classic or operant) that best describes tolerance is still debatable, a useful conceptual framework has been proposed in which tolerance is subdivided into environmental-dependent (ED) and environmental-independent (EI) forms (103). ED tolerance is defined as decreased response (to a drug) that is dependent upon cues derived from the environment in which the drug has been administered, i.e., room, odors, and route of administration. In other words, if there is a significant change in the environmental cues associated with the drug administration, tolerance will no longer be exhibited. This form of tolerance is a learned response (see discussion below). EI tolerance is demonstrated only when the diminished response to the drug still occurs, even though all environmental conditions are different in the tolerant test environment as compared with the drug administration environment. Although it is not difficult to envision ED tolerance as having a functional CNS component, recent observations have suggested ED tolerance may also have a dispositional component (103). The general framework for the different forms of tolerance is depicted in Fig. 1.

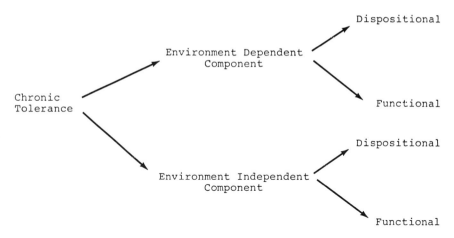

FIG. 1. Flow chart of various forms of tolerance. (Modified from Tabakoff et al., ref. 103.)

Although it is theoretically possible to discuss pure ED and pure EI tolerance, practically, it would be difficult to sufficiently alter the environmental cues to eliminate ED tolerance completely. This is particularly significant if one considers that it is not presently known which cues are significant and which cues are irrelevant to the organism being tested. In the future it should be possible, by systematically varying environmental cues in a multivariant design, to determine the influence of each cue. Until such parametric studies are carried out, one can only assume that ED and EI tolerance each contribute to the altered response to a drug, and the relative contribution of each is dependent upon the number of significant cues in common between the drug administration environment and the tolerance test environment.

The following formula indicates the components that contribute to tolerance or the altered response (ΔR) to a drug in a given situation:

	ΔR	$=$	$(\alpha \text{FED} + \text{FEI}) + (\alpha \text{DED} + \text{DEI})$
where:	FED	$=$	functional environmental-dependent tolerance;
	FEI	$=$	functional environmental-independent tolerance;
	DED	$=$	dispositional environmental-dependent tolerance;
	DEI	$=$	dispositional environmental-independent tolerance;
	α	$=$	number of significant cues in common.

As previously stated, it is practically impossible to eliminate ED tolerance completely. However, an experimental procedure such as a multiple-injection program, during which tolerance to a given effect of the drug is determined on successive injections, would have a greater α and, therefore, a greater ED tolerance than inhalation or liquid diet techniques in which the drug is administered by one route of administration and the organism is thereafter challenged by an alternative route of drug administration. The different relative contribution of ED and EI tolerances generated by different experimental procedures may account for the different results found by different laboratories, as is discussed later. These factors may be particularly important, since these different forms of tolerance may be mediated by different neural mechanisms, and these mechanisms may be differentially changing during aging (90,91). Therefore, the ability to develop or maintain various types of tolerance should also change with age.

ROLE OF LEARNING IN TOLERANCE
AND PHYSICAL DEPENDENCE

A parallel has often been noted between learning and tolerance. This observation is based on the fact that manipulations that interfere with learning, such as frontal cortical lesions (66,113) or the administration of protein synthesis inhibitors, such as cycloheximide (66,70,80), also disrupt tolerance. While this relationship was first suggested to occur with tolerance to morphine (16), similar experiments demonstrate that the same parallels can also be drawn between learning and tolerance to ethanol [see review, (62)].

The first attempt to show that tolerance to ethanol could be learned employed a "before and after" design. Chen (13,14) injected rats with ethanol, either before or after a daily test session of performance in a circular maze. After repeated injections, the group that had been receiving ethanol after their daily sessions were tested in the circular maze under the influence of ethanol. This group was far more impaired in their performance than the animals that had an opportunity to practice this task under the influence of ethanol. It was concluded that tolerance was a learned phenomenon that need not be related to a physiological adaptation to ethanol. LeBlanc and co-workers (63–66) replicated these experiments. However, they found that the group receiving ethanol after the daily test sessions did eventually develop tolerance to the same extent as the "before" group. They suggested that learning merely enhanced the rate of development of tolerance, and termed the phenomenon "behaviorally augmented" tolerance. More recently, Wenger and his colleagues (115,116) addressed this issue. Using the same "before and after" design, they eliminated the occasional days in which the "after" group was assessed for performance on the task under the influence of ethanol during the time in which tolerance was being developed. By testing the "after" group only at the end of the experiment, they eliminated any practice effects in this group. They also eliminated any evidence of tolerance. In conclusion, Wenger et al. (115) assert that tolerance occurs only with practice with the effects of ethanol.

In contrast to the operant learning approach to tolerance, Siegel (94–97) has popularized a model of tolerance based on classic, or Pavlovian, conditioning. Here, the ritual of administering a drug and the environment in which this procedure takes place become conditioned stimuli signaling the unconditioned stimulus, the presence of the drug. The unconditioned response is the drug effect. Repeated pairings of these environmental stimuli with the effects of the drug lead to the development of a conditioned response that, in this case, is "compensatory," that is, opposite in direction to the effect of the drug. The combination of the drug effect and this compensatory response results in an attenuated response to the drug, i.e., tolerance. We have referred to this type of tolerance as "environment-dependent." Although Siegel provided evidence in support of this idea primarily with research on morphine, both he and other researchers have recently demonstrated that this type of tolerance can be developed to the hypothermic (12,24,59,73,76) and hypnotic effects of ethanol (76).

The Pavlovian conditioning paradigm has also been used to explain withdrawal symptomatology, "craving," and relapse. As indicated above, repeated pairings of environmental stimuli with the effect of a drug can lead to the development of a conditioned compensatory response. When the appropriate stimuli are present, but a placebo instead of the drug is administered, the compensatory response occurs. Like the compensatory response, withdrawal symptoms tend to be opposite to the drug effect (40,96,97). Thus, when an alcoholic enters an environment previously associated with drinking, a conditioned compensatory response, which can be seen as withdrawal distress, occurs. Since this response, which is presumably uncomfortable, can be attenuated by ethanol, it may be interpreted as "craving" (40, 71,72,75,97,119,120). A learned response can be retained for a long period of time and may not be readily eliminated without an extinction procedure. Thus, an alcoholic who has been abstinent for a long interval may relapse because he experiences the conditioned response when faced with cues previously associated with drinking.

In a large number of studies, performance on tests of learning and memory has been reported to decline with age (57). Many variables can influence this effect, including genetic differences (36,57). Thus, one would predict that aged animals would become tolerant to ethanol more slowly than younger animals in a learning paradigm. However, since perseveration problems, as well as slower extinction rates, have been noted in older animals, one would also predict that older animals would extinguish learned tolerance at a slower rate.

INTERACTIONS WITH INITIAL SENSITIVITY

Tolerance

Although a relationship between initial sensitivity and tolerance and physical dependence has been suggested (62), there are few studies indicating the nature of this relationship. Tolerance is associated with initial sensitivity by definition, since tolerance is expressed as the difference between initial sensitivity and subsequent measures of sensitivity. Kalant et al. (50) proposed a mathematical formula indicating that the extent of development of tolerance is dependent upon initial sensitivity, whereas Tabakoff et al. (107) have provided evidence that initial sensitivity influences the rate of tolerance development.

One factor that has clearly been shown to affect initial sensitivity is genetic. Inbred strains of mice and rats differ in their initial response to ethanol. Breeding studies in which animals were selected for the magnitude of their response to ethanol on a particular measure, or for their preference for ethanol, have subsequently been shown to differ on many measures of sensitivity to ethanol (8). Some investigators have utilized the genetically determined differences in initial sensitivity to assess the relationship to tolerance. The inbred strains of mice, C57Bl and DBA, differ in their initial sensitivity to ethanol, with C57Bl being less responsive than DBA (8,89). Tabakoff and Ritzmann (105) demonstrated that C57Bl mice develop acute tolerance, while DBA mice do not. Similarly, Grieve et al. (37) showed that C57Bl, but not DBA, mice developed tolerance within 2.5 hr with continuous inhalation of ethanol. Using hypothermia instead of the hypnotic response as an index of the effect of ethanol, Moore and Kakihana (79) also reported that C57Bl mice developed tolerance, while DBA mice did not. In using the lines of mice selectively bred for their response to the hypnotic effects of ethanol, the short-sleep (SS) and long-sleep (LS) mice, Tabakoff et al. (107) showed that the SS mice developed tolerance to the hypnotic effects of ethanol faster than the LS mice.

The behavioral data from the few studies that addressed the question of the affect of age on initial sensitivity would all seem to indicate that old animals are more sensitive to various effects of ethanol, including the hypnotic (1,2,18,86), hypothermic (2,122), motor impairing (1,2), and lethal (117,118) effects of ethanol. However, in most of these reports, the differences in response with age can be attributed to alterations in the metabolism and/or distribution of ethanol, which result in higher or longer lasting peak levels of ethanol. In most cases, the level of ethanol for a given response was the same across all age groups. Only two studies provide evidence of greater sensitivity with age for a given level of ethanol. Abel and York (2) showed that 18- to 20-month-old female Sprague-Dawley rats regained righting reflex at lower blood ethanol levels than rats aged 2 to 3 or 11 to 12 months. Similarly, Ritzmann and Springer (86) found that 24-month-old C57Bl mice lost righting reflex at lower brain ethanol levels than 6- or 12-month-old mice. Since mice of all age groups regained righting reflex at the same brain ethanol level, which was a higher brain ethanol level than those at which they lost righting reflex, all age groups demonstrated acute tolerance.

One other study considers the influence of age on the development of tolerance. The groups examined include TO Swiss mice 18 to 20, 35 to 40, and 150 to 200 days of age. Using an ethanol inhalation procedure, Grieve and Littleton (38) showed that the 35- to 40-day-old mice demonstrated a twofold decrease in sensitivity to ethanol within 3 to 5 hr, but that the 18- to 20- and 150- to 200-day-old mice developed no tolerance in 6 to 7 hr. Although the oldest group employed cannot be considered "old," the pattern observed suggests that the ability to become tolerant develops after weaning and declines with maturity.

Physical Dependence

A few studies have utilized the inbred strains to examine differences in withdrawal severity. Using either a vapor inhalation technique (34) or a liquid diet procedure (49) to render the animals dependent, the studies showed that mice of the DBA and BALB strains were more susceptible to withdrawal reactions than the C57Bl mice. Under conditions in which blood ethanol concentrations were maintained at similar levels in both strains during 10 days of exposure to ethanol vapor, DBA mice exhibited more severe withdrawal than C57Bl mice.

In considering these interactions, we see that animals showing the lowest initial sensitivity develop tolerance more rapidly and have the least severe withdrawal. Grieve et al. (32) suggested that an animal with the ability to adapt rapidly to the presence of ethanol may also adapt rapidly to its absence, thus accounting for this relationship.

Kalant et al. (50) have pointed out that the rate of elimination of a drug may play an important role in the development of tolerance and dependence. With slower elimination of a drug, an organism has more time to adapt to its presence and disappearance. Increasing the rate of removal of a drug should exacerbate the withdrawal response.

In the one animal study examining the effect of age on severity of withdrawal, Wood et al. (123) made several interesting observations. They exposed 3-, 14-, and 25-month-old C57Bl mice to a liquid diet containing 5% ethanol for 14 days. Blood ethanol levels did not differ between groups when measured on the 4th and 12th day of presentation of the ethanol-containing diet. However, the young mice consumed more ethanol than the older groups, and the older mice were noted to be more intoxicated. This supports other reports indicating that the elimination rate of ethanol is slower in older C57Bl mice (18,86) and suggests that the older mice are more sensitive to ethanol. Withdrawal was more severe and of longer duration in the older groups. As seen with the inbred strains, with apparently similar exposure to ethanol, the more sensitive animals had the most severe withdrawal. Differences in ethanol elimination rates probably accounted for the similar blood ethanol levels across groups in the face of different ethanol consumption, but the slower elimination rate in the older animals was not sufficient to ameliorate their withdrawal.

Preference for Ethanol

It is intrinsically obvious that an organism must be exposed to ethanol in order to develop tolerance and physical dependence. The critical, though unanswered, question is: why does one consume large quantities of ethanol? One popular hypothesis suggested that preference for ethanol is related to initial sensitivity. Using genetically determined differences, it was noted that in inbred strains of mice, the C57Bl/6 strain voluntarily consumes more ethanol solution than water, whereas the BALB/c and DBA/2 mice avoid ethanol and prefer water. The ethanol-preferring C57Bl mice have a low sensitivity to ethanol, and the ethanol-avoiding BALB mice have a high sensitivity to ethanol. Unfortunately, the ethanol-avoiding DBA mice are not consistently more sensitive to ethanol than the ethanol-preferring C57Bl mice, depending on the task (8).

In the two selective breeding studies where lines of rats were bred for their preference for ethanol, the ethanol-preferring line was found to be less sensitive to ethanol than the nonpreferring line (8,25,67). However, in studies in which animals were selectively bred for their sensitivity to ethanol on a given measure, there was no difference between the high- and low-sensitivity lines in preference for ethanol (6,17). Thus, it does not appear that ethanol preference is closely related to initial sensitivity to ethanol. Studies of the influence of age on preference for ethanol have provided divergent results [see review, (122)]. Based on the genetic studies discussed above, resolution of the issue of the effect of age on preference for ethanol will not necessarily be relevant to the effect of age on sensitivity to ethanol and its consequent relationship to tolerance and dependence.

NEUROCHEMISTRY

Neurotransmitters and Tolerance

Although many theories proposed some alterations in neurotransmitter activity as a probable underlying mechanism for the effects of ethanol, there is not, as yet, a consistent pattern of ethanol-induced changes in transmitter metabolism. Although many different neurotransmitters are altered by ethanol (see Freund, *this volume*), we will focus on catecholamines (CA) as one example of a possible interaction between aging and ethanol on a possible mechanism by which tolerance and physical dependence develop. Hunt and Majchrowicz (46) reported, after an acute injection of ethanol, an initial increase in turnover of norepinephrine (NE) followed by a decrease, 2 hr postinjection, and a second rise as blood ethanol levels returned to normal. These findings are in agreement with those of Pohorecky (82), who reported a decrease in turnover 1 hr after injection. The initial rise found in the study of Hunt and Majchrowicz (46) may be a stress reaction, since the turnover rates are compared with untreated controls. There is also considerable agreement on the effect of acute ethanol on dopamine (DA). Several investigators have reported a decrease in DA turnover 2 hr after a single injection of ethanol (46,82). Seeman and Lee (93) have shown a potentiation of the spontaneous release of DA from synaptosomes by anesthetic doses of ethanol *in vitro*. If such a release occurs *in vivo*, there is a possibility that through transsynaptic inhibition, the result of this release could be a decrease in DA turnover.

A number of biochemical changes in brain have been shown to correlate roughly with the development of tolerance (50). However, it has been difficult to establish an exact relationship between the development of tolerance and neurochemical processes. It is, therefore, unclear which changes are causative and which are consequences of tolerance or which are related to some other aspect of the drug's action. Some support for the involvement of NE systems in the physiologic events that display tolerance has, however, been gathered. One such event is the slowing of alpha rhythm in the electroencephalogram (EEG) (7) and a characteristic "beta buzz," which is produced by ethanol. These EEG phenomena are believed to be adrenergic in origin (7), and tolerance to these ethanol-induced phenomena has been shown to develop following repeated ethanol exposure (81). It is possible that this tolerance is due to changes in adrenergic activity.

The involvement of certain neurotransmitter systems in tolerance to ethanol becomes clearer in studies that examine the effect on tolerance of manipulating different systems. Intraventricular administration of the CA neurotoxin, 6-hydroxydopamine (6-OHDA), inhibits the development of tolerance to the hypnotic and hypothermic effects of ethanol in C57Bl mice exposed to a liquid diet containing ethanol, without altering withdrawal (104). If 6-OHDA is given after tolerance has been established, the ability to express tolerance is unaffected. It is the depletion of NE, not DA, that influences the development of tolerance, since selective depletion of DA did not interfere with the development of tolerance (104). In using rats, Wood and Laverty (121) were unable to replicate these findings. However, they did note that 6-OHDA treatment altered the animals' response to the hypnotic effects of ethanol. Le et al. (60) provide support for a role of NE in tolerance in the rat by finding that depletion of both serotonin and NE prevented the development of tolerance instead of merely retarding it, as occurs with serotonin depletion alone.

In examining ED tolerance in C57Bl mice, Melchior and Tabakoff (76) found that 6-OHDA-treated mice developed tolerance to the hypnotic effects of ethanol at a slower rate. The degree of decrease in rate of development of tolerance was related to the amount of NE depletion. The same effect on tolerance was observed when α-methyl-p-tyrosine (α-MPT), a CA synthesis inhibitor, was used to decrease CA levels instead of 6-OHDA.

In studies of rats involving the "moving belt" task, body temperature and sleep duration, administration of the serotonergic neurotoxin, 5,7-dihydroxytryptamine (5,7-DHT), or the serotonergic synthesis inhibitor, p-chlorophenylalanine (PCPA), retarded the development of tolerance to ethanol (27,28,33,59). Parametrically, the administration of tryptophan to increase whole brain serotonin content increased the rate of development of tolerance (58,61).

Similar data have been obtained from C57Bl mice given a low dose of 5,7-DHT and exposed to the ethanol-containing liquid diet (Melchior and Tabakoff, *unpublished observations*). However, when an ED tolerance paradigm was used, low doses of 5,7-DHT caused a substantial increase in initial sensitivity to the hypnotic effect of ethanol and increased the rate of development of tolerance (76). At higher doses of 5,7-DHT, these effects diminished. Interestingly, Khanna et al. (54) have noted that low doses of 5,6-DHT, which produce only a 20% reduction of serotonin, facilitated the development of tolerance in their studies with rats. This may be due to the supersensitivity that results from this treatment. Using 5,7-DHT or PCPA, a reduction of serotonin levels of more than 75% was necessary to effectively retard the development of tolerance (54). The results of these studies indicate that species, type of tolerance, and degree of change in certain neurotransmitter systems can all influence the rate of development of tolerance.

Neurotransmitters and Physical Dependence

The behavioral and physiological aspects of the alcohol-withdrawal syndrome have been well described. In humans, it includes such behavioral symptoms as tremors, hallucinations, and convulsive seizures (38,39). However, the neurochemical mechanisms that mediate these systems are not well understood. Evidence that catecholaminergic activity is altered during withdrawal in humans comes from reports that there is an increase in the levels of CA metabolites in the urine of chronic alcoholics undergoing withdrawal (68). It is not clear from these studies if this increase in metabolites reflects an increase in CNS activity or that of some other system, i.e., hormonal, peripheral nervous system, etc.

Support for the involvement of CNS catecholamines in the ethanol withdrawal syndrome comes from pharmacological attempts to alter these systems during withdrawal in animals. Goldstein (32) has shown that drugs that interfere with the CNS catecholamine system tend to aggravate the withdrawal reaction. In addition, Blum and Wallace (10) have shown that α-MPT, which inhibits CA synthesis, results in a potentiation of ethanol-induced withdrawal. It has also been shown that similar treatment will potentiate audiogenic (48) and electroconvulsive seizures (15). Until recently, the majority of animal studies have relied upon seizures as the primary index of withdrawal, either rating the severity of seizures (29,35) or measuring alterations in seizure threshold to convulsive agents such as pentylenetetrazol (99) or sound (30). We have reported that hypothermia in animals is an additional index of ethanol withdrawal (88). These findings are particularly significant in light of the proposed role of adrenergic transmitters in temperature regulation. Models for body temperature control provide a well-circumscribed area of brain, as well as defined interactions between neurotransmitters, which are useful tools for understanding the physiological manifestation of ethanol-induced alteration in neurotransmitter activity on an objective quantitative response.

The changes in transmitter turnover that occur during chronic intoxication appear to continue during withdrawal (3). The increase in NE turnover (13,45,82) is of particular interest, since most models proposed for temperature regulation involve NE-containing neurons, either directly activating heat loss (77) or as inhibitors of both heat loss and heat production (9). If the observed alteration in NE turnover has a significant role in the symptomatology of the withdrawal syndrome, it should be apparent in the organism's thermal response during withdrawal, and the response should be altered by drugs that alter NE activity. On the other hand, although DA is not yet incorporated in most of the models of temperature regulation, several recent reports have indicated a DA role in temperature regulation (100). In addition, alterations in DA have been demonstrated to be involved in several symptoms associated with morphine withdrawal, including a hypothermic response (20,39,114). It is possible that DA may also have a significant role in some aspects of ethanol withdrawal.

Decreases in brain levels of CA have been found during aging (26,29,99,100). The activity of the enzymes necessary for the production of CA—tyrosine hydroxylase (TH) (9,78) and DOPA decarboxylase (DDC) (69)—have been shown to decrease with age. The greatest decreases have been reported to occur in regions high in DA content (78). Coupled with this decrease in the ability to synthesize CA, there has also been reported an increase in monoamine oxidase (MAO), the enzyme responsible for the breakdown of CA (19,110). This decrease in the ability to synthesize CA along with the increase in MAO has been implicated in physical dependence, and many of the theories of dependence have been based upon this assumption (33,47,74). If these CA systems do, in fact, mediate some of the effects of chronic ethanol consumption, one would expect, at some point during the age-induced decreases in their activity, that those effects mediated by these systems would become impaired.

Neurohypophyseal Peptides

Age Changes in Hypothalamic Function and the Response to Ethanol

The hypothalamus is important, both in homeostatic control of the organism as a whole and in producing shifts in the metabolism and function of individual cells. In a recent review of age-induced changes in hypothalamic function, Frolkis (31) has pointed out several parameters of hypothalamic aging that might provide considerable potential for an interaction between ethanol and aging that would result in a change in the organism's response to ethanol at different ages. There is considerable evidence that the activity of neurosecretory processes declines with age (31), and there is particularly strong evidence that this is the case for arginine vasopressin (AVP) (31). This is exemplified by an increase in the amount of neurosecretory material found in the CNS and has been interpreted as a decrease in the release of this material (31).

There is also, at this time, an increase in the response of the hypothalamus to intracerebroventricular (i.c.v.) administration of NE (31), which is similar to the response observed in denervated preparations (47) and would be consistent with the hypothesis that the release of neurosecretory material is, in part, controlled by NE-containing neurons (43). As already mentioned, data from our laboratory have shown that lesions of NE neurons inhibit the development of tolerance to ethanol (87,104), and lesions that result in reduction of hypothalamic NE content result in a loss of the ability to develop tolerance to barbiturates (68). We have also shown that AVP has the ability to maintain ethanol tolerance [as discussed below (45)]. If endogenous AVP, which is released by hypothalamic NE neurons, plays a role in maintaining ethanol tolerance, the age-induced reduction in the activity of these systems would lead to a loss in the ability to establish or maintain functional tolerance to ethanol in old organisms. It is significant that the target organ for AVP in the body remains reactive to AVP; therefore, if the CNS receptor for AVP also remains intact, administration of this compound could reverse any age-induced deficits resulting from a reduction in AVP release.

There has also been reported a decrease in the ability of the hypothalamic-pituitary-adrenal system in aged animals to control enzyme activity and protein synthesis. This effect appears to be due to a decrease in adrenocorticotrophic hormone (ACTH) secretion, which is particularly observable in the response to stress in aged rats. Our studies (102) have shown an increase in the circulating levels of corticosterone in mice during withdrawal from chronic ethanol. Sze (98) has proposed that ACTH has a "permissive" function in the development of physical dependence on ethanol. "Permissive" is used to indicate that the hormone does not, by itself, initiate the effect, but its presence is necessary if the response to ethanol is to occur (98). The observed decreases in ACTH in aged animals would suggest the possibility that aged animals would differ in their response to chronic ethanol when compared with young animals.

It has been proposed that neurohypophyseal peptides (NHPs), e.g., AVP, oxytocin (OXT), Pro-Leu-GlyNH$_2$ (MIF, the C-terminal tripeptide of OXT), or cyclo (Leu-Gly) (cLG, a structural analog of MIF) may act as neuromodulators, that is, they modify ongoing neuronal processes rather than initiate new responses (56). Data gathered thus far on the effect of these NHPs on response to a number of behaviors, including the effects of chronic drug exposure (see below), appear consistent with this hypothesis. Since the release of these peptides is altered during aging (31), it is possible that these systems may also mediate age-induced changes in the development of tolerance to and dependence on ethanol.

Effects of NHP on the Acute Response to Ethanol

Prior to evaluating effects of NHP on an organism's response during chronic drug exposure, it is essential to determine the effect of the peptides on the initial response to the drug, as well as any direct action the peptides may have on the dependent variables used to assess the effects of the drug. Several experiments conducted to determine the influence of various NHPs on blood and brain levels of ethanol following acute injection of ethanol (3-5 g/kg) led to the conclusion that these NHPs did not alter the distribution of ethanol in brain or blood (42–45). Of the peptides tested, only AVP had any action on the dependent variables used to assess effects of ethanol, i.e., a decrease in body temperature, maximal 30 min postinjection, and returning to base line within 2 hr. Administered 2 hr prior to ethanol, neither AVP, MIF, or cLG altered the hypothermic response to ethanol (43). However, cLG (40 nmoles/kg) significantly increased the duration of the sedative effects of ethanol. Other doses of cLG or AVP did not alter this response. In the studies cited above, the peptides were given 2 hr prior to ethanol treatment. Crabbe et al. (21–23) administered [des-glycinamide[9]] (DG)-AVP immediately after injection of ethanol and compared its influence on the reaction of strains of mice differing in their hypothermic response to ethanol. The results of these studies indicated the peptide attenuated the strain differences in the initial sensitivity to ethanol (21,22). Therefore, it may be premature to dismiss the possibility that there may be a direct effect of some of these peptides on acute responses to ethanol.

Effects of NHP on Tolerance to Ethanol

NHP has been shown to alter tolerance that developed after chronic administration (45). In these experiments, mice were chronically treated with ethanol via liquid diets, as previously described (88). Using this model, tolerance to the hypothermic and sedative effects of ethanol were evident after 7 days and persisted for up to 6 days postwithdrawal (88). In the initial experiments, AVP or OXT (10 μg/g) was injected once a day throughout the period of ethanol exposure, as well as during the subsequent 9-day postwithdrawal period. Tolerance was assessed at 3-day intervals, starting 24 hr after onset of the withdrawal period, by injecting ethanol 3 g/kg, intraperitoneal (i.p.) and monitoring the intensity of the hypothermic response and duration of sedation (sleep time) of the drug. As previously stated, mice given ethanol, but not peptide, were tolerant to ethanol on both response measures; this tolerance was found to dissipate, the half-life being about 3 days (45). Injection of AVP, but not OXT, maintained tolerance at the same level, as was exhibited on the first day of testing, throughout the 9-day postwithdrawal period. In other words, there was no decay in the amount of tolerance that had developed as long as AVP injections were continued. Once the peptide treatment was discontinued, tolerance disappeared at the same time-rate as in the nonpeptide-treated mice, a half-life of 3 days. In subsequent experiments, AVP was also found to maintain the level of tolerance, even if it was administered only after chronic ethanol treatment was terminated, i.e., daily during the postwithdrawal-tolerance testing period (44). These data again support the initial observation (45) that the level of tolerance remained constant as long as the peptide AVP was administered; whereas, if AVP administration was terminated, the rate of decay was similar to that of ethanol-treated mice not receiving peptide. Structure-activity studies indicated that OXT, MIF, and cLG were devoid of activity in these tests. AVP, as well as [des-glycinamide⁹] lysine vasopressin (DG-LVP), administration maintained tolerance to ethanol with AVP being more potent (41,44). Since, in these experiments, ethanol was administered by the liquid diet method and the level of tolerance was determined by i.p. injection, one would assume that the major portion of tolerance that would be demonstrated by this procedure would be EI tolerance. Furthermore, it has been repeatedly shown that dispositional tolerance does not develop during the 7-day diet method; therefore, the tolerance that is maintained by these peptides is most likely FEI tolerance.

Because of the numerous reports of the effects of AVP on learning and memory (111,112), one might expect an even more dramatic effect of these peptides on FED tolerance. However, the results of preliminary studies testing this hypothesis were somewhat surprising. To assess FED tolerance, ethanol was administered using a multiple-injection paradigm. Each injection of ethanol was preceded by injection of AVP or DG-LVP. Both peptides delayed the development of tolerance rather than facilitating the onset of tolerance, as would be predicted from the learning studies. It might be argued that the effect of AVP and DG-LVP on development of tolerance to ethanol is based on the liquid diet technique, rather than on a particular form of tolerance. However, using an inhalation technique, Rigter et al. (83) administered ethanol and employed pyrazole to maintain blood ethanol levels of male Swiss mice. Following 72 hr of ethanol exposure, mice were both physically dependent and tolerant to ethanol. Tolerance to the hypothermic effects of ethanol was assessed 1, 2, and 3 days postwithdrawal.

Although all mice were tolerant on the first day postwithdrawal, tolerance produced by this method was found to have dissipated by the second day of testing. Administration of DG-AVP (0.08–0.80 μg/hr, subcutaneously via osmotic minipumps) throughout ethanol exposure and during the 3-day tolerance testing period was found to increase the degree of tolerance obtained in these mice. However, even the highest dose (0.80 μg/hr) did not alter the rate at which tolerance abated (22). On the other hand, in subsequent studies, the same group of investigators reported a single dose of DG-AVP (0.1 μg/g) injected one-half hour prior to the injection of a challenge dose of ethanol enhanced tolerance to the hypothermic effects of ethanol in animals previously exposed to ethanol (22). In addition, Khanna et al. (52) induced tolerance in rats by oral administration of ethanol (5 g/kg) over a 25-day period. In these experiments, DG-AVP (10 μg) was found to maintain tolerance to the effects of ethanol on both the hypothermic response and the moving belt test (66). It, therefore, appears that under certain circumstances, AVP and several analogs can either increase or maintain FEI tolerance to ethanol. The effects of these peptides on FED tolerance is, as yet, unclear. However, as previously stated, the observation that NHP release declines with aging would suggest that if they regulate some or all forms of tolerance, these phenomena should change during aging.

Effects of NHP on Physical Dependence on Ethanol

AVP or OXT was administered to mice once each day during a 7-day exposure to a liquid diet containing 7% ethanol (88). On the morning of the eighth day, the ethanol diets were replaced with control diets (equicaloric, with sucrose replacing ethanol), and the mice were monitored for signs of withdrawal. Measurements were made both of seizures, using the rating scale developed by Goldstein and Pal (35), and of withdrawal hypothermia (88). In addition, the seizure threshold was determined for mice using the convulsant drug, pentylenetetrazole. During all of these studies, peptide injections were discontinued 24 hr prior to the start of the ethanol withdrawal period, or pentylenetetrazole injection (43). Ethanol-treated mice exhibited withdrawal reaction as determined by occurrence of seizures and loss of body temperature. Treatment with either AVP or OXT (45) did not alter these parameters. Similarly, the ethanol-treated mice were more sensitive to pentylenetetrazole, exemplified by the low dose required to induce a clonic-tonic seizure (43). Administration of AVP or OXT did not alter the increased sensitivity of ethanol-treated mice to pentylenetetrazole, nor did the peptides alter seizure threshold of control mice, which had been pair-fed the control diet (43). Using an osmotic minipump, Crabbe and Rigter (21) administered DG-AVP (0.08 μg/hr/mouse) during the withdrawal period and found that peptide increased the intensity of ethanol-induced convulsions, as well as the period of time during which convulsions were evident. In these experiments, only the dose of 0.08 μg/hr/mouse was effective in exacerbating the withdrawal syndrome, and neither higher nor lower doses had an effect. If DG-AVP was injected subcutaneously at intervals during the withdrawal period (rather than infused by the minipumps), the highest dose tested (10 μg/ mouse) significantly extended the duration of seizure activity in ethanol-treated mice. Crabbe and Rigter (21) concluded that the influence of the peptide on seizure activity was not due to a direct effect on seizure threshold, since DG-AVP did not produce seizures in nonethanol-treated mice. This is consistent with the observation that the peptide did not alter the ED_{50} for pentylenetetrazole-induced seizures in nonethanol-treated mice (43). On the other hand, Kastin et al. (51) reported that multiple i.c.v. injections of relatively high doses of AVP resulted in myoclonic-myotonic convulsions. It was suggested that AVP may act by producing a kindling-like process. Ethanol withdrawal has also been proposed to be similar to the kindling phenomenon (4). Although no convulsive effects were reported by Crabbe and Rigter (22) using DG-AVP, nor were there any changes in seizure threshold observed using AVP (44). It is possible that the relatively low doses used in these studies may have produced subliminal changes in seizure threshold, which may have altered the ethanol withdrawal syndrome. Until more detailed studies are performed using these peptides, the mechanism by which they affect ethanol-induced physical dependence remains unanswered.

Interaction of NHP with Neurotransmitters

In previous studies, it was observed that lesions of brain noradrenergic pathways prevented development of tolerance to ethanol (87,104,106,108). In these studies, mice were treated with 6-OHDA so that NE, but not DA, levels were significantly reduced. Subsequently, lesioned and sham-lesioned mice were exposed to ethanol by the liquid diet method (88). The lesion itself did not alter the acute response to ethanol; however, those mice that had been lesioned failed to develop tolerance to ethanol (87). If similar lesions were made after tolerance had already developed, the expression of tolerance was unaltered (104). Therefore, it was concluded that an intact noradrenergic system was necessary for the development of tolerance, rather than the display of that tolerance (104). Since AVP administration stabilizes the level of tolerance that develops to ethanol, in an experimental paradigm similar to the one in which 6-OHDA lesions block development of tolerance, several experiments were conducted to determine if AVP could still be active in maintaining tolerance in lesioned mice (42,85). In these experiments, after tolerance was induced, mice were lesioned with 6-OHDA. As previously observed, the 6-OHDA lesion does not alter the expression of tolerance that had developed prior to the lesion (104). Subsequent to the lesion, the mice were withdrawn from ethanol, and AVP was administered to lesioned and sham-lesioned mice. Figure 2 summarizes the results. Comparing sham-lesioned mice with lesioned mice, which had both received AVP injections, it was found that although AVP maintained the same level of tolerance to ethanol in the sham-lesioned group, it failed to alter the disappearance rate of tolerance in the NE-depleted mice (42,85). These data indicate not only that an intact noradrenergic system is necessary for the development of tolerance, but that, in addition, AVP may act through a noradrenergic system to maintain tolerance

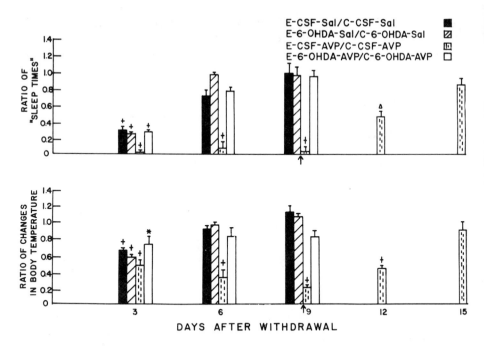

FIG. 2. Response of male C57Bl/6 mice to a challenge dose of ethanol (3 g/kg) as determined by duration of the loss of righting reflex (sleep time) or decrease in body temperature. Data are presented as the ratio of the response of experimental animals to the response of appropriate controls. When tolerance is present in experimental animals but not in controls, the ratio is less than 1.0; as tolerance disappears, the ratio approaches 1.0. Significance was determined by t-test. Individual groups were ethanol-fed, i.c.v. injection of vehicle, i.p. injection of saline (E-CSF-Sal); control-fed, i.c.v. injection of vehicle, i.p. injection of saline (C-CSF-Sal); ethanol-fed, i.c.v. injection of 6-OHDA, i.p. injection of saline (E-6-OHDA-Sal); control-fed, i.c.v. injection of 6-OHDA, i.p. injection of saline (C-6-OHDA-Sal); ethanol-fed, i.c.v. injection of vehicle, i.p. injection of arginine vasopressin (E-CSF-AVP); control-fed, i.c.v. injection of vehicle, i.p. injection of arginine vasopressin (C-CSF-AVP); ethanol-fed, i.c.v. injection of 6-OHDA, i.p. injection of arginine vasopressin (E-6-OHDA-AVP); control-fed, i.c.v. injection of 6-OHDA, i.p. injection of arginine vasopressin (C-6-OHDA-AVP). The i.c.v. injections were performed on the sixth day of chronic ethanol treatment and AVP injections (40 nmole/kg) were given once a day, starting 24 hr after the withdrawal from ethanol. Control animals received similar treatments at appropriate times ($+$, $p<0.01$; Δ $p<0.05$).

to ethanol. In support of this, AVP can alter CA turnover in various brain regions (109). On the other hand, Khanna et al. (53) has shown that electrolytic lesions of the median raphe nucleus blocked the ability of DG-AVP (10 μg) to maintain tolerance to ethanol in rats. In these studies, ethanol was administered orally (5 g/kg) for 25 days, and tolerance to ethanol was determined using the hypothermic response, as well as the moving belt test. The authors concluded that an intact serotonergic mesolimbic pathway is necessary both for the development of tolerance and for the peptide DG-AVP to maintain that tolerance (53). It has been suggested that both noradrenergic and serotonergic pathways are involved in development of tolerance to ethanol and that the relative importance of these systems may be species-dependent (60,101,103).

SUMMARY

The little available data on the development of physical dependence on ethanol by aged organisms indicate that there is an increase in the dependence liability with increasing age. Although these data are in agreement with clinical observations, clearly, more information is necessary before any conclusion can be made concerning the interrelationship between ethanol and aging in regard to the development of physical dependence. Although little data are presently available on the development of tolerance to ethanol in aged organisms, a number of observations provide circumstantial evidence that some alterations in the development or manifestation of tolerance should occur. If the postulations that ED tolerance is analogous to learning are correct, along with the studies indicating learning deficits occur during ontogeny, one would expect a similar loss of FED tolerance during aging. Similarly, those neurotransmitter systems that have been implicated in the development of FEI tolerance are also known to decay with increasing age; therefore, a loss in the ability to establish this form of tolerance probably is also altered.

The demonstration that NHPs are capable of maintaining FEI tolerance, coupled with the observation that their release declines with age, would also suggest, if their endogenous role is similar to their pharmacological effect, that what tolerance did develop might decay at an accelerated rate in old compared with young individuals. One study has indicated a decreasing ability to develop tolerance with increasing age; however, the oldest group was not old enough to be considered aged. Clearly, more information is necessary before the relationship proposed above can be readily accepted. To this end, some difficult methodological problems need to be overcome. However, considering the growth in the elderly segment of our society, the need to pursue these goals is self-evident. In addition, from a purely scientific viewpoint, since the various mechanisms that have been hypothesized to play a role in tolerance and physical dependence decline at different rates, the study of these phenomena in an aging-ethanol model might provide a useful tool for further analysis of the underlying mechanism(s) mediating the development of these addictive states.

Finally, although the data on the development of tolerance to and physical dependence on ethanol must be considered preliminary, the observation that aged organisms do not develop tolerance to ethanol as efficiently as young organisms plus the data that suggest that old subjects develop a greater physical dependence on the drug than young subjects, provides further evidence that these two aspects of chronic ethanol exposure may be dissociated.

ACKNOWLEDGMENTS

C. L. Melchior is the recipient of an ADAMHA Fellowship, NIDA DA–5172. The authors thank Margaret Tyler-Albert for help in preparation of the manuscript.

REFERENCES

1. Abel, E. L. (1978): Effects of ethanol and pentobarbital in mice of different ages. *Physiol. Psychol.*, 6:366–368.
2. Abel. E. L. (1979): Age-related differences in response to ethanol in the rat. *Physiol. Psychol.*, 7:391–395.
3. Ahtee, L., and Svartstrom-Fraser, M. (1975): Effects of ethanol dependence and withdrawal on the catecholamines in rat brain and heart. *Acta Pharmacol. Toxicol.*, 36:289–298.
4. Ballanger, J. C., and Post, R. M. (1978): Kindling as a model for alcohol withdrawal syndromes. *Brit. J. Psychiatry*, 133:1–14.
5. Barnes, G. M., and Russell, M. (1977): *Drinking Patterns Among Adults in Western New York*, Research Institute on Alcoholism, Buffalo, NY.
6. Bass, M. B., and Lester, D. (1981): Selective breeding for ethanol sensitivity: Least affected and most affected rats. In: *Development of Animal Models as Pharmacogenetic Tools*, edited by G. E. McClearn, R. A. Deitrich, and V. G. Erwin, pp. 193–202, U.S. Government Printing Office, Washington, DC.
7. Begleiter, H., and Platz, A. (1972): The effect of alcohol on the central nervous system. In: *Biology of Alcoholism*, edited by B. Kissin and H. Begleiter, pp. 293–343, Plenum Press. NY.
8. Belknap, J. D. (1980): Genetic factors in the effects of alcohol: Neurosensitivity, functional tolerance and physical dependence. In: *Alcohol Tolerance and Dependence*, edited by H. Rigter and J. C. Crabbe, Jr., pp. 157–180, Elsevier/North-Holland Biomedical Press, NY.
9. Bligh, J., Cottle, W. H., and Maskrey, M. (1971): Influence of ambient temperature on the thermoregulatory response to 5-hydroxytryptamine, noradrenaline and acetylcholine injected into the lateral cerebral ventricles of sheep, goats and rabbits. *J. Physiol.*, 212:377–392.
10. Blum, K., and Wallace, J. E. (1974): Effect of catecholamine synthesis inhibition on ethanol induced withdrawal symptoms in mice. *Br. J. Pharmacol.*, 51:109–111.
11. Calahan, P., and Cisin, I. H. (1968): American drinking practices: Summary of findings from a national probability sample. *Q. J. Stud. Alcohol.*, 29:130–151.
12. Cappell, H., Roach, C., and Poulos, C. X. (1981): Pavlovian control of cross-tolerance between pentobarbital and ethanol. *Psychopharmacology*, 74:54–57.
13. Chen, C. S. (1968): A study of the alcohol-tolerance effect and an introduction of a new behavioral technique. *Psychopharmacologia*, 12:433–440.
14. Chen, C S. (1972): A further note on studies of acquired behavioral tolerance to alcohol. *Psychopharmacologia*, 27:265–274.
15. Chen, G., Ensor, C. R., and Bohner, B. (1968): Drug effects on the disposition of active biogenic amines in the CNS. *Life Sci.*, 7(1):1063–1074.
16. Cohen, M., Keats, A. S., Krivoy, W., and Ungar, G. (1965): Effect of actinomycin D on morphine tolerance. *Proc. Soc. Exp. Biol. Med.*, 119:381–384.
17. Collins, A. C. (1981): A review of research using short-sleep and long-sleep mice. In: *Development of Animal Models as Pharmacogenetic Tools*, edited by G. E. McClearn, R. A. Deitrich, and V. G. Erwin, pp. 161–170, U.S. Government Printing Office, Washington, DC.
18. Collins, A. C., Yeager, T. N., Leback, M. E., and Panter, S. S. (1975): Variations in alcohol metabolism: Influences of sex and age. *Pharmacol. Biochem. Behav.*, 3:973–978.
19. Cote, L. J., and Kremzner, L. T. (1974): Changes in neurotransmitter systems with increasing age in human brain. *Trans. Am. Soc. Neurochem.*, 5:83.
20. Cox, B., Ary, M., and Lomax, P. (1975): Dopaminergic mechanisms in withdrawal hypothermia in morphine dependent mice. *Life Sci.*, 17:4–42.
21. Crabbe, J. C., and Rigter, H. (1980): Learning and the development of alcohol-tolerance and dependence: The role of vasopressin-like peptides. *TINS*, 1:20–23
22. Crabbe, J. C., and Rigter, H. (1980): Hormones, peptides and ethanol responses. In: *Alcohol Tolerance and Dependence*, edited by H. Rigter, and J. C. Crabbe, pp. 293–316, Elsevier/North-Holland Biomedical Press, Amsterdam.
23. Crabbe, J. C., Rigter, H., and Kerbusch, S. (1980): Genetic analysis of tolerance to ethanol hypothermia in recombinant inbred mice: Effects of desglycinamide-9-arginine-8-vasopressin. *Behav. Genetics*, 10:139–152.
24. Crowell, C. R., Hinson, R. E., and Siegel, S. (1981): The role of conditional drug responses in tolerance to the hypothermic effects of ethanol. *Psychopharmacology, 73:51–54.*
25. Eriksson, K., and Rusi, M. (1981): Finnish selection studies on alcohol-related behaviors: General

outline. In: *Development of Animal Models as Pharmacogenetic Tools*, edited by G. E. McClearn, R. A. Deitrich, and V. G. Erwin, pp. 87-117, U.S. Government Printing Office, Washington, DC.

26. Finch, C. E. (1973): Catecholamine metabolism in the brain of aging male mice. *Brain Res.*, 52:261–276.
27. Frankel, D., Khanna, J. M., Kalant, H., and LeBlanc, A. E. (1974): Effects of acute and chronic ethanol administration on serotonin turnover in rat brain. *Psychopharmacology*, 37:91–100.
28. Frankel, D., Khanna, J. M., LeBlanc, A. E., and Kalant, H. (1975): Effect of p-chlorophenyla-lanine on the acquisition of tolerance to ethanol and pentobarbital. *Psychopharmacologia*, 44:247–252.
29. Freund, G. (1969): Alcohol withdrawal syndrome in mice. *Arch. Neurol.*, 21:315–320.
30. Freund, G., and Walker, D. W. (1971): Sound-induced seizures during ethanol withdrawal in mice. *Psychopharmacology*, 22:45–49.
31. Frolkis, V. V. (1976): The hypothalamic mechanisms of aging. In: *Hypothalamus, Pituitary and Aging*, edited by A. V. Everritt, and J. A. Burgess, pp. 614–633, Charles C. Thomas, Springfield, IL.
32. Goldstein, D. (1973): Alcohol withdrawal reactions in mice: Effects of drugs that modify neu-rotransmission. *J. Pharmacol. Exp. Ther.*, 186:1–9.
33. Goldstein, A., and Goldstein, D. (1968): Enzyme expansion theory of drug tolerance and physical dependence. In: *The Addictive States. Res. Publ. Assoc. Res. Nerv. Ment. Dis.*, 46:265–267.
34. Goldstein, D. B.,and Kakihana, R. (1974): Alcohol withdrawal reactions and reserpine effects in inbred strains of mice. *Life Sci.*, 15:415–425.
35. Goldstein, D., and Pal, N. (1971): Alcohol dependence produced in mice by inhalation of ethanol: Grading the withdrawal reaction. *Science*, 172:288–289.
36. Goodrick, C. L. (1975): Behavioral differences in young and aged mice: Strain differences for activity measures, operant learning, sensory discrimination and alcohol preference. *Ex. Aging Res.*, 1:191–207.
37. Grieve, S. J., Griffiths, P. J., and Littleton, J. M. (1979): Genetic influences on the rate of development of ethanol tolerance and dependence in mice. *Drug Alcohol Depend.*, 4:77–86.
38. Grieve, S. J., and Littleton, J. M. (1979): Age and strain differences in the rate of development of cellular tolerance to ethanol in mice. *J. Pharm. Pharmacol.*, 31:696–700.
39. Gross, M. M., Lewis, E., Best, S., Young, N., and Feuer, L. (1975): Quantitative changes of signs and symptoms associated with acute alcohol withdrawal: Incidences, severity and circadian effects in experimental studies of alcoholics. In: *Alcohol Intoxication and Withdrawal—Experi-mental Studies,*, edited by M. M. Gross, *Adv. Exp. Med. Biol.*, 59:615–631.
40. Hinson, R. E., and Siegel, S. (1980): The contribution of Pavlovian conditioning to ethanol tolerance dependence. In: *Alcohol Tolerance and Dependence*, edited by H. Rigter, and J. C. Crabbe, pp. 181–199, Elsevier/North-Holland Biomedical Press, NY.
41. Hoffman, P. L., Melchior, C. L., Ritzmann, R. F., and Tabakoff, B. (1981): Structural require-ments for neurohypophyseal peptide effects on ethanol tolerance. *Alcohol Clin. Exp. Res.*, 5:154.
42. Hoffman, P. L., Melchior, C. L., and Tabakoff, B. (1983): Vasopressin maintenance of ethanol tolerance requires intact brain noradrenergic systems. *Life Sci.*, 32:1065–1071.
43. Hoffman, P. L., Ritzmann, R. F., and Tabakoff, B. (1979): The influence of arginine vasopressin and oxytocin on ethanol dependence and tolerance. In: *Currents in Alcoholism*, edited by M. Galanter, pp. 5–15, Grune and Stratton, NY.
44. Hoffman, P. L., Ritzmann, R. F., and Tabakoff, B. (1980): Neurohypophyseal peptide influences on ethanol tolerance and acute effects of ethanol. *Pharmacol. Biochem. Behav.*, 13(1):279–284.
45. Hoffman, P. L., Ritzmann, R. F., Walter, R., and Tabakoff, B. (1978): Arginine vasopressin maintains ethanol tolerance. *Nature*, 276:614–616.
46. Hunt, W. A., and Majchrowicz, E. (1974): Alterations in the turnover of brain norepinephrine and dopamine in alcohol-dependent rats. *J. Neurochem.*, 23:549–552.
47. Jaffe, J., and Sharpless, S. (1968): Pharmacological denervation supersensitivity in the central nervous system: A theory of physical dependence. In: *The Addictive States. Res. Publ. Assoc. Res. Nerv. Ment. Dis.*, 46:226–243.
48. Jube, P. C., Picchioni, A. L., and Chin, L. (1973): Role of brain norepinephrine in audiogenic seizures in the rat. *J. Pharmacol. Exp. Ther.*, 184:1–20.
49. Kakihana, R. (1979): Alcohol intoxication and withdrawal in inbred strains of mice: Behavioral and endocrine studies. *Behav. Neural. Biol.*, 26:97–105.

50. Kalant, H., LeBlanc, A. E., and Gibbins, R. R. (1971): Tolerance to and dependence on some non-opiate psychotropic drugs. *Pharmacol. Rev.*, 23(3):135–191.
51. Kasting, N. W., Veale, W. L., and Cooper, K. E. (1980): Convulsive and hypothermic effect of vasopressin in the brain of the rat. *Can. J. Physiol. Pharmacol.*, 58:316–319.
52. Khanna, J. M., Kalant, H., Le, A. D., and LeBlanc, A. E. (1979): Effect of modification of brain serotonin (5-HT) on ethanol tolerance. *Alcohol Clin. Exp. Res.*, 3:353–358.
53. Khanna, J. M., Le, A. D., and Kalant, H. (1981): Interaction between des-Gly-9-Arg-8-vasopressin (DGAVP) and 5-HT in the retention of ethanol tolerance. *Alcohol Clin. Exp. Res.*, 5:157.
54. Khanna, J. M., LeBlanc, A. E., and Le, A. D. (1979): Role of serotonin in tolerance to ethanol and barbiturates: Evidence for a specific vs. non-specific concept of tolerance. *J. Drug Alcohol Dep.*, 4:1–13.
55. Kissin, B. (1973): The pharmacodynamics and natural history of alcoholism. In: *The Biology of Alcholism*, edited by B. Kissin, and H. Begleiter, pp. 1–37, Plenum Press, NY.
56. Krivoy, W. A., Lane, M., and Kroeger, D. (1963): The action of certain polypeptides on synaptic transmission. *Ann. N.Y. Acad. Sci.*, 104:312–325.
57. Kubanis, P., and Zornetzer, S. F. (1981): Age-related behavioral and neurobiological changes: A review with an emphasis on memory. *Behav. Neural. Biol.*, 31:115–172.
58. Le, A. D., Khanna, J. M., Kalant, H., and LeBlanc, A. E. (1979): Effect of L-tryptophan on the acquisition of tolerance to ethanol-induced motor impairment and hypothermia. *Psychopharmacology*, 61:125–129.
59. Le, A. D., Khanna, J. M., Kalant, H., and LeBlanc, A. E. (1980): Effect of 5,7-dihydroxytryptamine on the development of tolerance to ethanol. *Psychopharmacology*, 67:143–146.
60. Le, A. D., Khanna, J. M., Kalant, H., and LeBlanc, A. E. (1981): The effect of lesions in the dorsal median and magnus raphe nuclei on the development of tolerance to ethanol. *J. Pharmacol. Exp. Ther.*, 218:525–529.
61. Le, A. D., Poulos, C. S., and Cappell, H. (1979): Conditioned tolerance to the hypothermic effect of ethyl alcohol. *Science*, 206:1109–1110.
62. LeBlanc, A. E., and Cappell, H. (1977): Tolerance as adaptation: Interactions with behavior and parallels to other adaptive processes. In: *Alcohol and Opiates*, edited by K. Blum, pp. 65–77, Academic Press, NY.
63. LeBlanc, A. E., Gibbins, R. J., and Kalant, H. (1973): Behavioral augmentation of tolerance to ethanol in the rat. *Psychopharmacologia*, 30:117–122.
64. LeBlanc, A. E., Gibbins, R. J., and Kalant, H. (1975): Generalization of behaviorally augmented tolerance to ethanol and its relation to physical dependence. *Psychopharmacologia*, 44:241–246.
65. LeBlanc, A. E., Kalant, H., and Gibbins, R. J. (1975): Acute tolerance to ethanol in the rat. *Psychopharmacologia*, 41:43–46.
66. LeBlanc, A. E., Matsunaga, M., and Kalant, H. (1976): Effects of frontal polar cortical ablation and cycloheximide on ethanol tolerance in rats. *Pharmacol. Biochem. Behav.*, 4:175–179.
67. Li, T.-K., Lumeng, L., McBride, W. J., and Waller, M. B. (1981): Indiana selection studies on alcohol-related behaviors. In: *Development of Animal Models as Pharamcogenetic Tools*, edited by G. E. McClearn, R. A. Deitrich, and V. G. Erwin, pp. 171–191, U.S. Government Printing Office, Washington, D.C.
68. Liacolini, E., Izekowitz, S., and Wegnan, A. (1960): Urinary epinephrine and norepinephrine excretion in delirium tremors. *Arch. Gen. Psychiat.*, 3:289–296.
69. Lloyd, K. G., and Hornykiewicz, O. (1972): Occurrence and distribution of aromatic L-amino acid (L-DOPA) decarboxylase in the human brain. *J. Neurochem.*, 19:1549–1559.
70. Loh, H. H., Shen, F.-H., and Way, E. L. (1969): Inhibition of morphine tolerance and physical dependence development and brain serotonin synthesis by cycloheximide. *Biochem. Pharmacol.*, 18:2711–2721.
71. Ludwig, A. M., and Stark, L. H. (1974): Alcohol craving: Subjective and situational aspects. *Q. J. Stud. Alcohol*, 35:899–905.
72. Lynch, J. J., Fertziger, A. P., Teitelbaum, H. A., Cullen, J. W., and Gantt, W. H. (1973): Pavlovian conditioning of drug reactions: Some implications for problems of drug addiction. *Cond. Ref.*, 8:211–223.
73. Mansfield, J. G., and Cunningham, C. L. (1980): Conditioning and extinction of tolerance to the hypothermic effect of ethanol in rats. *J. Comp. Physiol. Psychol.*, 94:962–969.
74. Martin, W. (1968): A homeostatic and reduncancy theory of tolerance to and dependence on narcotic analgesic. In: *The Addictive States. Res. Publ. Assn. Res. Nerv. Ment. Dis.*, 4:206–223.

75. Matthew, R. J., Claghorn, J. L., and Largen, J. (1979): Craving for alcohol in sober alcoholics. *Am. J. Psychiat.*, 136:603–606.

76. Melchior, C. L., and Tabakoff, B. (1981): Modification of environmentally cued tolerance to ethanol in mice. *J. Pharmacol. Exp. Ther.*, 219:175–180.

77. Myers, R. D. (1974): Temperature regulation. In: *Handbook of Drug and Chemical Stimulation of the Brain: Behavioral, Pharmacologic and Physiologic Aspects*, edited by R. D. Myers, pp. 237–301, Van Nostrand Reinhold, Cincinnati, OH.

78. McGeer, E. G., and McGeer, P. L. (1975): Age changes in the human for some enzymes associated with metabolism of catecholamines, GABA and acetylcholine. In: *Neurology of Aging*, edited by J. M. Ordy, and K. Brizzee, pp. 287–305, Plenum Press, NY.

79. Moore, J. A., and Kakihana, R. (1978): Ethanol-induced hypothermia in mice: Influence of genotype on development of tolerance. *Life Sci.*, 23:2331–2338.

80. Nakajima, S. (1976): Cycloheximide: Mechanisms of its amnestic effect. *Curr. Dev. Psychopharmacol.*, 3:26–53.

81. Perrin, R. G., Kalant, H., and Livingston, K. E. (1975): Electroencephalographic studies of ethanol tolerance and physical dependence in the cat. *Electroencephalogr. Clin. Neurophysiol.*, 39:157–162.

82. Pohorecky, L. A. (1974): Effects of ethanol on central and peripheral noradrenergic neurons. *J. Pharmacol. Exp. Ther.*, 189:380–391.

83. Rigter, H., Rijk, H., and Crabbe, J. C. (1980): Tolerance to ethanol and severity of withdrawal in mice are enhanced by a vasopressin fragment. *Eur. J. Pharmacol.*, 64:53–68.

84. Ritchie, J. M. (1975): The aliphatic alcohols. In: *The Pharmacological Basis of Therapeutics*, edited by L. S. Goodman, and A. Gilman, 4th ed., pp. 137–150, MacMillan, NY.

85. Ritzmann, R. F., Hoffman, P. L., and Tabakoff, B. (1978): Neurohypophyseal peptides, norepinephrine and ethanol tolerance. *Neurosci. Abstr.*, 4:413.

86. Ritzmann, R. F., and Springer, A. (1980): Age-induced alterations in CNS sensitivity to ethanol in mice. *Age*, 3:15–17.

87. Ritzmann, R. F., and Tabakoff, B. (1976): Dissociation of alcohol tolerance and dependence. *Nature*, 263:418–420.

88. Ritzmann, R. F., and Tabakoff, B. (1976): Body temperature in mice: A quantitative measure of alcohol tolerance and physical dependence. *J. Pharmacol. Exp. Ther.*, 199:158–170.

89. Ritzmann, R. F., and Tabakoff, B. (1979): Strain differences in the development of tolerance to ethanol. In: *Advances in Experimental Medicine and Biology*, edited by H. Begleiter, and B. Kissen, pp. 197–210, Plenum Press, NY.

90. Samorajski, T., Friede, R. L., and Ordy, J. M. (1971): Age differences in the ultrastructure of axons in the pyramidal tract of the mouse. *J. Geront.*, 26:542–551.

91. Samorajski, T., and Rolsten, C. (1973): Age and regional differences in the chemical composition of brains of mice, monkeys and humans. *Prog. Brain Res.*, 40:253–266.

92. Schuckitt, M. A., and Miller, P. L. (1978): Alcoholism in elderly men: A survey of a general ward. *Ann. N.Y. Acad. Sci.*, 273:558–571.

93. Seeman, P., and Lee, T. (1974): The dopamine-releasing actions of neuroleptics and ethanol. *J. Pharmacol. Exp. Ther.*, 190:131–140.

94. Siegel, S. (1977): Learning and psychopharmacology. In: *Psychopharmacology in the Practice of Medicine*, edited by M. E. Jarvik, pp. 61–70, Appleton-Century-Crofts, NY.

95. Siegel, S. (1978): A Pavlovian conditioning analysis of morphine tolerance. In: *Behavioral Tolerance: Research and Treatment Implications*, edited by N. A. Krasnegor, pp. 27–53, U.S. Government Printing Office, Washington, DC.

96. Siegel, S. (1979): The role of conditioning in drug tolerance and addiction. In: *Psychopathology in Animals: Research and Treatment Implications*, edited by J. D. Keehn, pp. 143–168, Academic Press, NY.

97. Siegel, S. (1982): Classical conditioning, drug tolerance and drug dependence. In: *Research Advances in Alcohol and Drug Problems*, edited by Y. Israel, F. B. Glaser, H. Kalant, R. E. Popham, W. Schmidt, and R. G. Smart, Plenum Press, NY.

98. Sze, P. Y., Yanai, J., and Ginsburg, B. E. (1976): Effects of early ethanol input on the activities of ethanol-metabolizing enzymes in mice. *Biochem. Pharmacol.*, 25:215–217.

99. Tabakoff, B., and Boggan, W. O. (1974): Effects of ethanol on serotonin metabolism in brain. *J. Neurochem.*, 22:759–764.

100. Tabakoff, B., Hoffman, P. L., and Ritzmann, R. F. (1972) Integrated neuronal model for devel-

opment of alcohol tolerance and dependence. In: *Currents in Alcoholism*, Vol. 3, edited by F. Seixas, pp. 97–118. Grune and Stratton, NY.

101. Tabakoff, B., Hoffman, P. L., and Ritzmann, R. F. (1978): Dopaminergic receptor function after chronic ingestion of ethanol. *Life Sci.*, 23:643–648.

102. Tabakoff, B., Jaffe, R. C., and Ritzmann, R. F. (1978): Corticosterone concentration in mice during ethanol drinking and withdrawal. *J. Pharm. Pharmacol.*, 30(6):371–374.

103. Tabakoff, B., Melchior, C. L., and Hoffman, P. L. (1982): Commentary on ethanol tolerance. *Alcohol Clin. Exptl. Res.*, 6(2):252–259.

104. Tabakoff, B., and Ritzmann, R. F. (1979): The effect of 6-hydroxydopamine on tolerance to and dependence on ethanol. *J. Pharmacol. Exp. Ther.*, 204:319–331.

105. Tabakoff, B., and Ritzmann, R. F. (1979): Acute tolerance in inbred and selected lines of mice. *Drug Alcohol Depend.*, 4:87–90.

106. Tabakoff, B., Ritzmann, R. F., and Oltmans, G. A. (1979): The effect of selective lesions of brain noradrenergic systems on the development of barbiturate tolerance. *Brain Res.*, 176:327–336.

107. Tabakoff, B., Ritzmann, R. F., Raju, T. S., and Deitrich, R. A. (1980): Characterization of acute and chronic tolerance in mice selected for inherent differences in sensitivity to ethanol. *Alcohol. Clin. Exp. Res.*, 4:70–73.

108. Tabakoff, B., Yanai, J., and Ritzmann, R. F. (1978): Brain noradrenergic systems as a prerequisite for development of tolerance to barbiturates. *Science*, 200:149–151.

109. Tanaka, M., Versteeg, D. H. G., and de Wied, D. (1977): Regional affects of vasopressin on rat brain catecholamine metabolism. *Neurosci. Lett.*, 4:321–325.

110. Tryding, N., Tufvesson, G., and Illsson, S. (1972): Aging, monoamines and monoamine oxidase levels. *Lancet*, 1:489.

111. van Ree, J. M., and de Wied, D. (1976): Propyl-leucyl-glycinamide (PLG) facilitates morphine dependence. *Life Sci.*, 19:1331–1340.

112. Walter, R., Ritzmann, R. F., Bhargava, H. M., Rainbow, T. C., Flexner, L., and Krivoy, W. A. (1978): Inhibition by Z-Pro-D-Leu of the development of tolerance to and physical dependence on morphine in mice. *Proc. Natl. Acad. Sci., USA*, 75:4573–4576.

113. Warren, J. M., and Akert, K. (1964): *The Frontal Granular Cortex and Behavior*, McGraw-Hill, NY.

114. Way, E. L., Loh, H. H., and Shen, F. (1969): Simultaneous quantitative assessment of morphine tolerance and physical dependence. *J. Pharmacol. Exp. Ther.*, 167:1–8.

115. Wenger, J. R., Berlin, V., and Woods, S. C. (1980): Learned tolerance to the behaviorally disruptive effects of ethanol. *Behav. Neural. Biol.*, 28:418–430.

116. Wenger, J. R., Tiffany, T. M., Bombardier, C., Nicholls, K., and Woods, S. C. (1981): Ethanol tolerance in the rat is learned. *Science*, 213:575–577.

117. Wiberg, G. S., Samson, J. M., Maxwell, W. B., Coldwell, B. B., and Trenholm, H. L. (1971): Further studies on the acute toxicity of ethanol in young and old rats: Relative importance of pulmonary excretion and total body water. *Toxicol. Appl. Pharmacol.*, 20:22–29.

118. Wiberg, G. S., Trenholm, H. L., and Caldwell, B. B. (1970): Change in LD_{50}, *in vivo* and *in vitro* metabolism, and liver alcohol dehydrogenase activity. *Toxicol. Appl. Pharmacol.*, 16:718–727.

119. Wikler, A. (1973): Conditioning of successive adaptive responses to the initial effects of drugs. *Cond. Ref.*, 8:193–210.

120. Wikler, A. (1973): Dynamics of drug dependence: Implications of a conditioning theory for research and treatment. *Arch. Gen. Psychiatry*, 28:611–616.

121. Wood, J. M., and Laverty, R. (1979): Effect of depletion of brain catecholamines on ethanol tolerance and dependence. *Eur. J. Pharmacol.*, 58:285–293.

122. Wood, W. G., and Armbrecht, H. J. (1982): Behavioral effects of ethanol in animals: Age differences and age changes. *Alcohol Clin. Exp. Res.*, 6:3–12.

123. Wood, W. G., Armbrecht, H. J., and Wise, R. W. (1982): Ethanol intoxication and withdrawal among three age groups of C57Bl/6 NNIA mice. *Pharmacol. Biochem. Behav.*, 17:1037–1041.

Alcoholism in the Elderly, edited by
J. T. Hartford and T. Samorajski.
Raven Press, New York © 1984.

Aging and the Effects of Ethanol: The Role of Brain Membranes

W. Gibson Wood, H. James Armbrecht, and Ronald W. Wise

Geriatric Research, Education, and Clinical Center, Veterans Administration Medical Center; and Departments of Medicine and Biochemistry, St. Louis University School of Medicine, St. Louis, Missouri 63125

In this chapter, the role of brain membranes as an explanation for age-related differences in response to ethanol will be examined. The studies that are included are those that primarily have used an animal model as a means of understanding the effects of ethanol on the aging individual. In addition, we review studies that have used, for the most part, animals that are *representative* of the life-span of the particular species and strain.

The effects of ethanol are age-related (38,41). Studies employing human subjects have reported that aging individuals differ in their responses to ethanol for measures such as blood ethanol levels (36) and cognitive performance (17) as compared with younger individuals. Brain tissue from human autopsy specimens taken from old individuals has been found to be more sensitive to the effects of ethanol than tissue from younger individuals (32). This sensitivity was demonstrated by the greater inhibition of synaptosomal $(Na^+ + K^+)$-adenosine triphophatase (ATPase) activity in response to ethanol for the tissue samples from old individuals.

ACUTE AND CHRONIC ADMINISTRATION OF ETHANOL

A general conclusion of the above-mentioned human studies is that aged subjects are more affected by ethanol than younger subjects. This conclusion also applies to animal studies on ethanol and aging with respect to both acute and chronic administration of ethanol (38). Studies (21,39) on the acute administration of ethanol have found that old C57BL/NNIA mice (24–28 months) lose the righting response at lower brain and blood ethanol levels than younger mice (6–8 months). Moreover, the old mice are impaired longer and regain the righting response at lower brain and blood ethanol levels than do younger mice (21,39).

When ethanol is administered chronically, old animals show a greater effect than younger animals. We reported recently (40) that old C57BL/NNIA male mice (25 months) administered an ethanol liquid diet (Bio-Serv®) for 14 days showed more severe signs of intoxication and withdrawal as compared with younger age groups (3 and 14 months). The 3-month group was least affected by ethanol in spite of the findings that they consumed significantly more of the ethanol diet and had higher blood ethanol levels than the two older groups. Samorajski et al. (26) have observed that old C57BL/6J mice maintained on a 10% (vol/vol) ethanol solution for approximately 16 months showed greater changes on measures such as passive avoidance learning and choline acetyltransferase activity in corpus striatum and cerebellum than younger mice.

MECHANISMS

The mechanism for age-related differences in response to both acute and chronic ethanol administration has not been determined. Mechanisms that have been proposed include metabolism (21), percentage of body water to body weight (9,37,42), and central nervous system sensitivity (2,32,33).

Metabolism

Metabolism of ethanol has been found to be related to age (21). Young C57BL/ NNIA mice (6 months old) cleared ethanol [intraperitoneal (i.p.) 3 g/kg] at a rate of 0.53 μmol/min/g, whereas the clearance for older mice (12 and 24 months) was 0.46 and 0.37 μmol/min/g. It was concluded, however, that age differences in metabolism could not account for the greater effects of ethanol on aging organisms (21). Vestal et al. (36) administered ethanol (0.57 g/kg) to human subjects ranging in age from 21 to 81 years and found that rates of ethanol elimination were not related to age. It would seem that metabolism of ethanol is not the primary mechanism that accounts for age-related differences in response to ethanol.

Body Water

The distribution of ethanol in body water has been proposed as an explanation for age-related differences in response to ethanol (9,37,42). This hypothesis is based on the finding that the percentage of body water to body weight and lean body mass decreases with increasing age (8). York (42) has tested directly the body water hypothesis by first determining the amount of body water in two age groups (5–7, 24–26 months) of CD female rats. Animals were injected (i.p.) with different doses of ethanol based on estimated body water. Blood ethanol levels were similar generally, and the rate of elimination did not differ between young and old animals. York also observed that the distribution of ethanol in blood and brain was similar within young (7 months) and old (28 months) female CD-strain rats. Age differences in ethanol-induced hypothermia were not observed when young and old rats were injected with ethanol based on estimated amount of body water.

The percentage of body water to body weight does contribute to age differences in response to ethanol. However, this explanation does not fully account for effects of acute and chronic ethanol administration. As discussed previously, old animals lose the righting response at lower brain and blood ethanol levels as compared with younger animals (21,39). When ethanol is administered chronically, signs of intoxication and withdrawal are more severe for aged animals even though ethanol consumption and blood ethanol levels are lower than those for younger animals (40).

Central Nervous System

The third major explanation that has been proposed to account for age-related differences in response to ethanol is the role of the central nervous system; specifically, the differential effect of ethanol on the biophysical and biochemical activity of brain membranes (2,32,33). Both ethanol administration and increasing age are associated with changes in brain membrane structure and function. Deterioration of membrane components has been suggested as a prime factor in the aging process. It also has been proposed that the membrane is the primary site for the effects of ethanol and the development of tolerance (5,6,13). Thus, age-related differences in response to ethanol may be the result of changes in brain membranes that occur with aging. This chapter examines the relationships among aging, ethanol, and brain membranes.

BIOLOGICAL MEMBRANES

Before discussing membranes and aging, we would like to discuss briefly some structural characteristics of biological membranes and how these characteristics are measured. For a detailed discussion of biological membranes, the reader is referred to the excellent reviews by Seeman (28) and Singer (29).

The current membrane model proposes that membranes are a lipid bilayer with proteins that penetrate into or protrude through the membrane (30). The lipids of brain membranes are composed mostly of phospholipids, sphingolipids, and cholesterol. In general, these lipids determine the fluidity of the lipid bilayer. Fluidity refers to the viscosity of the lipid environment. Changes in fluidity occur with changes in the cholesterol content and the degree of unsaturation of the fatty acyl chains. Changes in the fluidity of the lipid bilayer can affect the activity of membrane proteins (27).

Several different methods have been used to measure fluidity of membranes, e.g., spin-labeling, nuclear magnetic resonance, and fluorescent probes (31). Spin-labeling is a method that has been used frequently in studies on the effects of ethanol (12) and is the method that we have employed for our work on aging, ethanol, and brain membranes (1,2). This method uses a spin-labeled probe (fatty acid or cholesterol analog) that is inserted into the membrane. One of the probes used commonly is the 5-nitroxide stearic acid. This probe orients itself parallel to the acyl chains of the phospholipids. The motion of the probe in the membrane is detected using electron spin resonance (ESR). The ESR spectrum can be used to calculate an average membrane fluidity assessed by that probe. Probes having nitroxide groups at different positions in the fatty acyl chain will report on the fluidity at different depths within the membrane (12). Although this method is a sophisticated measure of lipid motion in the membrane, it has its drawbacks. The average fluidity calculated assumes that the probe is distributed evenly throughout the lipid environment and that the lipid environment is homogeneous. However, the membrane can contain regions of both fluid- and gel-phase lipids, which may result in an underestimation of membrane fluidity.

AGING AND BRAIN MEMBRANES

This section will cover some of the work that has been accomplished with respect to membranes and aging. The emphasis of the chapter is on brain membranes. However, because of the paucity of data, studies that have examined membranes from other organs will be included.

There have been very few studies that have examined the biophysical and biochemical properties of brain membranes from different age groups of animals. Most studies have concentrated on whole brain homogenate, or on different regions of brain (10). Therefore, this section includes studies that have examined organs in addition to the brain.

In a study of whole brain homogenate and myelin fractions from three age groups (3, 8, 26 months) of C57BL/10J mice, it was found that the protein content of the whole brain homogenate did not differ among the three age groups, whereas the lipid content was higher in the older animals (35). This difference in lipid content would seem to be due to the nearly threefold increase in myelin between 3 and 26 months. In the myelin fractions, the percent protein did not differ among the three age groups. The ratio of cholesterol to phospholipid was greater for myelin from old mice, and the ratio of galactolipid to phospholipid was lower for the older mice. In addition, a decrease in unsaturated acyl groups of membrane phosphoglycerides with increasing age was reported.

Age differences in myelin protein have not been observed for Sprague-Dawley rats 3, 13, and 19 months of age (19). The cholesterol/phospholipid ratio did increase with age. Also, there was found an increase in unsaturation in the acyl chains of major myelin glycosphingolipids. The increase in unsaturated acyl groups differs from results reported with mice (35). It was concluded in the study that the compositional changes observed with increasing age suggested that fluidity of myelin increased with age. Fluidity was not measured in the study.

We have measured (2) the fluidity of synaptic plasma membranes, brain microsomes, and erythrocytes from C57BL/NNIA male mice of three different age groups (3–5, 11–13, 22–24 months). Membranes were labeled with a 5-nitroxide stearic acid probe that reports motion close to the surface of the membrane; motion was recorded using a Varian E109E ESR spectrometer. All measurements were made at 37°C. Table 1 contains the fluidity data for the three membranes expressed as the order parameter S for each age group. Significant age differences in fluidity were not observed for any of the membranes using this spin-labeled probe. However, these results are restricted to that part of the membrane close to the surface; differences may exist deeper in the bilayer, which could be tested using a different probe.

TABLE 1. *Base-line order parameter for membranes from three age groups of mice*

Age group (months)	Synaptic plasma membranes	Brain microsomes	Erythrocytes
3–5	0.591 ± 0.002	0.577 ± 0.001	0.607 ± 0.001
11–13	0.594 ± 0.001	0.578 ± 0.004	0.603 ± 0.002
22–24	0.593 ± 0.001	0.573 ± 0.002	0.604 ± 0.001

Data are the mean ($\pm$ SE) of the order parameter in the absence of ethanol (base line). Order parameter was calculated as previously described (2). In model membranes, the order parameter can vary between completely ordered (1.0) and completely fluid (0) (12).

Some studies that have examined membranes from organs other than brain have reported age-related differences in fluidity. Fluidity, as measured by ESR of hepatic microsomal membranes, was greater for CFN male rats 24 to 27 months as compared with rats 3 and 12 months of age (1). A phase transition at 24°C was observed in membranes from rats 24 to 27 months of age but not from the younger age groups. Whereas fluidity of hepatic microsomes was greater for old animals, a decline in fluidity of lymphocytes with increasing age has been observed for mice and humans (22,23). Fluidity was measured by fluorescence depolarization at a temperature of 22°C. It also was observed that the ratio of cholesterol to phospholipids was greater for lymphocytes from old organisms than from younger individuals. Fluidity of erythrocytes did not differ for young (<25 years) or old (>65 years) subjects (4). ESR was used to measure fluidity near the membrane surface. Age differences were noted in the physical state of membrane proteins using a probe that is protein-specific, and it was concluded that membrane proteins may be involved in changes occurring with aging (4).

Using indirect methods to measure membrane function, the membrane properties of mitochondria from Wistar male rats, 2 to 4 months and 24 months of age, were examined (11). The osmotic properties of mitochrondria were analyzed using potassium chloride (KCl). Mitochondria from young animals were found to show a linear relationship between KCl concentration and swelling, whereas mitochondria from aged animals showed an impairment in response to hypo-osmotic conditions. The decreased diffusion of ions across the membrane suggests that the membranes from old animals may be more "rigid." These findings are similar to the results for lymphocytes that were discussed above.

From this brief review of the biophysical properties of membranes from different age groups, it is apparent that this is a topic that has not received a great amount of attention. There would appear to be differences depending on the membrane being examined and the method of investigation employed. It is possible that not all membranes demonstrate the same change in fluidity and composition with increasing age. However, the majority of the studies have observed age differences in membrane properties regardless of the source of the membrane.

ETHANOL AND BRAIN MEMBRANES

Interest in the effects of ethanol on membranes has been increasing over the past few years (e.g., 5,6,12–16). Ethanol's effect on membranes is viewed by some investigators as being nonspecific and resulting in a physical, as compared with a chemical, effect. In a recent review, it was proposed that the pharmacological effects of ethanol are caused by ethanol "acting on the lipids of cell membranes in a physical, rather than chemical, manner and that tolerance develops by changes in the chemical composition of the membrane lipids" (13). Ethanol-induced changes in membrane structure and composition may result in changes in the activity of membrane-bound enzymes, e.g., $(Na^+ + K^+)$-ATPase, adenylate cyclase (31). Many membrane-bound enzymes have been shown to require a specific membrane fluidity and composition for optimal function (27). Neurotransmitter release and uptake, which is altered by ethanol consumption, may also be modulated by changes in membrane fluidity (31).

Membrane fluidity is affected by ethanol (5). Several investigators have reported that when membranes—e.g., synaptic plasma membranes, erythrocytes, liver mitochondria—are perturbed with ethanol, fluidity increases. This increase in membrane fluidity is thought to be due to the partitioning of the ethanol into the hydrocarbon region of the membrane (31). Increased fluidity may alter the mobility of membrane lipids and thus modify the function of membrane proteins. Alternatively, ethanol may interact directly with the hydrophobic regions of membrane proteins. Whereas, fluidity is increased when ethanol is administered *in vitro*, membranes from animals who received ethanol *in vivo* chronically are resistant to this fluidizing effect of ethanol. This resistance has been attributed to increased cholesterol content (6), changes in other lipids (14–16), and reduced membrane binding of ethanol (24).

It has been reported that cholesterol is increased in brain membranes from young mice and rats as a result of chronic ethanol administration *in vivo* (6). This increase has been correlated with tolerance to ethanol. However, the exact role of cholesterol with respect to tolerance and membrane fluidity has not been established. Brain lipid extracts from synaptosomal membranes from ethanol-tolerant and control mice differed in base-line fluidity (i.e., in the absence of ethanol *in vitro*) and when perturbed with ethanol. Following removal of cholesterol, differences in fluidity were not observed when bilayers were perturbed with ethanol (15). In addition, base-line differences in fluidity were no longer detectable. When cholesterol was added back to equalize the amount of cholesterol to phospholipid, ethanol-induced differences in fluidity were observed (i.e., membranes from ethanol animals were less fluid) but not base-line differences. The investigators concluded that although the presence of cholesterol was required for ethanol tolerance, other changes in lipid composition must be involved.

Changes in lipids other than cholesterol have been found to be affected following chronic ethanol administration (14). A decrease in unsaturation of synaptosomal phospholipids during chronic ethanol administration has been observed (14). Animals on a diet high in saturated fats lost the righting response at a higher blood ethanol level as compared with controls and a group on a highly unsaturated diet. Koblin and Deady (18) also have reported that mice fed an unsaturated diet had longer sleep times and lower blood ethanol levels at awakening as compared with animals on a fatty-acid-deficient (saturated) diet or Purina Lab Chow®. However, these results are interpreted with caution because pair-feeding procedures were not used, and the animals receiving the diet devoid of unsaturated fatty acids had double the weight of the other groups.

Recent evidence indicates that myelin lipids isolated from rats chronically administered ethanol show a decrease in phospholipid-to-protein ratio and changes in phospholipid acyl group composition (34). There was an increase in 16:0, 18:0, and 18:1 acyl groups, and a decrease in 20:1, 20:4, and 22:6 acyl groups, resulting in an overall decrease in unsaturation. It also has been reported that ethanolamine plasmalogen increased while phosphatidylethanolamine decreased in myelin from rats treated chronically with ethanol *in vivo*. These compositional changes might also be expected to decrease fluidity of the membrane (20).

Changes in cholesterol and other lipids have been proposed as explanations for the tolerance resulting from chronic administration of ethanol. In addition, it has been observed that there is a reduced partitioning of ethanol into the membrane of ethanol-tolerant animals. This effect was found in synaptosomes and liver mitochondria from rats administered ethanol for 35 days (24). The change in partitioning may be caused by a change in lipid composition, which, in turn, makes the membranes resistant to the disordering effects of ethanol (24).

AGING, ETHANOL, AND BRAIN MEMBRANES

In this chapter we have reviewed studies that have reported that biological membranes are affected by perturbation with ethanol and show changes with increasing age. A reasonable hypothesis to account for age-related differences in response to ethanol is that these differences are due to changes in membranes that occur with aging.

Sun and Samorajski (32) studied the effects of ethanol on $(Na^+ + K^+)$-ATPase activity of synaptic plasma membranes from different age groups of C57BL/10 male mice (3, 8, and 26–29 months) and from human brain obtained at autopsy. Synaptic plasma membranes from different age groups of mice were incubated with ethanol ranging in concentrations from 1 to 5% vol/vol. The incubation resulted in greater inhibition of ATPase activity in synaptic plasma membranes from old animals than from that of younger animals. Similar results were reported using synaptic plasma membranes from human brains. It was concluded that the age-related difference in ATPase activity in response to ethanol may be caused by changes in the membrane cholesterol content that occur with increasing age or changes in the ratio of saturated to unsaturated acyl groups (32).

Ethanol fluidizes biological membranes *in vitro*. We examined whether this fluidization is related to age (2). Synaptic plasma membranes, brain microsomes, and erythrocytes were prepared from C57BL/NNIA male mice of three different age groups (3–5, 11–13,22–24 months). Details concerning the methods for measurement of membrane fluidity are described in the section "Biological Membranes." Briefly, fluidity was measured using the 5-nitroxide stearic acid probe. Motion of the probe was determined by ESR. Membranes were incubated with either 250 mM or 500 mM ethanol. These ethanol concentrations are higher than ethanol concentrations found *in vivo* (20–40 mM) during moderate-to-severe intoxication. However, it was our intention to demonstrate clearly age-related differences in membrane fluidity in response to ethanol. Figure 1 shows the order parameter for synaptic plasma membranes at base line and following incubation with ethanol for each age group. Fluidity at base line did not differ among the three groups. When perturbed with ethanol, the largest change in the order parameter (i.e., an increase in fluidity) occurred in the synaptic plasma membranes from young animals. Changes in ethanol-induced fluidity were small for the old animals at both ethanol concentrations. Figure 2 describes the order parameters for erythrocytes at base line and when

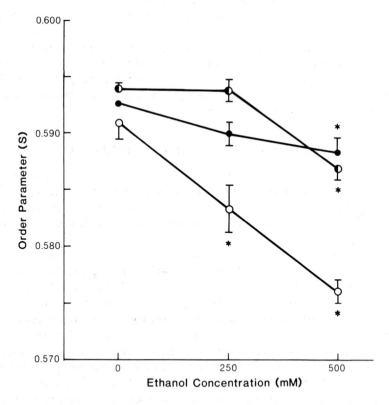

FIG. 1. Mean (±SE) order parameter of synaptic plasma membranes at base line and at two concentrations of ethanol for each of three age groups of mice (3–5 months, ○——○; 11–13 months, ●——●; and 22–24 months, ●——●). A decrease in the order parameter indicates an increase in membrane fluidity. Asterisk indicates significant differences (*t*-test $p < 0.05$) for age-matched comparisons between base line and the two ethanol concentrations.

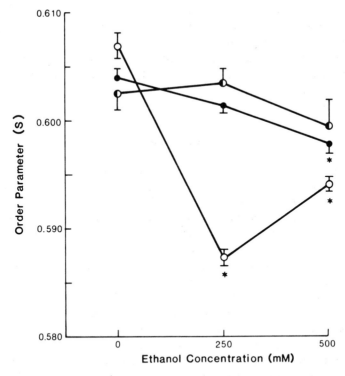

FIG. 2. Mean ($\pm$ SE) order parameter of erythrocyte membranes at base line and at two concentrations of ethanol for each of three age groups of mice (3–5 months, ○——○; 11–13 months, ●——●; and 22–24 months, ●——●). A decrease in the order parameter indicates an increase in membrane fluidity. Asterisk indicates significant differences (*t*-test $p<0.05$) for age-matched comparisons between base line and the two ethanol concentrations.

perturbed with ethanol. The changes in fluidity were similar to those observed using synaptic plasma membranes. Membranes from old animals were least affected by ethanol. Brain microsomes from old animals also did not show an increase in fluidity when perturbed with ethanol.

In a study that measured indirectly the physical properties of membranes, differences were found in terms of the effects of ethanol and among different age groups (11). Male Wistar rats of two age groups (2–4 months, 24 months) were administered a liquid diet (Sustacal®) with or without ethanol for 14 days. Mitochondrial respiration and KCl-induced swelling of mitochondria were determined. Ethanol had a greater effect on mitochondrial respiration of old animals as compared with younger animals. The osmotic properties of mitochondria were examined to determine indirectly if there were age- or ethanol-related membrane differences among the groups. Changes in osmotic properties of mitochondria may reflect changes in membrane structure and function. Mitochondria were incubated with different concentrations of KCl. The response of mitochondria from young control animals to KCl was linear, i.e., with increasing concentration there was an increase in swelling. The young ethanol group showed less response to KCl as compared with the younger control group. The old ethanol and control groups did not differ in response to KCl. Differences were noted between the old groups and the young control group but not between the young ethanol group. The reduced responsiveness of the old control group to perturbation with KCl is similar to the change in ethanol-induced fluidity of membranes from old mice.

CONCLUSIONS

The most obvious conclusion that can be reached from this review is that very little information is available on the effects of ethanol on brain membranes with respect to aging. Of the few studies that have been reported, age-related differences in response to acute and chronic administration of ethanol have been observed for $(Na^+ + K^+)$-ATPase activity, membrane fluidity, and respiration and permeability of mitochondria. It is unclear at this time whether or not the greater sensitivity to the *in vivo* effects of ethanol for old as compared with young organisms is caused by changes in membranes with increasing age. However, the studies to date indicate clearly that there is a relationship between aging and the effects of ethanol *in vitro* on the biophysical and biochemical properties of biological membranes.

Ethanol-induced fluidity was less in membranes isolated from old mice as compared with that of younger mice. This age difference in fluidity was observed for synaptic plasma membranes, erythrocytes, and brain microsomes. Resistance to the fluidizing effect of ethanol has been seen in membranes from animals that have chronically been administered ethanol. It has been suggested that this resistance may be related to increased tolerance (5). At first glance, the findings of very little change in membrane fluidity for old animals would appear to be contrary to the membrane hypothesis because old animals are more affected by ethanol *in vivo* as compared with younger animals [see (38) for a review]. However, the *in vitro* findings are limited to the probe that was used as an indicator of fluidity and the ethanol concentrations. We used a probe that measures lipid motion close to the membrane surface, and although changes in fluidity caused by increased cholesterol should be observable, changes due to decreased unsaturation of acyl groups might not be. It is possible that use of a probe that monitors motion deeper in the membrane would be a better indicator of ethanol and age changes. The dose of ethanol in our experiments exceeded *in vivo* concentrations that occur during moderate-to-moderately severe intoxication. Although our findings indicate clearly that there are age differences, further studies are needed using doses within *in vivo* physiological limits. In addition, membranes should be examined from animals who have received ethanol both *in vitro* and *in vivo*. The effects of chronic *in vivo* administration of ethanol on membranes from different age groups of animals have not been examined.

It has been hypothesized that alcoholism may accelerate the aging process, e.g. (3,7,25). Support for this hypothesis, i.e., premature aging hypothesis, has been largely from neuropathological and neuropsychological studies comparing young alcoholics with old nonalcoholics. Such information gained from these studies is limited because of life-history variables—e.g., health status, poly drug use, psychosocial problems—that may affect both biological and behavioral responses. Interestingly, our studies of membrane fluidity and the results with mitochrondria permeability (11) do support the so-called premature aging hypothesis. Whether or not alcoholism accelerates the aging process or processes has not been determined because there is no agreement as to what the aging process(es) is. Presumably, the causes of changes in membranes with aging and changes with alcoholism are very different.

As we indicated earlier, there has been very little work in the area of aging, ethanol, and membranes. Thus, any results and conclusions should be viewed cautiously. Future work in this area should examine composition of membranes, e.g., protein, cholesterol, phospholipid, and fatty acid profiles. In addition, it needs to be determined if there is an age-related difference in binding of ethanol to the membrane. Finally, it should be ascertained whether or not changes in diet, e.g., saturated and unsaturated fats, can affect age differences in response to both *in vivo* and *in vitro* ethanol administration. Obviously there is a large amount of work that needs to be done in an area that has potential benefit for understanding the effects of ethanol and the aging process.

ACKNOWLEDGMENTS

This work was supported by the Medical Research Service of the Veterans Administration and the Geriatric Research, Education, and Clinical Center of the VA Medical Center, St. Louis, Missouri. Appreciation is extended to Cheryl Duff, Britt Thomas, and Judy Walsh for expert technical assistance.

REFERENCES

1. Armbrecht, H. J., Birnbaum, L. S., Zenser, T. V., and Davis, B. B. (1982): Changes in hepatic microsomal membrane fluidity with age. *Exp. Gerontol.*, 17:41–48.
2. Armbrecht, H. J., Wood, W. G., Wise, R. W., Walsh, J. B., Thomas, B. N., and Strong, R. (1983): Ethanol-induced disordering of membranes from different age groups of C57BL/6NNIA mice. *J. Pharmacol. Exp. Ther.*, 226:387–391.
3. Blusewicz, M. J., Dustman, R. E., Schenkenberg, T., and Beck, E. C. (1977): Neuropsychological correlates of chronic alcoholism and aging. *J. Nerv. Ment. Dis.*, 165:348–355.
4. Butterfield, D. A., Ordaz, F. E., and Markesbery, W. R. (1982): Spin-label studies of human erythrocyte membranes in aging. *J. Gerontol.*, 37:535–539.
5. Chin, J. H. and Goldstein, D. B. (1977): Drug tolerance in biomembranes: A spin label study of the effects of ethanol. *Science*, 196:684–685.
6. Chin, J. H., Parsons, L. M., and Goldstein, D. B. (1978): Increased cholesterol content of erythrocyte and brain membranes in ethanol-tolerant mice. *Biochim. Biophys. Acta.*, 513:358–363.
7. Courville, C. B. (1955): *Effects of Alcohol on the Nervous System of Man.* San Lucas Press, Los Angeles, CA.
8. Edelman, I. S., Haley, H. B., Schloerb, P. R., Sheldon, D. B., Friis-Hansen, B. J., Stoll, G., and Moore, F. D. (1952): Further observations on total body water I. Normal values throughout the life span. *Surg. Gynecol. Obstet.*, 95:1–12.
9. Ernst, A. J., Dempster, J. P., Yee, R., St. Dennis, C., and Nakano, L. (1976): Alcohol toxicity, blood alcohol concentration and body water in young and adult rats. *J. Stud. Alcohol*, 37:347–356.

10. Finch, C. E. (1977): Neuroendocrine and autonomic aspects of aging. In: *Handbook of the Biology of Aging*, edited by C. E. Finch and L. Hayflick, pp. 262–280. Van Nostrand Reinhold, NY.
11. Fitzgerald, G. A., and Balcavage, W. X. (1979): Consequences of dietary ethanol on permeability and respiration of mitochondria and liver ADH in young and aged rats. In: *Currents in Alcoholism, Biomedical Issues and Clinical Effects of Alcoholism*, Volume 5, edited by M. Galanter, pp. 91–99. Grune and Stratton, NY.
12. Goldstein, D. B. (1981): Uses of electron paramagnetic resonance in alcohol research. *Alcohol. Clin. Exp. Res.*, 5:137–140.
13. Goldstein, D. B., and Chin, J. H. (1981): Interaction of ethanol with biological membranes. *Fed. Proc.*, 40:2073–2076.
14. John, G. R., Littleton, J. M., and Jones, P. A. (1980): Membrane lipids and ethanol tolerance in the mouse. The influence of dietary fatty acid composition. *Life Sci.*, 27:545–555.
15. Johnson, D. A., Lee, N. M., Cooke, R., and Loh, H. H. (1979): Ethanol-induced fluidization of brain lipid bilayers: Required presence of cholesterol in membranes for the expression of tolerance. *Mol. Pharmacol.*, 15:739–746.
16. Johnson, D. A., Lee, N. M., Cooke, R., and Loh, H. (1980): Adaptation to ethanol-induced fluidization of brain lipid bilayers: Cross-tolerance and reversibility. *Mol. Pharmacol.* 17:52–55.
17. Jones, M. K., and Jones, B. M. (1980): The relationship of age and drinking habits to the effects of alcohol on memory in women. *J. Stud. Alcohol*, 41:179–186.
18. Koblin, D. D., and Deady, J. E. (1981): Sensitivity to alcohol in mice with an altered brain fatty acid composition. *Life Sci.*, 28:1889–1896.
19. Malone, M. J., and Szoke, M. C. (1982): Neurochemical studies in aging brain. I. Structural changes in myelin lipids. *J. Gerontol.*, 37:262–267.
20. Moscatelli, E. A., and Demedink, P. (1980): Effects of chronic consumption of ethanol and low-thiamin, low protein diets on the lipid composition of rat whole brain and brain membranes. *Biochim. Biophys. Acta*, 596:331–337.
21. Ritzmann, R. F., and Springer, A. (1980): Age differences in brain sensitivity and tolerance to ethanol in mice. *Age*, 3:15–17.
22. Rivnay, B., Bergman, S., Shinitzky, M., and Globerson, A. (1980): Correlations between membrane viscosity, serum cholesterol, lymphocyte activation and aging in man. *Mech. Ageing Dev.*, 10:119–126.
23. Rivnay, B., Shinitzky, M., and Globerson, A. (1979): Viscosity of lymphocyte plasma membrane in aging mice and its possible relation to serum cholesterol. *Mech. Ageing Dev.*, 10:71–79.
24. Rottenberg, H., Waring, A., and Rubin, E. (1981): Tolerance and cross-tolerance in chronic alcoholics: Reduced membrane binding of ethanol and other drugs. *Science*, 213:583–585.
25. Ryan, C., and Butters, N. (1980): Learning and memory impairments in young and old alcoholics: Evidence for the premature-aging hypothesis. *Alcohol. Clin. Exp. Res.*, 4:288–293.
26. Samorajski, T., Strong, R., Volpendesta, D., Miller-Soule, D., and Hsu, L. (1982): The effects of aging, ethanol, and dihydroergotoxine mesylate (Hydergine) alone and in combination on behavior, brain neurotransmitter and receptor systems. In: *Alcoholism and Aging: Advances in Research*, edited by W. G. Wood and M. F. Elias, pp. 115–129. CRC Press, Boca Raton, FL.
27. Sandermann, H. (1978): Regulation of membrane enzymes by lipids. *Biochim. Biophys. Acta*, 515:209–237.
28. Seeman, P. (1975): The actions of nervous system drugs on cell membranes. In: *Cell Membranes, Biochemistry, Cell Biology and Pathology*, edited by G. Weissmann and R. Claiborne, pp. 239–247. HP Publishing, NY.
29. Singer, S. J. (1975): Architecture and topography of biologic membranes. In: *Cell Membranes, Biochemistry, Cell Biology and Pathology*, edited by G. Weissmann and R. Claiborne, pp. 35–44. HP Publishing, NY.
30. Singer, S. J., and Nicolson, G. L. (1972): The fluid mosaic model of the structure of cell membranes. *Science*, 175:720–731.
31. Sun, A. Y. (1979): Biochemical and biophysical approaches in the study of ethanol-membrane interaction. In: *Biochemistry and Pharmacology of Ethanol*, Volume 2, edited by E. Majchrowicz, and E. P. Noble, pp. 81–100. Plenum Press, NY.
32. Sun, A. Y., and Samorajski, T. (1975): The effects of age and alcohol on $(Na^+ + K^+)$-ATPase activity of whole homogenate and synaptosomes prepared from mouse and human brain. *J. Neurochem.*, 24:161–164.
33. Sun, A. Y., Samorajski, T., and Ordy, J. M. (1975): Alcohol and aging in the nervous system.

In: *Neurobiology of Aging*, edited by J. M. Ordy and K. R. Brizzee, pp. 505–520. Plenum Press, NY.

34. Sun, G. Y., Danopoulos, V., and Sun, A. Y. (1980): The effect of chronic ethanol administration on myelin lipids. In: *Currents in Alcoholism*, Volume VII, edited by M. Galanter, pp. 83–91. Grune and Stratton, NY.

35. Sun, G. Y., and Samorajski, T. (1972): Age changes in the lipid composition of whole homogenates and isolated myelin fractions of mouse brain. *J. Gerontol.*, 27:10–17.

36. Vestal, R. E., McGuire, E. A., Tobin, J. D., Andres, R., Norris, A. H., and Mizey, E. (1977): Aging and ethanol metabolism. *Clin. Pharmacol. Ther.*, 21:343–354.

37. Wiberg, G. S., Trenholm, H. L., and Coldwell, B. B. (1970): Increased ethanol toxicity in old rats: Changes in LD50, *in vivo* and *in vitro* metabolism and liver alcohol dehydrogenase activity. *Toxicol. Appl. Pharmacol.*, 16:425–434.

38. Wood, W. G., and Armbrecht, H. J. (1982): Behavioral effects of ethanol in animals: Age differences and age changes. *Alcohol. Clin. Exp. Res.*, 6:3–12.

39. Wood, W. G., and Armbrecht, H. J. (1982): Age differences in ethanol-induced hypothermia and impairment in mice. *Neurobiol. Aging*, 3:243–246.

40. Wood, W. G., Armbrecht, H. J., and Wise, R. W. (1982): Ethanol intoxication and withdrawal among three age groups of C57BL/6NNIA mice. *Pharmacol. Biochem. Behav.*, 17:1037–1041.

41. Wood, W. G., and Elias, M. F., editors (1982): *Alcoholism and Aging: Advances in Research.* CRC Press, Boca Raton, FL.

42. York, J. L. (1982): Body water content, ethanol pharmacokinetics, and the responsiveness to ethanol in young and old rats. *Dev. Pharmacol. Ther.*, 4:106–116.

Alcoholism in the Elderly, edited by
J. T. Hartford and T. Samorajski.
Raven Press, New York © 1984.

Age Effects on Alcohol Metabolism

David L. Garver

*Department of Psychiatry, Pharmacology, and Cell Biophysics, University of Cincinnati
College of Medicine, Cincinnati, Ohio 45267*

It has generally been observed that the elderly are relatively intolerant to the effects of alcohol (ethanol). Quantities of ethanol that appear to cause few problems in younger adults are tolerated poorly by the elderly; as age increases, so does the sensitivity to ethanol and its effects. Indeed, blood levels of ethanol are *higher* in the elderly following comparable (mg/kg or mg/body surface area) ingestion or infusion of ethanol. But such elevated ethanol levels are generally not the result of age-related metabolic changes in the breakdown of ethanol by the body. Elevated ethanol levels and their consequent effects are rather the result of age-related differences of distribution of ethanol within the body. In this chapter, we review evidence indicating that elevated blood ethanol levels exist in the elderly despite rates of ethanol elimination that are similar to those of younger individuals. We also review evidence concerning age-related changes in ethanol distribution within the body, which result in higher ethanol blood levels in the elderly. In addition, we briefly review the effects of the metabolic oxidation of ethanol in altering the rates of other metabolic processes and other effects of elevated ethanol levels in the elderly which result in a series of clinical problems related to ethanol use/abuse by the elderly.

ABSORPTION

Ethyl alcohol (ethanol) is readily absorbed through the mucous membranes of the stomach and small intestine mucosa following ingestion (5). Peak blood levels of ethanol are generally reached 30 to 90 min following imbibing, depending upon the quantity of ethanol ingested (Fig. 1) (2). The ultimate distribution of ethanol within the body is rapid, but selective.

DISTRIBUTION

Ethanol is not distributed evenly throughout the body. The polarity of the ethanol molecule makes ethanol water misable, but *not* fat misable. *Ethanol does not distribute to fatty tissues.* The volume of distribution (V_d) of ethanol is then the V_d of body water.

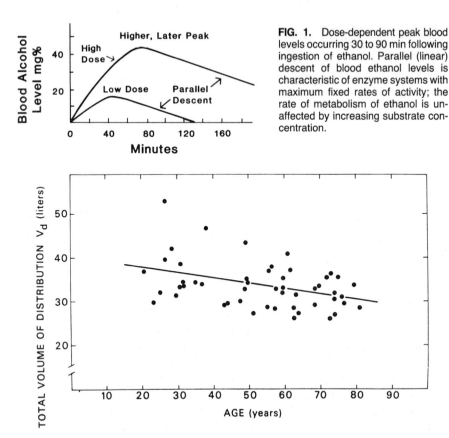

FIG. 1. Dose-dependent peak blood levels occurring 30 to 90 min following ingestion of ethanol. Parallel (linear) descent of blood ethanol levels is characteristic of enzyme systems with maximum fixed rates of activity; the rate of metabolism of ethanol is unaffected by increasing substrate concentration.

FIG. 2. Total volume of distribution (V_d) of ethanol as a function of age. (Reproduced from Vestal, R. E., et al., ref. 6, with permission.)

Women are known to have lesser body water per kilogram total body weight than men; a greater percentage of women's total body weight is fatty tissues. At age 20, females have approximately 33% of their total body weight in lipids. In contrast, males at age 20, have only 15% of their total body weight in lipids (4).

What is not generally appreciated is that by the age of 55, there is a relative increase in the lipid content of the body. In males, age 55, fat has increased from 15 to 36% of total body weight. In females at age 55, fat has increased from 33 to 48% of total body weight (1,4).

Accompanying the aging process is then a redistribution of lipid and water compartments of the body: more lipid and less water in both males and females. Since the distribution of ethanol is limited to only the body water compartment, which is decreasing with age, the V_d of ethanol, therefore, decreases with age (Fig. 2) (6).

When similar amounts of ethanol are administered to a series of subjects ranging from age 20 to age 80, such quantities of ethanol are introduced into relatively smaller body water compartments as subjects' ages increase. Similar amounts of ethanol, therefore, result in higher peak plasma ethanol concentrations in the elderly; introduction of similar amounts of ethanol into the relatively larger water body compartments of younger subjects results in lower peak plasma ethanol levels (Fig. 3) (6).

The mean kinetic curve of plasma ethanol concentrations following an ethanol infusion to a group of men over the age of 57 is contrasted to the similar mean curve for a group of men less than 57 years of age in Fig. 4 (6). Although the data in Fig. 4 are on males, one would expect that females both below and above the age of 57, because of greater body lipids relative to smaller body water compartments, would have even higher peak levels of ethanol following similar ethanol infusions. The key points here are that (a) accompanying aging is a relative decrease in the total water body compartment and that (b) since ethanol distributes only to the body water compartments, the consequence of such a decrease in body water is greater concentrations of ethanol in the blood of the elderly as compared with young adults following comparable amounts of ethanol.

METABOLISM

Ethanol is metabolized (oxidized) in the liver primarily by the enzyme alcohol dehydrogenase to acetaldehyde (Fig. 5).

Alcohol dehydrogenase is a relatively unusual oxidizing enzyme in that it is fully saturated [has reached its maximum velocity (V_{max}) of conversion of ethanol to

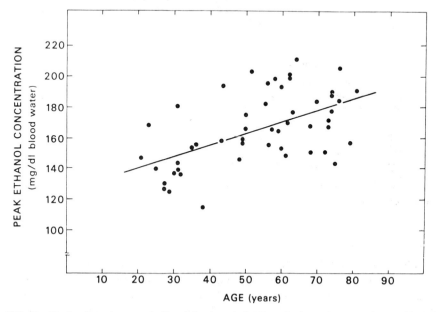

FIG. 3. Peak ethanol concentration following similar (per body surface area) quantities of infused ethanol as a function of age. (Reproduced from Vestal, R. E., et al., ref. 6, with permission.)

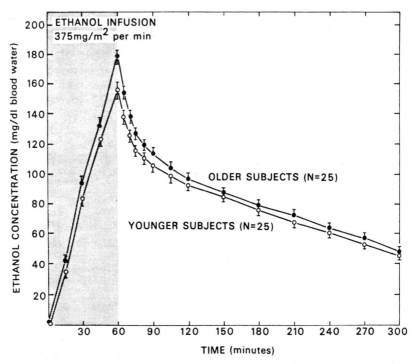

FIG. 4. Mean peak ethanol concentrations and parallel decline of blood ethanol levels following ethanol infusions in younger (aged 21–56) and older (aged 57–81) subjects. (Reproduced from Vestal, R. E., et al., ref. 6, with permission.)

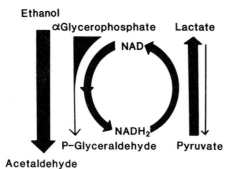

FIG. 5. The metabolic conversion of ethanol to acetaldehyde utilizing the coenzyme nicotinamide-adenine dinucleotide (NAD). Ethanol successfully competes with α-glycerophosphate for NAD, resulting in accumulation of nonmetabolized α-glycerophosphate. The task of reoxidizing $NADH_2$ to NAD falls to the reduction of pyruvate to lactate, resulting in accumulation of excessive lactate.

acetaldehyde] at relevant plasma ethanol concentrations. The maximum fixed rate of ethanol metabolism is therefore the breakdown of about 10 g of ethanol/hr, regardless of blood ethanol concentrations. This fixed rate of metabolism results in a steady, linear fall of blood ethanol of 10 to 20 mg%/hr; the rate of descent of plasma ethanol is unaffected by initial peak ethanol concentrations (Figs. 1 and 4) (2,5).

Though real genetic differences of alcohol dehydrogenase activity exist between individuals and races—and nongenetic differences can be induced by chronic alcohol use—*there is no evidence that the activity of the enzyme alcohol dehydrogenase changes as a function of age in man.* The slopes for ethanol elimination (Fig. 4) are linear, parallel, and quantitatively identical in older and younger subjects; the elimination time of ethanol is not related to age (6). Such findings are consistent with earlier studies, which also failed to find an effect of age on rates of ethanol elimination within a large group of geriatric patients (3).

SECONDARY EFFECTS OF THE METABOLISM OF ETHANOL

Gout and Fatty Liver

The oxidation of ethanol to acetaldehyde by alcohol dehydrogenase is accompanied by the reduction of its coenzyme nicotinamide-adenine dinucleotide (NAD) to $NADH_2$ (Fig. 5). The reoxidation of nicotinamide-adenine dinucleotide, reduced form ($NADH_2$) falls partly to the accompanying reduction of pyruvate to lactic acid (Fig. 5). Following excessive ethanol use, the metabolic attempt to reoxidize $NADH_2$ to NAD results in elevated levels of lactic acid. Such prolonged, excessive elevations in lactic acid, in turn, inhibit the secretion by the kidney of urates. The consequent hyperuricemia underlies clinial attacks of gout (2).

α-Glycerophosphate, ordinarily oxidized to glyceraldehyde by the cofactor NAD, also accumulates when α-glycerophosphate needs to compete with ethanol for NAD (Fig. 5). The result is an increase of α-glycerophosphate, which, in turn, stimulates the esterification of fatty acids with consequent accumulation of fat in the liver (2).

OTHER EFFECTS OF INCREASED ETHANOL LEVELS IN THE ELDERLY

Diuresis and Decreased Sexual Function

Ethanol is known to decrease the release of antidiuretic hormone (ADH) from the posterior pituitary (2,5). The consequence of such inhibition of ADH is a decrease of water uptake by the kidney with often relatively sudden increased urine formation—a particular problem in elderly males whose urinary flow may already be compromised by prostatic hypertrophy. Precipitous urinary obstruction may result.

Ethanol decreases the release of lutenizing hormone (LH) from the anterior pituitary (2,5). The consequence of such neurohormonal loss is a further reduction of testosterone synthesis and release, accompanied clinically by a decline in hormonally dependent sexual interests and performance.

Additive/Supraadditive Sedation in Drug Interactions

Unlike many other drugs, plasma concentrations of ethanol are generally not altered by concomitant medication, nor does ethanol alter the concentrations of other drugs given at the same time. But ethanol does appear to interact with a variety of sedative-hypnotic drugs in a manner that lowers the threshold at which effects of apparent intoxication occur. The concomitant use of barbiturates. benzodiazepines, and other sedative-hypnotics, such as chloral hydrate, shift to the left the levels of ethanol required for various degrees of intoxication.[1] While the "Mickey Finn" (chloral hydrate plus ethanol) may not be the "blackout drops" of mystery thrillers, the effect of such combinations nonetheless testifies to the sometimes supraadditive effects of combining sedatives with ethanol (2,5).

Ethanol Withdrawal Syndromes

Following a single intoxicating dose of ethanol, changes in neuronal excitatory patterns can be observed. Initially, ethanol causes a depression of neuronal firing rates. Such a period of neuronal depression is followed by a period of compensatory hyperactivity. The period of compensatory hyperactivity may correspond to the period of "hangover" irritability 8 to 10 hrs following substantial ethanol ingestion (2).

Following longer drinking periods, ethanol withdrawal or reduction of quantities of ethanol ingested can result in a prolonged period of neuronal hyperactivity that is manifested clinically by hyperirritability and sleeplessness. When the full-blown picture of delirium tremens is present, the diagnosis is not difficult to make. The sensitive clinician must be alert for milder stages of the ethanol withdrawal process—irritability and sleeplessness—which can often be misdiagnosed in the elderly as part of a gradual dementing process, especially when accompanied by at least mild degrees of confusion. It is frequently not recognized that *variations* in ethanol levels in such patients are the cause of the hyperactive, irritable, sleepless syndrome.

SUMMARY

There does appear to be a relative intolerance to ethanol among the elderly. One critical aspect of such intolerance is the presence of higher blood ethanol levels secondary to a decreased body water compartment into which ethanol distributes in the elderly. Higher ethanol blood levels result in metabolic alterations such as hyperuricemia and increased esterification of fatty acids in the liver, as well as changes in urinary output and sexual function. Although these secondary effects of ethanol are not unique to the elderly, they pose special considerations in the evaluation of medical and psychiatric problems of the older patient. Drinking histories are especially important in the evaluation of irritability, sleep disturbance, sexual dysfunction or disinterest, as well as in the evaluation of liver and kidney function.

Despite evidence that higher blood ethanol levels are found in the elderly following comparable ingestion/infusion of ethanol, there is *no* evidence to suggest

---

[1]Mild intoxication <50 mg%; frank intoxication with psychomotor impairment 50 to 150 mg%; profound intoxication with anesthesia/coma >250 mg%; death from respiratory depression >500 mg%.

that there are age effects on the rate of ethanol metabolism in man. The elimination rates of ethanol appear to be virtually identical across age groupings.

Of considerable interest are questions that ask if the elderly, apart from higher blood ethanol levels, have a true hypersensitivity to the effects of ethanol. Such true hypersensitivity of receptors or membranes of the elderly need be discriminated from the effects of higher ethanol blood and tissue levels alone. It is tempting to suppose that aged cells, membranes, and neurotransmitter systems may be uniquely susceptible to pharmacologic and metabolic effects of ethanol. The effect of ethanol on sodium conductance across membranes, on neuronal excitability, and on resultant states of consciousness and behavior may be quantitatively different in the aged than in the younger adult.

The evidence for such "true hypersensitivity" of the elderly to alcohol is scanty, impressionistic, and uncertain—but relevant to the understanding of the metabolic effects of alcohol in the aged. It is the subject for future research.

REFERENCES

1. Forbes, G. B., and Reina, J. C. (1970): Adult lean body mass declines with age: some longitudinal observations. *Metabolism*, 19:653–663.
2. Kalant, H., Khanna, J. M., and Israel, Y. (1980): The alcohols. In: *Principles of Medical Pharmacology*, 3rd ed., edited by P. Seemen, V. M. Sellers, and W. H. E. Roschlau, pp. 245–253. University of Toronto Press, Toronto.
3. Kurzinger, R. (1963): Der Alkoholabbau bei alten Menschen. *Dtsch. Gesundheitswesen*, 18:1224–1230.
4. Novak, L. P. (1972): Aging, total body potassium, fat-free mass, and cell mass in males and females between ages 18 and 85 years. *J. Gerontol.*, 27:438–443.
5. Ritchie, J. N. (1980): The aliphatic alcohols. In *The Pharmacologic Basis of Therapeutics, 6th ed.*, edited by A. G. Gilman, L. S. Goodman, and A. Gilman, pp. 376–390. McMillian, NY.
6. Vestal, R. E., McGuire, E. A., Tobin, J. D., Adres, R., Norris, A. H., and Mezey, E. (1977): Aging and ethanol metabolism. *Clin. Pharmacol. Ther.*, 21:343–354.

Alcoholism in the Elderly, edited by
J. T. Hartford and T. Samorajski.
Raven Press, New York © 1984.

Pharmacology of Alcoholism and Aging

H. Bruce Bosmann

*Departments of Pharmacology and Cell Biophysics and of Internal Medicine,
University of Cincinnati College of Medicine,
Cincinnati, Ohio 45267*

Use of ethanol in the elderly has, at best, modest therapeutic value; its toxicogenic potential, however, is enormous. Justifiable therapeutic uses in the elderly, though limited, include topical use as a skin coolant upon evaporation in fevers; as a topical bactericidal agent; and since ethanol hardens skin and prevents sweating, it can be useful for the prevention of decubitis ulcers (6). Relief of pain either alone or in a combination such as Brompton's mixture[1] administered every 4 hr 24 hr per day (94) has proven beneficial in terminal neoplastic disease (30). Probably the most efficacious use of ethanol is in the direct injection of ethanol at the time of diagnostic renal cyst aspiration (5) and the injection of ethanol into the pituitary fossa for relief of pain associated with malignancy (80,97).

Aside from these somewhat esoteric beneficial uses of ethanol, it has long been argued that ethanol has a general therapeutic effect in the elderly. Brooks (8) glamorously described it as "the greatest blessings of old age;" Galen [referred to in Davis (14)] called it the "nurse of old age;" and, recently, Leake and Silverman (53) said "there is scarcely a drug used in old age that has an overall beneficial effect equal to that of wine." Indeed, Hennekens et al. (37) have demonstrated that in a series of 568 married (and matched controls) men, daily consumption of small-to-moderate amounts of ethanol [2 oz (59.2 ml) or less daily] was inversely related to coronary death. However, it is clear that in spite of earlier claims of alcohol being of therapeutic value in the elderly as "a mild sedative" (53), a nutrient (53), in "circulatory defects" (8), and so on, unequivocally medical evidence indicates that ethanol is contraindicated in the elderly.

The short-term effects of ethanol on the cardiovasculature are minor (102), but long-term effects of ethanol on the heart muscle are negative (78). The vasodilator palliative effect ascribed to ethanol is unproven, and, in fact, high ethanol intake can lead to hypertension (not hypotension) (49); the use of ethanol (or any of the other putative unproven cerebral vasodilator drugs) as a cerebral vasodilator is

---

[1]Morphine, 15 mg; cocaine, 10 mg; ethanol (95%), 1.8 ml; simple syrup, 3.5 ml; chloroform water, NF, qs ad 10 ml.

contraindicated. Although ethanol may have the short-term effect of a stimulant acting on the central nervous system (CNS), its long-term (and chronic) effects are as a depressant and result in respiratory depression, sedative-hypnotic effects, pronounced disinhibition, ataxia, impaired psychomotor performance, unconsciousness, anesthesia, and ultimately death (dose-dependent). Long-term direct brain damage long thought to be associated with nutrient deprivation in fact now seems to be the result of direct ethanol neurotoxicity (95).

Long-term effects of ethanol on the stomach and intestinal tract (32,98), pancreas (60), and notably the liver (43,67) are all degenerative in the elderly. Finally, a multitude of other negative effects of ethanol have been recorded, including decreased sexual function (99), increased incidence of hematologic disorders (56), and even a case of ethanol allergy in a 76-year-old woman (38). Thus, although to some ethanol may have redeeming social value, the tremendous toxicity and abuse potential essentially make it the most dangerous "drug" taken by the elderly. Indeed, chronic ethanol intake appears to increase behavioral defects that normally accompany aging (25), although alcoholic "premature aging" seems unlikely (68), and there seems to be little hard data supporting a common "pathology" between aging and alcoholism (74).

PHARMACOKINETICS

Absorption of ethanol by any route except the skin is extremely rapid. This includes absorption after oral ingestion or inhalation of vapor. Ethanol is a small, neutrally charged, highly water-soluble molecule that requires no metabolism or digestion; absorption occurs in the stomach and more rapidly in the intestine by simple diffusion. Similarly, vaporized ethanol can be breathed into the lung where it is rapidly absorbed by simple diffusion; breathing of such vapor in high enough concentrations can be fatal.

In the elderly, ethanol is just as rapidly absorbed after oral ingestion because it is absorbed by simple diffusion and is not rate limited even though there generally is less surface area for absorption in the stomach and intestine of the elderly. Peak blood level time is slightly longer than in young adults, but the same or higher peak concentrations are achieved (91). Because the elderly adult is characterized by less total body water per unit mass (79), less extracellular fluid, and higher body fat, the same ingested dose of ethanol will result in a higher blood level in an elderly adult than in a young adult because of the lower effective fluid volume of distribution (96). Although males and females differ substantially in the amount of fat per body mass at any age, the principle of higher fat and less body water is relative for elderly males and females (66). Similarly, because ethanol is water soluble and the elderly are characterized by less tissue water per mass, local organ ethanol concentrations will be higher in the elderly for the same ingested dose (19,101).

Ethanol, when taken orally, is absorbed almost completely within 1 hr, with peak levels reached at 40 min in young adults and at about 45 min in elderly adults (27); after 10 hr the blood ethanol level is zero.

Distribution of ethanol in body tissues is fairly proportional to the amount of tissue water in the tissue. Small amounts of unchanged ethanol are excreted in the urine or exhaled by diffusion into the alveolar air; this accounts for only 2% of the ethanol of an orally ingested dose, the remaining 98% of the dose is metabolized. In the elderly, compromised kidney function is sometimes alluded to as the reason for elevated blood ethanol levels over young adults. As is evident, the amount of unchanged ethanol excreted is too small for this to be considered a valid explanation (101). (Interestingly, because of its molecular nature, ethanol forms a nearly perfect equilibrium with alveolar air; therefore, exhaled air is a much better measure of ethanol blood concentration than urine samples for medical-legal purposes.) Ethanol is widely held in the blood with plasma concentrations exceeding erythrocyte concentrations; blood levels of ethanol are routinely twice those of bone marrow (100). Because of the CNS implications of ethanol, brain and cerebrospinal fluid concentrations are important. Ethanol levels in the brain and cerebrospinal fluid do not seem to correlate with the age of an individual (e.g., levels in the elderly are not higher than those in young adults, as might be expected if meningeal penetration was higher); on autopsy following ethanol intoxication death, brain levels of ethanol are between 2 to 7 g/kg wet weight.

METABOLISM

After absorption, almost all of an oral dose of ethanol is enzymatically converted to acetaldehyde primarily in the liver (93). The acetaldehyde is then oxidized to acetyl-coenzyme A (acetyl-CoA), or acetate, and generally enters the tricarboxylic acid cycle or may be utilized for cholesterol or other lipid molecule synthesis (55). The first enzymatic reaction is catalyzed by a liver cytosolic enzyme, alcohol dehydrogenase, at zero-order kinetics. The final products of the ethanol in the tricarboxylic acid cycle are CO_2 and water; the energy (food) value of ethanol is about 7 kcal/g. Ethanol can be also enzymatically converted to acetaldehyde by the smooth microsomal mixed-function oxidases. This reaction is important since many drugs are metabolized by the hepatic smooth endoplasmic reticulum mixed-function oxidase system (73). In general, the metabolism of ethanol seems to be equivalent in older and younger patients; thus the higher blood levels observed in the elderly are more likely a function of lower volume of distribution than of decreased metabolism (91). Finally, although it seems paradoxical, in at least one study (29), alcohol metabolism as measured by serum lactate/pyruvate ratios was the same in control patients, alcoholics with cirrhosis, alcoholics without liver disease, and nonalcoholic cirrhotics. Thus it seems that ethanol may be metabolized efficiently in spite of extensive liver pathology.

METABOLIC EFFECTS

Ethanol has a wide variety of metabolic effects and, in fact, ethanol-induced organ damage adversely affects the metabolism of other xenobiotics. The metabolic effects of ethanol are of particular importance in the elderly because of the poly-pathology with which many elderly present. Many view aging as being characterized by a decline in the ability to adapt to environmental stress (59). The effects of ethanol on the metabolism of xenobiotics is also of importance because of the polypharmacy, which unfortunately is very high in the elderly.

Hypoglycemia can be induced by ethanol ingestion (50 ml) after a 2-day fast; these patients have lower liver glycogen because they do not have the characteristic glucagon response of increased blood sugar (21). Hyperlipidemia follows both acute and chronic alcohol ingestion and probably occurs by different mechanisms; for the chronic ethanol user, decreases in lipoprotein-degrading enzymes have been found (58). Fatty livers are, of course, common after excess prolonged ethanol ingestion and result from increased utilization of fat from lipid depots, increased esterification to triglycerides rather than to cholesterol esters and phospholipids, and decreased release of liver triglycerides. Significant elevations in high-density lipoprotein cholesterol have been found in male alcoholics without severe liver damage; the elevation seems to be offset by the development of alcoholic liver disease (16). Ethanol also enters all cell membranes and is intercalated between lipids of the membrane bilayer (23) and, as such, affects cellular fluidity, which has implications for carcinogenesis (23) and aging-atherosclerosis (23,13). Indeed, Freund and Forbes (26) have shown that at concentrations found in human blood, ethanol affects *in vitro* lymphocyte proliferation. Functioning of the reticuloendothelial system (RES) is severely impaired in patients with alcoholic liver cirrhosis, possibly owing to an effect of ethanol on the membranes of RES (52). Such RES impairment may, in part, be responsible for the frequency of infections seen in elderly alcoholics (52).

Effects of ethanol on the brain are numerous and profound. At the behavioral level, alcoholics differed from controls on 6 of 14 scales of the standardized Luria-Nebraska Neuropsychological Battery (11). Scales affected by ethanol were visual, receptive language, arithmetic, memory, intelligence, and pathognomonic (11). Chronic ethanol consumption accelerates age-related impairment of shuttle-box-avoidance learning in mice, and this acceleration is not caused at the molecular level by an increased lipofusion body deposition in the brain nor is it prevented by the antioxidant effect of vitamin E (24). Memory seems to be profoundly affected by ethanol: older women and moderate-drinking women given a moderate dose of ethanol retained less on two different types of memory tasks than did young women and women who were light ethanol drinkers (44). Similarly, in groups of 10 young men (20-25 years old) and 10 older men (35-45 years old), age and low doses of ethanol had a synergistic negative effect on the subjects' performance on a continuous tracking task (57).

At the biochemical level in brain, Cochran et al. (12) have reported no difference in regional levels of 5-hydroxytryptamine (5-HT) in alcoholic suicides and controls. Carlsson et al. (10), in an extensive joint effort by several Swedish laboratories, reported an age-related decrease in levels of dopamine in the nigrostriatal system, of norepinephrine in the hippocampus, and of 5-HT in the gyrus cinguli and an increase in 5-HT in the medulla oblongata and an increase in monoamine oxidase B (MAO-B) in several brain regions in patients with no known pathology. In contrast, in patients with senile dementia of nonvasculature type and in chronic alcoholics, all of the monoamines were reduced, choline acetyltransferase levels were reduced, and MAO-B was increased. Thus, there was a full separation of the normal brain neurotransmitter status between young and old and between young and senile dementia, or ethanol-using patients (10). This has led the Swedish authors (10) to conclude that chronic ethanol use can lead to a brain biochemical neuro-transmitter presentation similar to senile dementia of the nonvasculature type and that chronic ethanol consumption can accelerate the neuronal aging process in terms of neurotransmitter content of the brain (10). Earlier conflicting reports of lowered MAO activity in brains of alcoholic suicides from these same workers (33) were probably due to the fact that MAO-B was measured in the later study while total MAO level was measured in the earlier study (10). Similarly, Amir (2) reported that age affected both voluntary ethanol intake and lower aldehyde dehydrogenase activity in rats but did not significantly affect cerebral aldehyde dehydrogenase levels. Finally, it has been reported (90) that gamma-aminobutyric acid (GABA) receptor binding was increased in postmortem brain of chronic alcoholic patients with an increased number of binding sites but no change in receptor-GABA affinity. In the same study (90), muscarinic cholinergic, and benzodiazepine receptors were unaltered, but a modest reduction in β-adrenergic receptors was found. The data suggested that GABAergic receptors might play a role in the chronic ingestion of ethanol (90).

At the hemodynamic level, chronic exposure of rats of different ages to ethanol resulted in a redistribution of circulation which was detrimental to cardiac function (65); the alcohol-induced redistribution affected the cardiovascular system of older animals more severely than younger rats (65). Chronic ethanol ingestion is associated with reversible abnormal heme biosynthesis in peripheral hematopoietic cells with the rate-controlling enzyme of heme synthesis, delta aminolevulinic acid (ALA) synthetase being increased (62) while ALA dehydratase and uroporphyrinogen de-carboxylase activity are depressed (62).

Endocrine function is impaired following ethanol ingestion. In 42 patients with alcoholic liver cirrhosis and without recent ethanol ingestion, significant elevations of serum estrone, estradiol, follicle-stimulating hormone, luteinizing hormone, and prolactin were found; serum testosterone was not significantly different from con-trols (3). In this report, no significant signs of hypogonadism and feminization were found, and it was concluded that clinical and hormonal hypogonadism and fem-inization occurred without significant relation (3). An abnormal metabolism of thyroid hormones is present in chronic alcoholics with a blunted thyroid-stimulating hormone response and generally depressed T_3 levels (46). Alcohol ingestion can lead to calcific pancreatitis, but prognosis does not seem to correlate with age of patient or disease onset (61). Interestingly, in a study of 31 women (41), a normal postmenopausal hormonal profile was found in 77% of chronic alcoholics over 45 years of age. In contrast, 84% of patients of reproductive age had functional hypo-thalamic disorders (41). This suggests chronic consumption affects female sexual function at the hypothalamo-pituitary level chiefly during the reproductive period and not in older age (41).

Impairment of liver function, particularly hepatic drug metabolizing systems, is of major consequence in the elderly. Results showing longer half-lives and lesser clearance values of antipyrine in alcoholic males (35) implies impaired hepatic drug metabolizing capacity and decreased activity of hepatic microsomal enzymes (35). Vestal et al. (92), however, have shown that age, alcohol, caffeine, and smoking must be taken into account in assessing hepatic metabolism in man, although there is little doubt that age and ethanol consumption inhibit drug and xenobiotic metabolism.

Impaired elimination of caffeine in alcoholic cirrhosis has been reported by Desmond et al. (15). Frusemide has been shown to have decreased protein binding and increased apparent volume of distribution in alcoholic cirrhotics (1). Perry et al. (72) have demonstrated that acute alcoholism inhibits the elimination rate of chlordiazepoxide and alters its metabolism. Each of these examples demonstrates that in the chronic use of ethanol, liver metabolism is decreased although, in some instances, administration of microsome-inducing drugs (e.g., phenobarbital) can partially restore that activity (76). Indeed, in liver specimens from patients with alcoholic liver disease, specific proteins can be identified as being either elevated in content or decreased in content using specific antibodies (34). Reduction in enzymes necessary for drug metabolism after ethanol usage can have extreme consequences for the elderly patient.

Finally, the combination of aging and sustained use of ethanol can be fatal; 30 to 50% of all deaths of chronic alcoholics are due to hepatic failure (76). Sustained use of ethanol can lead to fatty infiltration, loss of membrane-bound detoxifying enzymes, cellular necrosis, and, finally, cellular death. Fortunately, life is compatible with a fraction of maximal liver function and hence the changes caused by ethanol, although irreversible, can be compatible with sustained life if the ethanol insult is removed before complete hepatic failure occurs. Metabolism of ethanol, like absorption and distribution, is not strikingly different in the young adult versus the older adult. Major problems are encountered in the older adult for two reasons. First, as a very function of age, the older alcoholic has insulted his organs for longer periods of time with the "toxin" and, hence, more chronic tissue damage has occurred. Moreover, each increment of added damage can be much more debilitating. Second, because the elderly have less maximal organ function and because they may have a polypathologic state and may be in a polypharmacy condition, the adverse metabolic effects of ethanol at various organ and cellular sites are much more toxic because the elderly patient must conserve and preserve as much of the remaining cellular and organ function as possible.

ADDICTION

Ethanol enjoys a rather special place in abuse pharmacology—it is the only drug easily available that causes acknowledged self-intoxication and the variety of adverse effects described above but is still socially acceptable. Indeed, early studies have found that users of illicit drugs will turn to ethanol when their "drug of choice" is unavailable, and, of course, ingestion of ethanol concurrent with administering almost every known drug of abuse has been reported (31).

Chronic maintenance of high concentrations of blood ethanol can produce a state of physical dependence and psychological craving. The consequences of withdrawal (discussed below) are the major contributor to physical dependence. The patient wants to drink ethanol to avoid the anxiety, sleep disturbances, nausea, and weakness that accompany nonmaintenance of the blood ethanol level. More serious clinical symptoms accompany withdrawal when dependence is chronic and serious (see below). Indeed, if ethanol levels are maintained for 3 to 4 days at levels greater than the metabolic rate (i.e., so ethanol levels are sustained), dependence can occur (63). Addiction can be a major problem in the elderly generally because of the length of time in which they have maintained ethanol levels (69). Approximately 2 to 10% of the elderly are alcoholic, and these are generally individuals beginning ethanol abuse after age 40 (81). Addiction to alcohol is quite similar to that seen with other sedative/hypnotics. In a study of previous alcohol consumers in Göteborg, Mellstrom et al. (64) have concluded that abstinence after ethanol abuse has negative consequences with regard to morbidity and mortality, for the negative effects of addiction are not reversible in the elderly (64).

TOLERANCE

Ethanol is a classic example of drug tolerance, for not only tolerance to ethanol occurs, but also cross-tolerance to several classes of drugs occurs (18). Tolerance can be so great that the inability to function may be the only sign of alcoholism in the older patient, and difficulty may arise in identifying the elderly "hidden" alcoholic (70). Chronic use of ethanol produces pharmacodynamic tolerance so that a higher blood concentration is necessary to provide intoxication than that in normal nonethanol users. Indeed, some alcoholics can perform normally with a blood ethanol level of 0.2%, twice the legal "significant intoxication" level in most states. This normal functioning is particularly distressing in the elderly as the ethanol consumption continues leading to irreversible hepatic, CNS, gastrointestinal, etc., pathology. In a study of 25 older male (mean age 58 ± 10.4 years) alcoholics versus 26 older abstaining males (mean age 61 ± 9.2 years), the ethanol intake caused both lower total caloric consumption and drastically lower food caloric consumption to occur leading to malnutrition (4). Tolerance does not extend the lethal concentration effect of ethanol; blood levels of 0.55% cause death in chronic alcoholics.

Cross-tolerance to several classes of drugs occurs with ethanol. Cross-tolerance probably is due to pharmacodynamic or receptor occupancy phenomena in the CNS, or to the accelerated or decelerated metabolism rate of the drug in question, depending on the particular effect the ethanol is having on the liver microsomal enzymes, i.e., activation or destruction. There is a great and dangerous cross-tolerance to other sedative-hypnotics, particularly the benzodiazepines, and to general anesthetics. Interestingly, there is no cross-tolerance to the opioid drugs (36,88). Tolerance and cross-tolerance can be difficult problems in the elderly because of the length of time an individual has been taking ethanol as well as the increased need for other medications.

WITHDRAWAL

The clinical manifestations of ethanol withdrawal in patients with severe dependence are complex and extreme. Magnesium replacement is sometimes indicated, and the benzodiazepines and other minor tranquilizers have been used to some good effect (77). The stages of withdrawal begin with tremulousness, which can occur as soon as the blood concentration drops below the tolerance level (i.e., within a few hours of the "last drink"). Tremors are evident (in some cases so pronounced that the patient cannot lift a glass to his mouth), and nausea, vomiting, anxiety, or sweating accompanies most syndromes. Orientation (psychological) seems to be maintained for several hours, generally directed toward getting another dose of ethanol.

In severe ethanol withdrawal, a period of hallucination follows and grand or petit mal seizures are common (63). The tremulous state peaks in severe withdrawal within 1 to 2 days, and if it progresses further, complete psychiatric collapse occurs, with disorientation, terrifying hallucinations, confusion, and agitation—all being described to varying degrees. The syndrome progresses to *tremulous delirium*, a condition described by Thomas Sutton in 1813 as hyperthermia and exhaustion; cardiovascular shutdown and death may follow. The condition is no better or worse in the elderly but may occur more commonly only because of the length of time of ethanol abuse and underlying organ deterioration of maximal function.

ADVERSE DRUG INTERACTIONS

As alluded to above in the discussion of cross-tolerance and metabolism, the combined intake of ethanol and certain drugs can have adverse effects in the general population and particularly in the elderly (48). For the year 1979, ethanol in combination with other drugs was reported to be the most frequent cause of drug-related medical crises in the U.S. [i.e., more reports of adverse reactions occurred with ethanol and another drug than any other drug toxicity or adverse reaction (17)].

Ethanol interacts, probably the most negatively and most prevalently, with the benzodiazepines and other minor tranquilizers (22). Indeed, it is virtually impossible to kill oneself by overdosage with diazepam (Valium®) alone; however, the combination of diazepam and ethanol can be lethal. Additive and synergistic adverse reactions have been noted for anesthetics, morphine and other opioids, and minor and major tranquilizers (83). Reports of ethanol adversely interacting with certain antidepressants, antihypertensives, anticonvulsants (7), and antibiotics have occurred (17,83). Ethanol can potentiate the adverse sedative effect of over-the-counter antihistamines (87) or potentiate the anticoagulant property of aspirin, leading to massive gastric hemorrhage in alcoholics (17).

"Blackouts" and a variety of behavioral and physical adverse reactions contrain-dicate the prescribing of tricyclic antidepressants to patients known to be taking ethanol; the reported cases of blackouts occurred in elderly adults (40). Theophylline clearance has been reported to be negatively affected by age and ethanol con-sumption—the combination of old age and ethanol would lead to potentially longer clearance times and toxicity (45). Diazepam is particularly sensitive to the com-bination of age and ethanol. Generally, dose levels of diazepam should be decreased in the elderly, and the drug is contraindicated in those patients taking ethanol (50). Unfortunately, several studies have confirmed the fact that the incidence of adverse reactions to drugs increases with age (9,42,82). Older people have more adverse reactions to drugs than do younger people (54) and adding ethanol to the equation only compounds these adverse reactions.

It is of interest that certain clinically active drugs give the "Antabuse®" (brand of disulfiram) effect (see below). This is especially true with drugs having active β-lactam rings such as the cephalosporins (75). Also, several of the newer antiar-rhythmic drugs, particularly lorcainide, must be used with caution in the elderly ethanol-using patient (51). Finally, interactions of several drugs (particularly the tranquilizers) and ethanol can be fatal (84); indeed the combination of the benzo-diazepine nitrazepam (correctly stated by the manufacturer not to have suicide potential alone) and ethanol has been used to commit suicide (89).

DRUG INTERVENTION IN ALCOHOLISM

A most interesting use of an adverse drug reaction and ethanol is in drug inter-vention. Disulfiram (Antabuse®) was a compound used in the rubber industry. Serendipitously, as it was being evaluated as an antihelmintic, its ability to produce ethanol intolerance was discovered. Thus, a drug that produced a reaction that made it absolutely intolerable to drink ethanol, the "Antabuse® reaction," is responsible for a drug intervention in alcoholism.

Disulfiram acts by inhibiting aldehyde dehydrogenase; thus, if ethanol is ingested, acetaldehyde accumulates and causes toxic reactions that make the patient extremely uncomfortable.

The extent of the reaction is to make the patient more than uncomfortable, perhaps best described by the Antabuse® package insert (Ayerst Laboratories, New York):

> The ANTABUSE®-ALCOHOL REACTION: ANTABUSE® plus alcohol, even small amounts, produces flushing, throbbing in head and neck, throbbing head-ache, respiratory difficulty, nausea, copious vomiting, sweating, thirst, chest pain, palpitation, dyspnea, hyperventilation, tachycardia, hypotension, syn-cope, marked uneasiness, weakness, vertigo, blurred vision, and confusion. In severe reactions there may be respiratory depression, cardiovascular collapse, arrhythmias, myocardial infarction, acute congestive heart failure, unconscious-ness, convulsions, and death.

There are a wide variety of other alcohol-sensitizing compounds and these have been listed by Sellers et al. (85). Although only disulfiram will be discussed here in detail, the drugs listed by Sellers et al. (85) plus procarbazine (86), which was omitted, are given here: *carbimide:* citrated calcium cyanamide; *hypoglycemic sulfonylureas:* chlorpropamide, tolbutamide; *other drugs:* chloramphenicol, griseofulvin, phentolamine, furazolidone, tolazoline, quinacrine, cefoperazone, metronidazole, pargyline; *alcohol-sensitizing mushrooms: Coprinus atramentarius, Clitocybe clavipes; other chemicals:* 4-bromopyrazole, hydrogen sulfide, tetraethyl lead, pyrogallol, and animal charcoal.

As pointed out above, grave consequences can result from the ethanol disulfiram reaction including esophagus rupture (20), shock and loss of consciousness (71), and severe behavioral deficits (71). Of even greater importance, however, is the fact that the previously held belief that disulfiram alone was innocuous is being questioned. Disulfiram-induced encephalopathy has been reported (39), disulfiram adverse (nonethanol) drug reactions have been demonstrated (47), and adverse behavioral effects have been implicated (28). Finally, it is the thesis of Sellers et al. (85) that the Antabuse® reaction is little more helpful than the threat of the reaction (placebo) and that pharmacologic intervention can only be useful, at best, as an adjunct to behavioral and social therapy.

REFERENCES

1. Allgulander, C., Beermann, B., and Sjögren, A. (1980): Frusemide pharmacokinetics in patients with liver disease. *Clin. Pharmacokinet.*, 5:570–575.
2. Amir, S. (1978): Brain and liver aldehyde dehydrogenase activity and voluntary ethanol consumption by rats: Relations to strain, sex, and age. *Psychopharmacology*, 57:97–102.
3. Bahnsen, M., Gluud, C., Johnsen, S. G., Bennett, P., Svenstrup, S., Micic, S., Dietrichson, O., Svendsen, L. B., and Brodthagen, U. A. (1981): Pituitary-testicular function in patients with alcoholic cirrhosis of the liver. *Eur. J. Clin. Invest.*, 11:473–479.
4. Barboriak, J. J., Rooney, C. B., Leitschuh, T. H., and Anderson, A. J. (1978): Alcohol and nutrient intake of elderly men. *J. Am. Diet. Assoc.*, 72:493–495.
5. Bean, W. J. (1981): Renal cysts: treatment with alcohol. *Radiology*, 138:329–331.
6. Beck, W. C. (1978): Handwashing substitute for degerming. *Am. J. Surg.*, 135:728–736.
7. Birkett, D. J., Graham, G. G., Chinwah, P. M., Wades, D. N., and Hickie, J. B. (1977): Multiple drug interactions with phenytoin. *Med. J. Aust.*, 2:467–468.
8. Brooks, H. (1928): The use of alcohol in the circulatory defects of old age. *Med. J. Rec.*, 127:199–206.
9. Caranasos, G. J., Stewart, R. B., and Cluff, L. E. (1974): Drug induced illness leading to hospitalization. *JAMA*, 228:713.
10. Carlsson, A., Adolfsson, R., Aquilonius, S. M., Gottfries, C. G., Oreland, L., Svennerholm, L., and Winblad, B. (1980): Biogenic amines in human brain in normal aging, senile dementia, and chronic alcoholism. *Ergot Compounds and Brain Function: Neuroendocrine and Neuropsychiatric Aspects*, edited by M. Goldstein, et al. Raven Press, NY.
11. Chmielewski, C., and Golden, C. J. (1980): Alcoholism and brain damage: An investigation using the Luria-Nebraska Neuropsychological battery. *Int. J. Neurosci.*, 10:99–105.
12. Cochran, E., Robins, E., and Grote, S. (1976): Regional serotonin levels in brain: A comparison of depressive suicides and alcoholic suicides with controls. *Biol. Psychiatry*, 11(3):283–294.
13. Cooper, R. A. (1977): Abnormalities of cell-membrane fluidity in the pathogenesis of disease. *N. Engl. J. Med.*, 297:371–377.
14. Davis, J. S. (1957): The medicinal benefits of beverage alcohol. *Va. Med.*, 84:3–9.
15. Desmond, P. V., Patwardhan, R. V., Johnson, R. F., and Schenker, S. (1980): Impaired elimination of caffeine in cirrhosis. *Dig. Dis. Sci.*, 25(3):193–197.
16. Devenyi, P., Robinson, G. M., Kapur, B. M., and Roncari, D. A. K. (1981): High-density lipoprotein cholesterol in male alcoholics with and without severe liver disease. *Am. J. Med.*, 71:589–594.

17. Drug Abuse Warning Network (1980): *DAWN Annual Report*. National Institute on Drug Abuse, Washington DC.
18. Eckardt, M. J., Hartford, T. C., Kaelber, C. T., Parker, E. S., Rosenthal, L. S., Ryback, R. S., Salmoiraghi, G. C., Vanderveen, E., and Warren, K. R. (1981): Health hazards associated with alcohol consumption. *JAMA*, 246(6):648–666.
19. Ernst, A. J., Dempster, J. P., Yee, R., St. Dennis, C., and Nahans, L. (1976): Alcohol toxicity, blood alcohol concentration and body water in young and adult rats. *J. Stud. Alcohol*, 37:347–356.
20. Fernandez, D. (1972): Another esophageal rupture after alcohol and disulfiram. *N. Engl. J. Med.*, 286:610.
21. Fields, J. B., Williams, H. E., and Mortimore, G. E. (1963): Studies on the mechanism of ethanol induced hypoglycemia. *J. Clin. Invest.*, 42:497–506.
22. Finkle, B. S. (1969): Drugs in drinking drivers: A study of 2,500 cases. *J. Safety Res.*, 1:179–183.
23. Freund, G. (1979): Possible relationships of alcohol in membranes to cancer. *Cancer Res.*, 39:2899–2901.
24. Freund, G. (1979): The effects of chronic alcohol and vitamin E consumption on aging pigments and learning performance in mice. *Life Sci.*, 24:145–152.
25. Freund, G. (1982): The interaction of chronic alcohol consumption and aging in brain structure and function. *Alcoholism*, 6:13–21.
26. Freund, G., and Forbes, J. T. (1976): Alcohol toxicity in cell culture. *Life Sci.*, 19:1067–1072.
27. Freund, G., and O'Hollaren, H. (1965): Acetaldehyde concentrations in alveolar air following a standard dose of ethanol in man. *J. Lipid Res.*, 6:473–480.
28. Fuller, R. K., and Roth, H. P. (1979): Disulfiram for the treatment of alcoholism: An evaluation of 128 men. *Ann. Intern. Med.*, 90:901–904.
29. Ginestal da Cruz, A., Correia, J. P., and Menezes, L. (1975): Ethanol metabolism in liver cirrhosis and chronic alcoholism. *Acta Hepato-gastroenterol.*, 22:369–374.
30. Glover, D. D., Lowry, T. F., and Jacknowitz, A. I. (1980): Brompton's mixture in alleviating pain of terminal neoplastic disease: Preliminary results. *South. Med. J.*, 73(3):278–282.
31. Goodwin, D. W., Davis, D. H., and Robins, L. N. (1975): Drinking amid abundant illicit drugs. *Arch. Gen. Psychiatry*, 32:230–233.
32. Gottfried, E. B., Korsten, M. A., and Lieber, C. S. (1976): Gastritis and duodenitis induced by alcohol: An endoscopic and histologic assessment. *Gastroenterology*, 70:890–898.
33. Gottfries, C. G., Oreland, L., Wiberg, A., and Winblad, B. (1975): Lowered monoamine oxidase activity in brains from alcoholic suicides. *J. Neurochem.*, 25:667–673.
34. Hahn, E., Wick, G., Pencev, D., and Timpl, R. (1980): Distribution of basement membrane proteins in normal and fibrotic human liver: collagen type IV, laminin, and fibronectin. *Gut*, 21:63–71.
35. Harman, A. W., Frewin, D. B., Priestly, B. G., and Alexander, C. B. J. (1979): Impairment of hepatic drug metabolism in alcoholics. *Br. J. Clin. Pharmacol.*, 7:45–48.
36. Hawkins, R. D., and Kalant, H. (1972): The metabolism of ethanol and its metabolic effects. *Pharmacol. Rev.*, 24:67–157
37. Hennekens, C. H., Willett, W., Rosner, B., Cole D. S., and Mayrent, S. L. (1979): Effects of beer, wine, and liquor in coronary deaths. *JAMA*, 242(18):1973–1974.
38. Hicks, R. (1968): Ethanol, a possible allergen. *Ann. Allergy*, 26:641–643.
39. Hotson, J. R., and Langston, J. W. (1976): Disulfiram-induced encephalopathy, *Arch. Neurol.*, 33:141–142.
40. Hudson, C. J. (1981): Tricyclic antidepressants and alcoholic blackouts. *J. Nerv. Ment. Dis.*, 169(6):381–382.
41. Hugues, J. N., Coste, T., Perret, G., Jayle, M. F., Sebaoun, J., and Modigliani, E. (1980): Hypothalamo-pituitary ovarian function in thirty-one women with chronic alcoholism. *Clin. Endocrinol.*, 12:543–551.
42. Hurwitz, N. (1969): Predisposing factors in reactions to drugs. *Br. Med. J.*, 1:536.
43. Jacobovits, A. W., Morgan, M. Y., and Sherlock, S. (1979): Hepatic siderosis in alcoholics. *Dig. Dis. Sci.*, 24:305–310.
44. Jones, M. K., and Jones, B. M. (1980): The relationship of age and drinking habits to the effects of alcohol on memory in women. *J. Stud. Alcohol.*, 41(1):179–186.
45. Jusko, W. J., Gardner, M. J., Mangione, A., Schentag, J. J., Koup, J. R., and Vance, J. W.

(1979): Factors affecting theophylline clearances: Age, tobacco, marijuana, cirrhosis, congestive heart failure, obesity, oral contraceptives, benzodiazepines, barbituates, and ethanol. *J. Pharm. Sci.*, 68(11):1358–1366.

46. Kallner, G. (1981): Assessment of thyroid function in chronic alcoholics. *Acta Med. Scand.*, 209:93–96.

47. Kiorboe, E. (1966): Phenytoin intoxication during treatment with Antabuse® (disulfiram). *Epilepsia*, 7:246–249.

48. Kissin, B. (1974): Interactions of ethyl alcohol and other drugs. In: *The Biology of Alcoholism: Clinical Pathology*, edited by Kissin, B. and H. Begleiter, pp. 109–161. Plenum Press, NY.

49. Klatsky, A. L., Friedman, G. D., Siegelaub, A. B., and Gerard, M. J. (1977): Alcohol consumption and blood pressure. Kaiser-Permanente multiphasic health examination data. *N. Engl. J. Med.*, 296:1194–1200.

50. Klotz, U., Avant, G. R., Hoyumpa, A., Schenker, S., and Wilkinson, G. R. (1975): The effects of age and liver disease on the disposition and elimination of diazepam in adult man. *J. Clin. Invest.*, 55:347–359.

51. Klotz, U., Fischer, C., Muller-Seydlitz, P., Schultz, J., and Muller, W. A. (1979): Alterations in the disposition of differently cleared drugs in patients with cirrhosis. *Clin. Pharmacol. Ther.*, 26(2):221–227.

52. Lahnborg, G., Friman, L., and Berghem, L. (1981): Reticuloendothelial function in patients with alcoholic liver cirrhosis. *Scand. J. Gastroenterol.*, 16:481–489.

53. Leake, C. D., and Silverman, M. (1967): The clinical use of wine in geriatrics. *Geriatrics*, 22:175–180.

54. Lee, P. V. (1978): Drug therapy in the elderly: The clinical pharmacology of aging. *Alcoholism*, 2 (1):39–42.

55. Lieber, C. S., Teschke, R., Hasumura, Y., and De Carli, L. M. (1975): Difference in hepatic and metabolic changes after acute and chronic alcohol consumption. *Fed. Proc.*, 34:2060–2074.

56. Lindenbawa, J. (1974): Hematologic effects of alcohol. In: *The Biology of Alcoholism, Vol. 3. Clinical Pathology* edited by B. Kissin, and H. Bigleiter, pp. 339–357. Plenum Press, NY.

57. Linnoila, M., Erwin, C. W., Ramm, D., and Cleveland, W. P. (1980): Effects of age and alcohol on psychomotor performance of men. *J.s36Stud. Alcohol.*, 41(5):488–495.

58. Losowsky, M. S., Jones, D. P., Davidson, C. S., and Lieber, C. S. (1963): Studies of alcoholic hyperlipidemia and its mechanism. *Am. J. Med.*, 35:794–804.

59. Makinodan, T., and Kay, M. M. B. (1980): Age influence on the immune system. *Adv. Immunol.*, 29:287–330.

60. Marks, I. N., Bank, S., and Barbezat, G. O. (1976): Alkoholpankreatitis Aetiologie Klinische Formen, Komplikationen. *Leber Magen Darm*, 6:257–270.

61. Marks, I. N., Girdwood, A. H., Bank, S., and Louw, J. H. (1980): The prognosis of alcohol-induced calcific pancreatitis. *S. Afr. Med. J.*, 19:640–643.

62. McColl, K. E., Moore, M. R., Thompson, G. G., and Goldberg, A. (1981): Abnormal haem biosynthesis in chronic alcoholics. *Eur. J. Clin. Invest.*, 11:461–468.

63. Mello, N. K., and Mendelson, J. H. (1977): Clinical aspects of alcohol dependence. In: *Drug Addiction: Morphine; Sedative Hypnotic and Alcohol Dependence*, edited by W. R. Marten. *Handbuch der experimentelen Pharmakologie*, 45:613–666. Springer-Verlag, Berlin.

64. Mellström, D., Rundgren, A., and Svanborg, A. (1981): Previous alcohol consumption and its consequences for ageing, morbidity, and mortality in men aged 70–75. *Age Ageing*, 10:277–286.

65. Morvai, V., and Ungvary, G. (1979): Effect of chronic exposure to alcohol on the circulation of rats of different ages. *Acta Physiol. Acad. Sci. Hung.*, 53(4):433–441.

66. Novak, L. P. (1972): Aging, total body potassium, fat free mass and cell mass in males and females between ages 18 and 85 years. *J. Gerontol.*, 27:438–450.

67. Orrego, H., Medline, A., Blendis, L. M., Rankin, J. G., and Kresden, D. A. (1979): Collogenisation of the Disse space in alcoholic liver disease. *Gut*, 20:673–679.

68. Parsons, O. A., and Leber, W. R. (1981): The relationship between cognitive dysfunction and brain damage in alcoholics: Causal, interactive or epiphenomense. *Alcoholism*, 5:326–343.

69. Pascarelli, E. F. (1974): Drug dependence: An age-old problem compounded by old age. *Geriatrics*, 29(12):109–115.

70. Pattee, J. J. (1982): Uncovering the elderly "hidden" alcoholic. *Geriatrics*, 37(2):145–146.

71. Peachey, J. E., Brien, J. F., Roach, C. A., and Loomis, C. W. (1981): A comparative review of the pharmacological and toxicological properties of disulfiram and calcium carbimide. *J. Clin. Psychopharmacol.*, 1:21–26.
72. Perry, P. J., Wilding, D. C., Fowler, R. C., Hepler, C. D., and Caputo, J. F. (1978): Absorption of oral and intramuscular chlordiazepoxide by alcoholics. *Clin. Pharmacol. Ther.*, 23(5):535–541.
73. Piriola, R. C. (1978): *Drug Metabolism and Alcohol.* University Park Press, Baltimore, MD.
74. Porjisz, B., and Begleiter, H. (1982): Evoked brain potential deficits in alcoholism and aging. *Alcoholism*, 6:53–63.
75. Portier, H., Chalopin, J. M., Freysz, M., and Tanter, Y. (1980): Interaction between cephalosporins and alcohol. *Lancet*, 2(8188):263.
76. Rautio, A., Sotaniemi, E. A., Pelkonen, R. O., and Luoma, P. (1980): Treatment of alcoholic cirrhosis with enzyme inducers. *Clin. Pharmacol. Ther.*, 28(5):629–637.
77. Redetzky, H. M. (1979): Treatment of ethanol intoxication. *Hosp. Formulary*, 71:934–940.
78. Regan, T. J., Ettinger, P. O., Haider, B., Ahmed, S., Oldewurtel, H. A., and Lyons, M. M. (1977): The role of ethanol in cardiac disease. *Ann. Res. Med.*, 28:393–409.
79. Ritschel, W. A. (1976): Pharmacokinetic approach to drug dosage in the aged. *J. Am. Geriatr. Soc.*, 24:344–354.
80. Roberts, M. T. S., and Henderson, R. S. (1981): Pituitary fossa injection with alcohol for widespread cancer pain. *N.Z. Med. J.*, 93(675):1–3.
81. Schuckit, M. A. (1977): Geriatric alcoholism and drug abuse. *Gerontologist*, 17(2):168–174.
82. Seidl, L. G., Thornton, G. F., Smith, J. W., and Cluff, L. E. (1966): Studies on the epidemiology of adverse drug reactions. III. Reactions in patients on a general medical service. *Bull. Johns Hopkins Hosp.*, 119:299.
83. Seixas, F. A. (1975): Alcohol and its drug interactions. *Ann. Intern. Med.*, 83:86–92.
84. Seixas, F. A. (1979): Drug/alcohol interactions: Avert potential dangers. *Geriatrics*, 34:89–102.
85. Sellers, E. M., Naranjo, C. A., and Peachey, J. E. (1981): Drugs to decrease alcohol consumption. *N. Engl. J. Med.*, 305:1255–1262.
86. Simmonds, M. A. (1982): (response to) Drugs to decrease alcohol consumption. *N. Engl. J. Med.*, 306:748.
87. Smiley, A. LeBlanc, A. E., French, I. W., et al. (1975): The combined effects of alcohol and common psychoactive drugs. In: *Alcohol Drugs and Traffic Safety.* Toronto Addiction Research Foundation, pp. 433–438.
88. Smith, C. M. (1978): *Alcoholism: Treatment*, Vol. 2. Eden Press, Montreal.
89. Torry, J. M. (1976): A case of suicide with nitrazepam and alcohol. *Practictioner*, 217:648–649.
90. Tran, V. T., Snyder, S. H., Major, L. F., and Hawley, R. J. (1981): GABA receptors are increased in brains of alcoholics. *Ann. Neurol.*, 9:289–292.
91. Vestal, R. E., McGuire, E. A., Tobin, J. D., Andres, R., Norris, A. H., and Mezey, E. (1976): Aging and ethanol metabolism. *Clin. Pharmacol. Ther.*, 21(3):343–354.
92. Vestal, R. E., Norris, A. H., Tobin, J. D., Cohen, B. H., Shock, N. W., and Andres, R. (1975): Antipyrine metabolism in man: Influence of age, alcohol, caffeine, and smoking. *Clin. Pharmacol. Ther.*, 18(4):425–432.
93. VonWartburg, J. P. (1971): The metabolism of alcohol in normals and alcoholics: Enzymes. In: *The Biology of Alcoholism. Vol. 1. Biochemistry*, edited by Kissin, B. and H. Begleiter, pp. 63–102. Plenum Press, NY.
94. Wade, A. (1977): *The Extra Pharmacopeia, 27th ed.* Pharmaceutical Press, London, p. 973.
95. Walker, D. W., and Hunter, B. E. (1978): Short term memory impairment following chronic alcohol consumption in rats. *Neuropsychologia*, 16:545–553.
96. Wiberg, G. S., Samson, J. M., Maxwell, W. B., Colwell, B. B., and Trenholm, H. L. (1971): Further studies on the acute toxicity of ethanol in young and old rats: Relative importance of pulmonary excretion and total body water. *Toxicol. Appl. Pharmacol.*, 20:22–29.
97. Williams, N. E., Miles, J. B., Lipton, S., Hipkin, L. J., and Davis, J. C. (1980): Pain relief and pituitary function following injection of alcohol into the pituitary fossa. *Ann. R. Coll. Surg. Engl.*, 62:203–207.
98. Wilson, F. A., and Hoyumpa, A. M. (1970): Ethanol and small intestinal transport. *Gastroenterology*, 76:338–403.
99. Wilson, G. T. (1977): Alcohol and human sexual behavior. *Behav. Res. Ther.*, 15:239–252.

100. Winek, C. L., and Jones, T. (1980): Blood versus bone marrow ethanol concentrations in rabbits and humans. *Forensic Sci. Int.*, 16:101–109.
101. Wood, W. G., and Armbrecht, H. J. (1982): Behavioral effects of ethanol in animals: Age differences and age changes. *Alcoholism*, 6:3–12.
102. Zsoter, T. T., and Sellers, E. M. (1977): Effect of alcohol on cardiovascular reflexes. *J. Stud. Alcohol.*, 38:1–10.

Alcoholism in the Elderly, edited by
J. T. Hartford and T. Samorajski.
Raven Press, New York © 1984.

Medical Issues in Alcoholism in the Elderly

*Steven R. Gambert, †Margaret Newton,
and †Edmund H. Duthie, Jr.

*Departments of Medicine; *New York Medical College, Valhalla, New York 10595, and
†The Medical College of Wisconsin, Wood Veterans Administration Medical Center,
Milwaukee, Wisconsin 53193*

Persons 65 years old and older represent an ever increasing percentage of the
U.S. population. At present they comprise 11 to 12% of the total population,
although by the year 2020, estimates place these numbers close to 20%. As people
age, not only normal aging processes are a consideration, but certain disease states
may be more prevalent.

As the number of aged individuals increases, health-care providers need to be
well aware of the problems specific to the elderly. Social, psychological, economic,
and health factors all influence quality of life and deserve careful consideration. It
is now being increasingly recognized that alcoholism is a problem not unique to
the younger population, but can manifest even for the first time late in life. The
elderly, for a variety of reasons, may start drinking either openly or, more commonly, in private. In addition, as the number of elderly increases, clinicians will
be faced with more patients who began drinking earlier in life and who continue
to do so late in life. Although a large number of persons will develop significant
health problems that preclude their reaching senescence, others will develop multiple
alcohol-related problems affecting many organ systems and, perhaps, leading to
premature physiological aging.

Another elderly group of patients who need to be evaluated are those who drank
to excess earlier in life with or without resultant health problems, but who gave up
abusing alcohol prior to reaching senescence.

This chapter discusses common medical issues that need to be considered in
caring for the elderly person who either drank to excess in the past or is presently
doing so. Psychological and social factors are discussed elsewhere in the text and
are not addressed in this chapter.

PHYSIOLOGICAL ACCOMPANIMENTS OF ACUTE
ALCOHOL INTOXICATION

Although alcohol has an immediate and readily observable effect on functions
of the central nervous system, it exerts little acute deleterious effect on other organ
systems. Alcohol has an acute direct effect on cardiac muscle, leading to increased

cardiac rate and output. Systolic blood pressure also is increased, and blood is preferentially shunted from the splanchnic circulation to the periphery with resultant cutaneous vasodilation. This latter phenomenon may result in a loss of body heat. This may be particularly harmful to the elderly who, for a variety of reasons, have a greater chance of developing accidental hypothermia. Even in low concentrations, alcohol increases acid production from the stomach's parietal cells. In the elderly, however, this may not be as significant a problem because of the decreased parietal cell mass that accompanies normal aging.

Following a large amount of alcohol ingestion, the gastric mucosa may become hyperemic with increased mucus and decreased acid secretion leading to acute gastritis. Nausea and vomiting may result because of local irritation. Acute pancreatitis may result from activation of proteolytic enzymes leading to autodigestion of pancreatic tissue. This latter phenomenon is thought to result from increased secretin production in response to alcohol's effect on increasing gastric acidity; secretin increases pancreatic enzymes. Another possible cause includes obstruction to pancreatic flow from inflammation of the duodenum with resultant edema and spasm at the sphincter of Oddi.

The patient with alcoholic ketoacidosis may exhibit symptoms along a continuum from alert, but ill appearing, to being in frank coma. Arterial blood pH is reduced with a high anion gap. In addition, the clinician may be misled as to diagnosis by noting only a weakly positive test for serum ketones. This occurs since betahydroxybutyrate is the predominant ketone present in this disorder, not detected by standard tests for ketones, i.e., nitroprusside test. Although the exact mechanism for all of the above manifestations is still unclear, data suggest that alcohol increases the lipolytic response to starvation, in addition to altering oxidative metabolic processes in cell mitrochondria.

The hypoglycemia in most cases is preceded by a period of starvation and/or vomiting, thereby depleting glycogen stores. Furthermore, alcohol inhibits hepatic gluconeogenesis from lactate, pyruvate, and amino acids by increasing nicotinamide adenine dinucleotide, reduced form (NADH), in the liver (37). Treatment rests on the repletion of glucose stores although the patient must be monitored closely and attention promptly given to correct any fluid or electrolyte abnormalities that may coexist.

There is a greater prevalence of gout among regular drinkers regardless of age (66). Acute alcohol intoxication results in transiently reduced renal urate clearance and hyperuricemia. This results from competitive inhibition of tubular urate secretion by betahydroxybutyrate and lactate generated from alcohol metabolism. This may be further compromised by a gradual drop in glomerular filtration rate (GFR) with normal aging, with resultant filtered load of urate. Dehydration, for whatever reason, also lowers GFR and hence filtered load of urate, further increasing the chance of developing hyperuricemia. Cirrhosis with its reduced "effective circulating volume" may also aggravate this condition. Diuretic usage may also lead to hyperuricemia.

In addition, the metabolic acidosis described previously may lead to negative calcium balance. Coupled with diets often deficient in calcium and a decreased intestinal absorption of calcium after the seventh decade of life, this further loss of calcium may lead to significant osteoporosis in the elderly alcoholic.

Alcohol also acutely affects body metabolism. Inhibition of antidiuretic hormone (ADH) from the posterior pituitary gland leads to prompt water diuresis. Dehydration may result with continued use providing a further stimulus to ADH release. Urinary ammonium excretion is increased as is titratable acidity following metabolic and respiratory acidosis. This may be even more of a problem in the elderly due to a decreased ability of the normal aged to excrete an ammonium load.

Neurologically, alcohol acutely serves as a central nervous system depressant acting at certain subcortical areas thought to control cerebral cortical activity. In addition, tendon reflexes may be hyperactive due to reduced inhibitory spinal motor neuronal activity. Large amounts of alcohol may lead to depression of central nervous system respiratory centers with eventual coma.

ALCOHOL-INDUCED METABOLIC ABNORMALITIES

Under normal circumstances, homeostatic mechanisms exist during periods of starvation to minimize body catabolism leading to ketone acid (betahydroxybutyrate and acetoacetate) formation and resultant metabolic acidosis (21). Both gluconeogenesis and glycogenolysis ensure proper maintenance of circulating glucose. Even after a period of total starvation for as long as several weeks, a healthy person can keep ketone acid accumulation to a minimum and serum bicarbonate and glucose fairly normal.

Alcoholic patients, however, usually owing to poor diet, vomiting, and concurrent illness, are particularly prone to developing a starvation-associated metabolic acidosis. In addition, they may develop hypoglycemia more readily.

As the chronic alcoholic develops compromised hepatic function, hydroxylation of vitamin D_3 to its more active 25-hydroxylated form by the liver may be compromised, leading to another form of metabolic bone disease, i.e., osteomalacia. This latter phenomenon is also made worse by a diet deficient in vitamin D, malabsorption of fat, and phenobarbital or phenytoin (Dilantin®) usage; both drugs increase conversion of 25-hydroxy vitamin D_3 to its inactive metabolites.

The liver is the main site of catabolism of testosterone and of the conjugation of its known metabolites with sulfuric or glucuronic acid. Although total plasma levels of androgens and estrogens may be normal in the alcoholic with cirrhosis, abnormalities of the globulin that binds them in plasma may lead to an increase in the ratio of physiologically free estrogen/free androgen, resulting in clinical manifestations including gynecomastia, testicular atrophy, spider angiomata, and palmar erythema.

It has been recently reported that patients with alcoholic liver disease have an increased rate of conversion of adrenocortical steroid precursors to estrogens (18,44,55). This may result from decreased uptake of androstenedione by the diseased liver with a resultant increase in estrone production (54).

A defect in hypothalamic-pituitary function has also been reported in chronic alcoholics. Plasma levels of follicle-stimulating hormone (FSH) and luteinizing hormone (LH) have been found to be low and prolactin levels abnormally high in alcoholic men (59,62). In addition, alcoholic men have a blunted response to a clomiphene challenge. Although these defects may result from increased circulating estrogens, other causes may also exist.

Since signs of feminization may occur in alcoholic men even prior to the development of significant liver pathology, alcohol has been implicated as having a direct effect on testicular function. Several investigators have reported a direct effect of alcohol on the testes. This seems only logical since alcohol dehydrogenase is present in testicular tissue (60,61). In a study reported in 1976, Gordon et al. (25) reported decreased concentrations of plasma testosterone, decreased testosterone production, and increased testosterone clearance in healthy men ingesting alcohol for short periods of time. This study also found a defect in the hypothalamic-pituitary axis; plasma LH did not increase in response to the lowering of plasma testosterone, despite only a short-term alcohol exposure. This implies a direct effect of alcohol on the axis. LH response to LH-releasing factor is also diminished by alcohol consumption.

Chronic alcohol ingestion is capable of inducing a lipemia despite adequate hepatic function. As alcohol is oxidized to acetate, fatty acids that enter the liver are diverted to triglyceride production. In addition, data suggest a decreased activity of lipoprotein lipase in chronic alcoholics. It is important to remember that alcohol may only be aggravating a preexisting primary lipid disorder. Clinically, the alcoholic may have hyperlipemia in the setting of pancreatitis. Although they may be causally related, no evidence has been shown to conclusively document this and either may occur as isolated entities. Since pancreatitis can result as a complication of certain primary hyperlipidemias (types I and V), the clinician must approach the differential diagnosis with an open mind. Although occurring in alcoholics, no data presently exist to conclusively implicate alcohol as a causative factor in Zieve's syndrome, consisting of hyperlipidemia, jaundice, and hemolytic anemia.

In moderation, alcohol has an effect on serum lipids. In both human and animal studies, alcohol has been shown to increase the high-density lipoprotein (HDL) portion of serum cholesterol with a comparable lowering of the low-density lipoprotein (LDL) portion (32). Since data suggest an inverse correlation between HDL cholesterol and coronary disease (5,26,42), moderate alcohol ingestion may prove beneficial to cardiovascular well-being.

ALCOHOL AND THE CARDIOVASCULAR SYSTEM

Chronic alcohol ingestion appears to have both direct as well as indirect effects on the cardiovascular system. Alcohol-induced cardiomyopathies have been described as well as many other alcohol-related problems (3,13), including alcoholic cardiomegaly, otherwise known as "München Bierherz" or "Munich beer heart" (12), cardiac fibrosis (4); microvascular infarcts and swelling (20,46); and altered subcellular myocardial components (2). In addition, changes have been noted in myocardial glycogen content as well as in lipid deposition (27,36,50). Clinically, tachycardia, decreased myocardial contractability, and altered cardiac output have all been noted in chronic alcoholics (1,7,12).

Previously, beer additives, including cobalt, have been implicated (3) in cardiac abnormalities. It now appears that alcohol itself has a direct toxic effect on the myocardium. Despite this, other etiologic factors have been suggested, including thiamin depletion, hypomagnesemia with hypokalemia, viral invasion, and autoimmune processes.

Although there is an apparent negative effect of alcohol on the heart itself and on its physiological functioning, several studies report reduced coronary artery disease in those subjects drinking moderate amounts of alcohol (5,67). Large epidemiological studies have also shown a reduced incidence of myocardial infarction in those with a moderate amount of alcohol intake (35,67). Taking this one step further, Barboriak et al. (9) reported significantly lower coronary occlusion scores as determined by coronary arteriography in those persons who consumed more than 1 oz. of alcohol per week as compared with those abstaining or imbibing less than this quantity. Preventing universal conclusion, however, all subjects in this study had a preexisting history of either unstable angina pectoris, moderate-to-severe angina, a previous myocardial infarction, or recurrent chest pain of unclear etiology. Since occlusion scores have a direct correlation to the incidence of myocardial infarctions, however, this study may have significant implications. It was particularly interesting that lower occlusion scores were noted in the higher alcohol-consuming group despite their higher prevalence of heavier smoking, higher serum triglycerides, and more hypertension. Unfortunately, no studies using less invasive techniques to assess coronary disease have yet been done in asymptomatic subjects consuming varying amounts of alcohol.

In another study, Barboriak et al. (8) compared coronary occlusion scores as determined by coronary arteriography to levels of HDL cholesterol. The HDL cholesterol/total cholesterol ratio universally correlated with extent of coronary disease. In addition, alcohol intake directly correlated with HDL levels. The authors concluded that alcohol intake and occlusion scores were significantly universally correlated even after factoring out age and HDL total cholesterol levels. Data suggest, therefore, that alcohol may exert an effect on coronary artery occlusion in addition to any effect mediated through a higher HDL level.

Additional work clearly needs to be done to better define whether or not alcohol has a protective effect on coronary disease in asymptomatic and nonaffected subjects. In addition, the clinician must be aware that problems resulting from chronic alcohol abuse place the person consuming more than moderate amounts of alcohol at a higher mortality risk from coronary heart disease. In addition, liver disease may result in lower HDL cholesterol levels because of problems in lipid synthesis. The older person, due to normal age changes in cardiovascular performance and a higher prevalence of certain diseases, may be particularly compromised if alcohol is allowed to further damage physiological cardiac reserve.

Alcoholic cardiomyopathy is most commonly seen in men. Although alcohol can have a direct effect on the cardiovascular system as mentioned above, the clinician must not forget "cardiac beriberi." This thiamine-responsive disorder is associated with a nutritional deficiency in vitamin B_1, and efforts should be made to provide an adequate diet as well as alcohol withdrawal.

The electrocardiogram in alcoholic cardiomyopathy can either be mostly normal, as in the case of beriberi described above, to significantly altered. Arrhythmias, especially atrial fibrillation, are common. The ventricular rate may be rapid and ectopic beats common. As the cardiac myopathy worsens, cardiomegaly and conduction disturbances become more significant and often difficult to treat despite the use of digitalis, diuretics, and other antiarrhythmic agents. Pathologically the heart develops areas of fibrosis and the left ventricle hypertrophies. Small areas of muscle degeneration can be seen microscopically and necrosis of tissue may also be found. Myocardial tissue shows varying degrees of mitochondrial damage and neutral lipid accumulation. Treatment rests on stopping alcohol consumption and continued medical management.

ALCOHOL AND THE GASTROINTESTINAL TRACT

The combined effects of both direct contact and systemic influences make the gastrointestinal tract unique in its response to both acute and chronic alcohol exposure. This subject has been reviewed recently (11,17,56,57,63), and the reader is referred to these treatises for greater detail.

The most proximal portion of the gastrointestinal tract is the oropharynx. With the application of alcohol to the oral mucosa, there is an increase in salivary flow. The increase appears to be short-lived and repeat administration results in a return of flow back toward base line. Clinicians have noted that chronic alcoholics may have parotid enlargement (12% prevalence in one series). This has led investigators to seek some physiological correlation. Stimulated salivary flow shows considerable inter- and intraindividual variations, making it difficult to draw sound conclusions. Dürr (16) and colleagues have reported a trend toward higher stimulated salivary flow rates and diminished protein composition of saliva with chronic alcoholism. More data are needed in this regard.

In the oropharynx, chronic alcohol abusers are known to have a higher incidence of glossitis and stomatitis. This is probably a function of poor nutrition and associated vitamin deficiencies. More important is the propensity with which chronic alcohol abusers develop squamous cell carcinoma of this region. Although it is difficult to separate the effects of coincident tobacco usage (upwards of 90% of alcoholics are smokers) in the genesis of head and neck neoplasms, it does seem that alcohol use does confer a higher risk for these lesions. In addition, heavy drinkers carry a greater risk than lighter drinkers. Clearly, the practitioner must carefully examine the oropharynx of every chronic alcoholic.

Esophageal disorders may accompany acute and chronic alcohol intake. Weber (65) has reported, in detail, the case of an alcoholic with dysphagia and pulmonary aspiration related to upper esophageal sphincter (UES) dysfunction and attributed to myopathic changes in the striated muscle of the pharynx. With abstinence from alcohol, the patient's symptoms resolved, as did the manometric findings of poor upper esophageal muscle function. Chronic alcoholics with polyneuropathy have normal UES and lower esophageal sphincter (LES) function with a decrease in distal esophageal peristalsis. Hogan (30), however, has shown impairment of UES and LES function as well as decreased secondary peristalsis in the distal one-third of the esophagus with acute administration of alcohol. This, coupled with the work of Kaufman and Kay (34) reporting gastroesophageal reflux following acute administration of alcohol, set the stage for a high incidence of reflux esophagitis following alcohol ingestion. Although clinical proof for this theory is lacking, acute and chronic esophagitis have been reported with chronic alcohol abuse.

Retching associated with an alcoholic debauch can induce a linear mucosal tear at the gastroesophageal junction. This has been termed the Mallory-Weiss tear and may result in gastrointestinal hemorrhage. An indirect effect of alcohol on the esophagus is the formation of esophageal varices. These dilated veins at the cardio-esophageal junction result from the portal hypertension due to hepatic cirrhosis. Upper gastrointestinal hemorrhage from this lesion is a source of serious morbidity and significant mortality in chronic alcoholics. Carcinoma of the esophagus has a higher frequency in alcoholics. Two-thirds of all patients with esophageal cancer report a history of heavy alcohol use. As is the case of oropharyngeal carcinoma, tobacco use appears to increase synergistically the chance of developing a cancer at this site.

The effects of acute alcohol ingestion on the stomach were alluded to earlier in this chapter. To reiterate, acute alcohol ingestion increases acid production and favors production of gastric juice with a lower than normal amount of pepsinogen. This effect appears to have some neurogenic mediation and some local mediation via the peptide hormone gastrin. Direct cellular effect of alcohol on the gastric mucosa with increase in intracellular cyclic adenosine monophosphate (AMP) is also contributory.

Barboriak (6) has reported delayed gastric emptying after the administration of alcohol to healthy volunteers. The effects of chronic alcohol usage on gastric physiology remain to be precisely defined. Chey (14) has reported a lower gastric basal acid output and maximal acid output in chronic alcoholics compared with controls. With alcohol usage there is a loss of the mucosa barrier function of the gastric mucosa and an increased permeability. Formation of erosive gastritis with the potential for subsequent upper gastrointestinal hemorrhage is common. Concomitant aspirin ingestion with alcohol use leads to a greater likelihood of acute erosive gastritis. Chronic alcoholics have an increased likelihood of developing chronic atrophic gastritis. It should also be noted that preexisting atrophic gastritis (felt to be common in old age) facilitates the formation of gastric mucosal lesions and subsequent upper gastrointestinal hemorrhage following alcohol ingestion.

Although it remains controversial as to whether or not alcohol ingestion per se is associated with peptic ulcer disease, cigarette smoking and hepatic cirrhosis are two conditions seen frequently in alcoholics which clearly are related to a higher incidence of peptic ulcer.

The small intestine is both morphologically and physiologically altered by alcohol ingestion. Acute ingestion of alcohol can cause duodenitis. Diminished glucose transport, a decline in active absorption of amino acids, and increased incorporation of fatty acids into triglycerides are noted in the intestinal mucosa with the acute administration of alcohol. Chronic alcohol administration can result in a diminished absorption of D-Xylose, a simple sugar whose absorption is a measure of small intestine mucosal integrity. This decreased absorption may be due to nutritional defects that accompany chronic alcohol use and not just alcohol administration. Although steatorrhea is commonly seen in alcoholics, it does not seem to be related to a primary mucosal defect. Rather, pancreatic exocrine dysfunction may be important in the pathogenesis of this problem. Intestinal mucosa shows a decreased ability to absorb sodium and water with chronic alcohol exposure.

Folic acid absorption is well known to decline in chronic alcoholics. This may result from changes in the small bowel rather than solely from the effect of alcohol. Vitamin B_{12} absorption declines in the chronic alcoholic, apparently because of malfunction of the ileum. The role of intrinsic factor abnormalities in this process remains in question.

Although iron deficiency is commonly found in alcoholics, the reason is more likely due to chronic gastrointestinal blood loss and poor iron intake rather than to an inability of the mucosa to absorb iron. In fact, studies have shown that alcoholics absorb the ferrous form of iron equally as well as controls and actually have a greater ability to absorb the ferric form of the mineral. Likewise, the propensity for chronic alcoholics to develop hypomagnesia is not due to abnormal mucosal absorption but rather to a combination of poor oral intake, excessive renal losses, and gastrointestinal losses via vomiting or diarrhea.

Brush border enzymes (lactase, sucrase, and alkaline phosphatase) have diminished activity after alcohol administration and may partially explain the diarrhea reported by alcohol abusers. Although not known for certain, the small bowel cellular transport system modulated by Na^+-K^+ adenosine triphosphatase (ATPase) may decline since the activity of this enzyme is inhibited by alcohol. *In vitro* data show an increase in small bowel mucosa cyclic AMP production via increased activity of adenylate cyclase. The effects of alcohol on these enzymes (Na^+-K^+ ATPase and adenylate cyclase) would also promote increased sodium and water secretion and its attendant diarrhea.

Alcohol ingestion affects the pancreas. Chronic ingestion results in pancreatic juice that has an increased protein and decreased bicarbonate concentration. Eventually there may be protein precipitation in the pancreatic ducts with subsequent calcification. These processes, combined with an increased ability of the zymogens to activate, underlie the clinical picture of chronic calcific pancreatitis. Affected patients have acute recurrent attacks of pain, exocrine and endocrine pancreatic insufficiency, and the presence of pancreatic calcifications. Acute alcoholic pancreatitis differs from the latter in its more dramatic clinical onset. These patients have disabling epigastric abdominal pain often with nausea and vomiting. Fever, tachycardia, and evidence of volume depletion may also be present. Old age adversely affects survival in patients with this fulminent illness. Therefore, elderly patients with acute alcoholic pancreatitis need careful medical management, at times requiring invasive hemodynamic monitoring to support their volume status and frequent laboratory determinations of glucose, electrolytes, and serum calcium.

The effects of alcohol ingestion on the liver are undoubtedly the most sought after and recognized effects of this agent on the gastrointestinal system. A spectrum of illness has been described (53), ranging from fatty metamorphosis to cirrhosis. A stepwise progression from one state to another has not been conclusively proven. Liver damage depends on the duration and dose of alcohol. The damage is a result of the alcohol itself so that even alcoholics with good nutrition are susceptible to hepatic damage. The fatty liver caused by alcohol ingestion shows lipid laden hepatocytes on microscopic section. Cessation of drinking at this stage results in a return of normal histology and apparently normal hepatic function.

Acute alcoholic hepatitis is a serious clinical disorder in which the patient has malaise, nausea, vomiting, abdominal pain and jaundice. There is fever, an enlarged tender liver, leukocytosis, and elevation in serum transaminases, alkaline phosphatase, and bilirubin. Histologic sections show irregular hepatocyte cytoplasm with clumps of highly refractile eosinophilic material, frequently perinuclear in location (Mallory bodies); polymorphonuclear leukocytes surround dying hepatocytes; Kupffer cell proliferation is noted and cholestasis is present. Although this illness has a clinical spectrum from mild to severe, its occurrence in an elderly patient requires cautious medical management most likely including hospitalization.

Cirrhosis is the other hepatic lesion induced by chronic alcohol ingestion. It is characterized microscopically by stellate fibrosis around portal zones with distortion of the vascular bed, loss of hepatocytes, and disorganization of lobular architecture. The consequences of this may include systemic complaints of fatigue, anorexia, weight loss, and jaundice. On examination, patients may show spider angiomata of the skin, icterus, ecchymoses related to abnormal hemostasis from nutritional deficiencies and poor hepatic function, gynecomastia, testicular atrophy, muscle wasting, palmar erythema, and Dupuytren's contracture. If there is portal hypertension, ascites, edema, esophageal varices, and splenomegaly may be noted. In far advanced disease, hepatic encephalopathy or altered renal function (hepatorenal syndrome) may occur and both are poor prognostic indicators. Therapy of cirrhosis requires total and absolute abstention from alcohol, a diet of sufficient calories possibly with some sodium and protein restrictions, and vitamin supplementation.

ALCOHOL AND ITS EFFECT ON NUTRITION AND BODY COMPONENTS

With advancing age, nutritional requirements for optimal health do not change drastically (22). However, there is a gradually declining caloric expenditure and hence need, so that an individual after 70 will require approximately 70% of the calories needed at age 40; the excess will be stored as fat. Protein requirements may be slightly increased with aging (23). This reduced need is in part due to reduced physical activity and reduced muscle mass. The percentage of body fat increases with advancing age, with a reduced lean body mass and concomitant lowering of total body water, extracellular and intravascular volumes. Bone mass and hence reserves of calcium, phosphate, and magnesium are reduced. Therefore, the aging body has contracted "reserves" of protein, water, sodium, potassium, magnesium, calcium, and phosphate. Normally the absorptive capacity of the gastro-intestinal tract remains adequate except for the suboptimal calcium transport, and the excretory capacity of the kidney, though reduced and slower to respond to acute changes, is adequate. Superimpose one or more chronic diseases, and multiple drug use common in the elderly, total body reserves and adaptability to sudden change are altered. Superimpose a variable pattern of alcohol use and the nutritional balance is further upset.

The studies of Vestal et al. (64) showed that normal aging does not alter the rate of elimination of intravenously administered alcohol. However, blood-water-ethanol levels were positively correlated with age. This they ascribed to the smaller volume of distribution and the lean body mass of normal elderly subjects. These experiments do not address the issue of tolerance in chronic alcohol users, nor the effect of concomitant food intake on rates of gastrointestinal alcohol absorption in elderly persons. Alcohol is absorbed directly through the stomach; but some passes into the intestine, and high concentrations are found in the duodenum and upper jejunum, with concentrations close to plasma levels being found in the distal jejunum and ileum.

Alcohol ingestion acutely or chronically affects nutrition by reducing intake as a result of altered cognitive function, appetite, absorption, metabolism, or excretion of nutrients, all of which may be especially deleterious in an old person with reduced functional reserves. Alcoholism is a major cause of malnutrition, resulting primarily from poor dietary intake. Because of the aforementioned body composition changes with aging and blunted homeostatic mechanisms, the elderly alcohol user is more susceptible to the nutritional consequences of alcoholism.

The nutritional consequences will depend on the extent to which normal nutrients are replaced by alcohol and on the direct toxic effects of alcohol on organ function. Although the ravages of malnutrition have been described in the skid row alcoholic, only about 3% of alcohol abusers in the United States are in this category. Under-nutrition is not rare in the elderly, even among nondrinkers. Among the elderly are the survivors of years of heavy imbibing with variable consequences (cirrhosis is among the eight leading causes of death in the over 65 population as well as in the 25–64-year-olds of both sexes), the social drinkers for whom the same or less alcohol has greater effects and may reflect a higher percentage of total caloric intake, and those who have found in alcohol a solace for late-life boredom and loneliness. A nutritional analysis of 58 middle-aged, middle-class alcoholics revealed that while drinking, 88% met or exceeded ideal body weight and had adequate intake of protein, carbohydrate, calcium, phosphate, sodium, potassium, iron, vitamins B and C. Calories consumed as alcohol varied widely but averaged approximately 30% of the total (31). In a survey of alcohol and nutrient intake of elderly men, Barboriak et al. (7) found a lower caloric intake from food in the imbibers than in the abstainers. In the elderly, with lower caloric needs, a given alcohol intake would replace a higher percentage of calories from other nutrients. Alcohol has a caloric value of 7.1 kcal/g; however, it does not supply net energy from its metabolism equivalent to its caloric value, and this results in the phenomenon of energy wastage. This is suggested by the studies of Pirola et al. (47,49). They demonstrated that in healthy volunteers, isocaloric substitution of ethanol for 50% of calories in otherwise balanced diets resulted in significant weight loss over a 2-week period. This finding has also been reported by other investigators who replaced 25% of food calories with alcohol in volunteers (40). Using a rat model, Pirola and Lieber have demonstrated that the increase in energy requirements during ethanol ingestion is accompanied by a higher rate of oxygen consumption (48). Numerous experiments in humans and in animals have demonstrated a marked increase in urinary epinephrine and a more modest increase in norepinephrine following acute alcohol ingestion. Alcohol withdrawal after heavy chronic consumption is also associated with high urinary catecholamines (24). Does this reflect increased energy expenditure during alcohol use? Could this exaggerate the "hyperadrenergic state in the elderly under normal circumstances" as postulated by Rowe and Troen (52)? The available data are inconclusive. In any case, clinicians should suspect alcohol as a possible cause for unexplained weight loss or "failure to thrive" in an elderly person.

Protein malnutrition may be seen in alcoholics as manifested by muscle wasting, hypoproteinemia, and edema. Alcohol intake in subjects on controlled isocaloric diets results in increased urinary nitrogen (uric acid and urea nitrogen) suggesting increased protein catabolism (40). Lack of adequate protein intake and coexistence of alcoholic liver disease contribute to the latter. Additionally, impaired hepatic albumin synthesis and loss of albumin into ascitic fluid contribute to the syndrome. The hypoalbuminemia may worsen malabsorptive syndromes often seen in this setting inasmuch as plasma proteins play a role in normal gastric motility, and their oncotic pressure is an essential component of passive intestinal transmucosal water and solute transport (in addition to the active transport of electrolytes which is enzymatically controlled). Thus, malabsorption accompanying severe protein depletion and hypoalbuminemia may contribute to further maldistribution of fluids and electrolytes, poorly tolerated by the elderly. Intravenous infusion of albumin to normal levels may correct the malabsorptive component owing to hypoalbuminemia (43). Protein malnutrition, if severe, may impair humoral and cellular immunity, leading to increased susceptibility to infections.

Carbohydrate malabsorption may occur as a result of direct ethanol-induced damage to the jejunal mucosa, which was alluded to earlier. It is important to remember that glucose and sodium transport are coupled so that acute and chronic effects on absorption of glucose will impair the efficiency of water and electrolyte movement across the mucosal surface. Such inhibition will aggravate diarrhea and external losses of all nutrients. Lactase-deficiency syndromes can be precipitated in genetically prone alcohol users. Perlow et al. (45) compared jejunal lactase activity (jejunal biopsies) in black and white males with and without a history of recent alcoholism and found markedly reduced lactase activity in the black drinkers, with improvement following 2 weeks of abstinence. Hence, transient lactose intolerance may contribute to the malabsorptive syndromes often observed, especially in the black population, which is genetically prone to lactase deficiency.

Mineral metabolism in elderly alcoholics depends on the adequacy of net body stores and the continuing effect of ethanol on intake, absorption, and excretion. Sodium deficit will be present in states of volume contraction for any of the usual reasons. Hyponatremic states are more common in the elderly, and the aging kidney has a reduced ability to excrete free water. This tendency could theoretically be worsened by the exaggerated ADH release to osmotic stimuli known to occur in the elderly. The resultant volume expansion will promote sodium diuresis even in the presence of hyponatremia (syndrome of inappropriate ADH release). Alcohol suppression of vasopressin release is more transient in the elderly (29). Hepatic cirrhosis, congestive failure, diabetes mellitus, and acute respiratory failure, more common in the aged patient, are associated with abnormal sodium and water balance and frequent hyponatremia.

Elevated plasma ADH levels are common in these settings and are thought to be caused, in part, by nonosmotic stimuli for vasopressin release (10,38,51,58). Thiazide diuretics impair free water clearance and may further aggravate the problem.

Potassium depletion is sometimes seen in the chronic alcoholic. Although urinary potassium increases acutely during ethanol feeding (41), poor intake, body protein catabolism, and malabsorptive syndromes in this setting account largely for the deficit. A direct effect of alcohol on renal potassium handling has not been demonstrated.

Hypomagnesemia and hypocalcemia are sometimes seen in chronic alcohol abusers. Body magnesium is primarily located in bone, with a smaller amount found in muscle and the remainder in extracellular fluid and erythrocytes. Deficits of magnesium under usual conditions are rare. Magnesium is abundant in the diet; renal conservation is efficient; and serum magnesium is partially bound to albumin. It is no surprise, therefore, that hypomagnesemic syndromes are observed most often in chronic alcoholics who have associated dietary deficiency. Malabsorptive states and hypoproteinemia may also contribute. Transient magnesiuria and calciuria have been demonstrated following experimental alcohol ingestion. This was accompanied by no change in glomerular filtration rate or renal blood flow and was independent of water loss (33). Although hypocalcemia would normally stimulate parathormone release and bone calcium mobilization, with resultant correction of the hypocalcemia, the associated hypomagnesia inhibits parathormone release and response. Whether or not increased renal loss of divalent cations is a major factor in the hypomagnesemia and hypocalcemia of chronic alcoholism is not known. Gastrointestinal absorption of calcium may be suboptimal in the elderly owing to impaired renal conversion of 25-hydroxycholecalciferol to $1,25(OH)_2D_3$, as demonstrated by Gray and Gambert in senescent rats (28). Impaired conversion of vitamin D to its 25-hydroxylated form by a liver damaged by alcohol would further impair intestinal Ca^{2+} absorption. Poor calcium intake, impaired absorption, as well as hypercalciuria associated with phosphate depletion, all contribute to the hypocalcemia and osteomalacia seen in heavy alcohol users.

Hypophosphatemic syndromes are another dramatic feature of advanced alcoholic states, of which proximal myopathy and generalized weakness, acute respiratory failure, congestive cardiomyopathy, and rhabdomyolysis may be manifestations. Acute hypophosphatemia may be precipitated by administration of intravenous glucose after hospitalization, because of rapid cellular uptake of PO_4^{3-}. The heavy use of antacids by some alcohol abusers in an attempt to relieve gastric distress serves to bind dietary phosphate and may contribute to the development of hypo-phosphatemic syndromes. Iron deficiency in elderly alcohol abusers may result from gastrointestinal blood loss although in the elderly population, achlorhydria must also be considered as a causative factor. An acid pH is essential to convert the dietary form of iron, ferric, to the form most readily absorbed by the gastrointestinal tract, ferrous.

Manifestations of vitamin deficiencies from reduced intake or altered metabolism may affect every organ system. Examples include Korsakoff-Wernicke psychosis, beriberi heart disease, pellagra, adult scurvy, osteomalacia, and the hematologic disorders noted below.

Hematologic consequences may be extensive. Iron-deficiency anemia may occur secondary to gastrointestinal blood loss, as noted above. Megaloblastic anemias in this setting are usually associated with folate deficiency, commonly occurring in malnourished alcoholics with reduced dietary intake and depleted stores. It is important to remember, however, that alcohol suppresses the hematologic response to folate therapy and prevents a normalization of a megaloblastic marrow despite continued folate intake (57); ethanol infusions cause transient drops in serum folate with no change in urine excretion (19). Serum folate is commonly low in alcoholics without anemia or megaloblastic changes in the erythroid or granulocyte series. Abstinence from alcohol plus a normal diet usually results in a normalization of serum folate and hematologic abnormalities. Malabsorption of both folate and vitamin B_{12} has been described in alcoholics.

Sideroblastic anemia is also common in malnourished alcoholic patients and is usually associated with the megaloblastic changes of folate depletion as well. Serum iron may be elevated. Pyridoxine deficiency appears to be essential in the pathogenesis; ethanol may cause the sideroblastic marrow changes secondary to an acetaldehyde-induced acceleration of the hydrolysis of pyridoxalphosphate (39).

Hemolytic anemias are also more common in chronic alcoholism. Many chronic alcoholics and cirrhotics have somewhat shortened red blood cell life spans even without anemia. Superimposed severe hypophosphatemic states, as noted earlier, may rapidly accelerate the hemolysis, leading to severe anemia. The hemodilution of cirrhosis or other edema-forming states may present as a normochromic normocytic anemia.

Although many types of anemia appear to be associated with alcohol use, anemia is not a normal aging phenomenon, and a thorough workup is always indicated.

Alcoholism has been alleged to be the most common cause of thrombocytopenia (15), with or without associated granulocytopenia. Folate deficiency may also contribute. Failure of these parameters to return to normal after a week of abstinence is usually indicative of another etiology. In fact, transient thrombocytosis often occurs following alcohol withdrawal, even when platelet counts are initially normal.

In summary, nutritional deficiencies have protean manifestations, which overlap with clinical presentations of alcoholism. Clinical manifestations of alcohol abuse may appear even with an adequate nutritional intake, such as in cirrhosis; in contrast, cirrhosis may develop secondary to severe malnutrition alone. Physical changes resulting from alcohol abuse may synergize nutritional deficiency states, as is the case with folate-induced megaloblastic anemia. Although gross damage may be limited to one organ system, alcohol abuse may result in multiple pathologies occurring simultaneously. Associated nutritional inadequacies may often present as impaired cellular or humoral immunity with severe infections. Alcohol abuse must be also considered in any elderly person with insidious weight loss or failure to thrive.

The physician must be aware that it is often difficult to obtain accurate information concerning nutrition or alcohol intake. A knowledge of the extent of alcohol use in the elderly, the wide variety of clinical presentations, and the great potential for reversal by abstinence and proper nutrition should heighten the efforts of health-care providers to identify and treat this serious and disabling problem.

SUMMARY

Alcohol has both acute and chronic effects on a variety of physiological functions. Because of poor detection of this problem in the elderly, many chronic disorders, including those resulting from alcohol abuse, may be falsely blamed on the aging process itself. The clinician must be careful to recognize signs of drinking early. As more and more people are living to their expected life-span, even those elderly who began drinking only late in life may develop problems from long-term alcoholism, previously noted only during middle-age. Normal aging processes may be hastened, making for more chronic disability and illness.

The elderly alcoholic may be mistaken as having dementia or a tumor, rather than a subdural hematoma resulting from a fall during a bout of drinking. The elderly alcoholic is particularly prone to falls, and the clinician must be well aware of the problems that may result.

Alcoholism is no longer a problem of the young. Efforts must be made to detect abuse early to minimize problems further complicating health status and to maintain a better quality of life. Although the elderly presently comprise 11 to 12% of the United States population, they expend almost one-third of the health-care dollar. Prevention is the best treatment for both acute and chronic medical problems resulting from alcohol abuse.

Continued research is necessary to further explore any potential benefit of mild-to-moderate alcohol intake. Whether or not alcohol has a beneficial effect on coronary artery disease remains to be determined. Despite studies suggesting this, numerous factors enter into one's life-style and the choice to imbibe, either in small or large amounts. Perhaps these are the factors that reduce coronary risk and not the alcohol itself. Until a well-designed, prospective study is done to address this problem, no answer exists. Even if alcohol is beneficial in moderate amounts, medically it is clear that alcohol abuse results in bodily harm, regardless of age.

REFERENCES

1. Ahmed, S. S., Levinson, G. E., and Regan, T. J. (1973): Depression of myocardial contractability with low doses of ethanol in normal man. *Circulation*, 43:378–385.
2. Alexander, C. S. (1967): Electron-microscopic observations in alcoholic heart disease. *Br. Heart J.*, 29:200–206.
3. Alexander, C. S. (1972): Cobalt beer cardiomyopathy. *Am. J. Med.*, 53:395–417.
4. Alexander, C. S. (1975): Alcoholic cardiomyopathy. *Postgrad. Med.*, 58:127–131.
5. Anderson, A. J., Barboriak, J. J., and Rimm, A. A. (1978): Risk factors and angiographically determined coronary occlusion. *Am. J. Epidemiol.*, 107:8–14.
6. Barboriak, J. J., and Meade, R. C. (1970): Effect of alcohol in gastric emptying in man. *Am. J. Clin. Nutr.*, 23:1151–1153.
7. Barboriak, J. J., Rooney, C. B., Leitschuh, T. H., and Anderson, A. J. (1978): Alcohol and nutrient intake of elderly men. *J. Am. Diet. Assoc.*, 72(5):493–495.
8. Barboriak, J. J., Anderson, A. J., and Hoffman, R. G. (1979): Interrelationship between coronary artery occlusion, high-density lipoprotein cholesterol, and alcohol intake. *J. Lab. Clin. Med.*, 94:348–353.
9. Barboriak, J. J., Anderson, A. J., Rimm, A. A., and Tristani, F. E. (1979): Alcohol and coronary arteries. *Clin. Exp. Research.*, 3:29–31.
10. Bichet, D., Szatolowicz, V., Chalmovitz, C., and Schrier, R. W. (1982): Role of vasopressin in abnormal water excretion in cirrhotic patients. *Ann. Intern. Med.*, 96:413–417.
11. Bode, J. D. (1980): Alcohol and the gastrointestinal tract. *Ergeb. Inn. Med. Kinderheilkd.*, 45:1–75.
12. Bollinger, O. (1884): Ueber die Häufigkeit und Ursachen der idiopathischen Herzhypertrophie in München. *Dtsch. Med. Wochenschr.*, 10:180–181.
13. Brigden, W. (1972): Alcoholic cardiomyopathy. *Cardiovasc. Clin.*, 4:187–201.
14. Chey, W. Y., Kusakcivglu, O., Dinoso, V., and Lorber, S. H. (1968): Gastric secretions in patients with chronic pancreatitis and in chronic alcoholics. *Arch. Intern. Med.*, 122:399–403.
15. Cowan, D. H., and Hines, J. D. (1973): Alcohol, vitamins and platelets. In: *Drugs and Hematologic Reactions*, edited by N. V. Bimitrov and J. H. Nodine, pp. 282–295. Grune and Stratton, NY.
16. Dürr, H. I., Bode, J. C., Bode, C., Figarella, C., and Sarles, H. (1980): Does chronic intake of alcohol cause changes in the secretory pattern of the parotid gland? In: *Alcohol and the Gastrointestinal Tract*, edited by C. Stock, J. C. Bode, and H. Sarles, pp. 257–262, INSERM, Paris.
17. Eckardt, M. J., Harford, T. C., Koelber, C. T., Parker, E. S., Rosenthal, L. S., Ryback, R. S., Salmoiraghi, G. C., Vanderveen, E., and Warren, K. R. (1981): Health hazards associated with alcohol consumption. *JAMA* , 246:648–666.
18. Edman, C. D., and MacDonald, P. C. (1975): Extraglandular production of estrogen in subjects with liver disease. *Gastroenterology*, 69:A-19, 819.
19. Eichner, E. R., and Hillman, R. S. (1973): Effect of alcohol on serum folate level. *J. Clin. Invest.*, 52:584–591.
20. Factor, S. M. (1976): Intramyocardial small vessel disease in chronic alcoholism. *Am. Heart J.*, 92:561–575.
21. Felig, P., Marliss, E., Owen, O. E., and Cahill, G. F., Jr. (1969): Blood glucose and gluconeogenesis in fasting man. *Arch. Intern. Med.*, 123:293–298.
22. Food and Nutrition Board, National Research Council. (1980): *Recommended Dietary Allowances*, 4th ed., rev. National Academy of Sciences, Washington, DC.
23. Gersovitz, M., Motil, K., Munro, H. N., Schrimshaw, N. S., and Young, V. R. (1982): Human

protein requirements: Assessment of the adequacy of the current recommended dietary allowance for dietary protein in elderly men and women. *Am. J. Clin. Nutr.*, 35:6–14.

24. Giacobini, E., Izekowitz, S., and Wegmann, A. (1960): Urinary norepinephrine and epinephrine excretion in delirium tremens. *Arch. Gen. Psychol.*, 3:289–296.

25. Gordon, G. G., Altman, K., Southren, A. L., Rubin, E., and Lieber, C. S. (1976): Effect of alcohol (ethanol) administration on sex-hormone metabolism in normal men. *N. Engl. J. Med.*, 295:793–797.

26. Gordon, T., Castelli, W. P., Hjortland, M. C., Kannel, W., and Dawber, T. (1977): High density lipoprotein as a protective factor against coronary heart disease. *Am. J. Med.*, 62:707–714.

27. Guozdjak, A., Bada, V., and Kruty, F. (1973): Effects of ethanol on the metabolism of the myocardium and its relationship to development of alcoholic cardiomyopathy. *Cardiology*, 58:290–297.

28. Gray, R. W., and Gambert, S. R. (1982): Effect of age on plasma 1,25-$(OH)_2$D in the rat. *Age*, 5(2):54–56.

29. Helderman, J. H., Vestal, R. E., Rowe, J. W., Tobin, J. D., Andres, R., and Robertson, G. L. (1978): The response of arginine vasopressin to intravenous ethanol and hypersonic saline in man: The impact of aging. *J. Gerontol.*, 33:39–47.

30. Hogan, W. J., Viegas de Androdi, S. R., and Winship, D. H. (1972): Ethanol-induced acute esophageal motor dysfunction. *J. Appl. Physiol.*, 32:755–760.

31. Hurt, R. D., Higgins, J. A., Nelwon, R. A., Morse, R. M., and Dickson, E. R. (1981): Nutritional status of a group of alcoholics before and after admission to an alcoholism treatment unit. *Am. J. Clin. Nutr.*, 34:386–393.

32. Johansson, B. G., and Medhus, A. (1974): Increase in plasma α-lipoproteins in chronic alcoholics after acute abuse. *Acta Med. Scand.*, 195:273–277.

33. Kalbfleisch, J. M., Lindeman, R. D., Ginn, H. E., and Smith, W. L. (1963): Effects of ethanol administration on urinary excretion of magnesium and other electrolytes in alcoholic and normal subjects. *J. Clin. Invest.*, 42:1471–1475.

34. Kaufman, S. E., and Kay, M. D. (1978): Induction of gastroesophageal reflux by alcohol. *Gut.*, 19:336–338.

35. Klatsky, A. L., Friedman, G. D., and Siegelaub, A. B. (1974): Alcohol consumption before myocardial infarction: results from the Kaiser–Permanente epidemiologic study on myocardial infarction. *Ann. Intern. Med.*, 81:294–301.

36. Klein, H., and Harmjanz, D. (1975): The effect of ethanol infusion on the ultrastructure of human myocardium. *Postgrad. Med. J.*, 51:325–329.

37. Levy, L. J., Duga, J., Girgis, M., and Gordon, E. E. (1973): Ketoacidosis associated with alcoholism and nondiabetic subjects. *Ann. Intern. Med.*, 78:213.

38. Linas, S. L., Anderson, R. J., Guggenheim, S. J., Robertson, G. L., and Berl, T. (1981): Role of vasopressin in impaired water excretion in conscious rats with experimental cirrhosis. *Kidney Int.*, 20:173–180.

39. Lumeng, L., and Li, T. (1974): Vitamin B_6 metabolism in chronic alcohol abuse. *J. Clin. Invest.*, 53:963–964.

40. McDonald, J. T., and Margen, S. (1976): Wine versus ethanol in human nutrition. 1. Nitrogen and calorie balance. *Am. J. Clin. Nutr.*, 29:1093–1101.

41. McDonald, J. T., and Margen, S. (1977): Effect of ethanol on human mineral metabolism. In: *Alcohol in nutrition, NIAA Research Monograph* edited by L. Ting-Kai, S. Schenkers, and L. Lumeng. U.S. Department of HEW.

42. Miller, G. J., and Miller, N. E. (1975): Plasma-high-density-lipoprotein concentration and development of ischemic heart disease. *Lancet*, 1:16–19.

43. Moss, G. (1982): Malabsorption associated with extreme malnutrition: Importance of replacing plasma albumin. *J. Am. Coll. Nutr.*, 1:89–92.

44. Olivo, J., Gordon, G. G., Rafii, F., and Southren, A. L. (1975): Estrogen metabolism in hyperthyroidism and in cirrhosis of the liver. *Steroids*, 26:47–56.

45. Perlow, W., Baraona, E., and Lieber, C. S. (1977): Symptomatic intestinal disaccharidase deficiency in alcoholics. *Gastroenterology*, 72:680–684.

46. Pintar, K., Wolanskyj, B. M., and Buggay, E. R. (1965): Alcoholic cardiomyopathy. *Can. Med. Assoc. J.*, 93:103–104.

47. Pirola, R. C., and Lieber, C. S. (1972): The energy cost of the metabolism of drugs, including ethanol. *Pharmacology*, 7:185–196.

48. Pirola, R. C., and Lieber, C. S. (1976): Energy wastage in rats given drugs that induce microsomal enzymes. *J. Nutr.*, 105(2):1544–1548.
49. Pirola, R. C., and Lieber, C. S. (1976): Hypothesis: Energy wastage in alcoholism and drug abuse: Possible role of hepatic microsomal enzymes. *Am. J. Clin. Nutr.*, 29:90–93.
50. Regan, T. J. (1971): Ethyl alcohol and the heart. *Circulation*, 44:957–963.
51. Rieger, G. A. J., Liebau, G. L., and Kochsiek, K. (1982): Antidiuretic hormone in congestive heart failure. *Am. J. Med.*, 72:49–52.
52. Rowe, J. W., and Troen, B. R. (1980): Sympathetic nervous system and aging in man. *Endocr. Rev.*, 1(2):167–179.
53. Sherlock, S. (1981): *Diseases of Liver and Biliary System.* Blackwell Scientific Publications, Oxford, Great Britain.
54. Siiteri, P. K., and MacDonald, P. C. (1973): Role of extraglandular estrogen in human endocrinology. In: *Handbook of Physiology*, Section 7, Volume 2, Part 1, edited by R. O. Greep, pp. 615–629, American Physiological Society, Washington, DC.
55. Southren, A. L., Gordon, G. G., Olivo, J., Rafii, F., and Rosenthal, W. S. (1973): Androgen metabolism in cirrhosis of the liver. *Metabolism.*, 22:695–702.
56. Stock, C., Bode, J. C., and Sarles, H., editors (1980): *Alcohol and the Gastrointestinal Tract.*, pp. 1–540. INSERM, Paris.
57. Sullivan, L. W., and Herbert, V. (1964): Suppression of hematopoiesis by ethanol. *J. Clin. Invest.*, 43:2048–2062.
58. Szatalowicz, V. L., Goldberg, J. P., and Anderson, R. J. (1982): Plasma antidiuretic hormone in acute respiratory failure. *Am. J. Med.*, 72:583–587.
59. Van Thiel, D. H., Lester, R., and Sherins, R. J. (1974): Hypogonadism in alcoholic liver disease: evidence for a double defect. *Gastroenterology.*, 67:1188–1199.
60. Van Thiel, D. H., Gavaler, J., and Lester, R. (1974): Ethanol inhibition of vitamin A metabolism in the testes: possible mechanism for sterility in alcoholics. *Science*, 186:941–942.
61. Van Thiel, D. H., and Lester, R. (1974): Sex and alcohol. *N. Engl. J. Med.*, 291:251–253.
62. Van Thiel, D. H., Gavaler, J. S., Lester, R., Loriaux, D. L., and Braunstein, G. D. (1975): Plasma estrone, prolactin, neurophysin, and sex steroid-binding globulin in chronic alcoholic men. *Metabolism*, 24:1015–1019.
63. Van Thiel, D. H., Lipsitz, H. D., Porter, L. E., Schade, R. R., Gottlieb, G. P., and Graham, T. O. (1981): Gastrointestinal and hepatic manifestations of chronic alcoholism. *Gastroenterology*, 81:594–615.
64. Vestal, R. E., McGuire, E. A., Tobin, J. D., Andres, R., Norris, A. H., and Megey, E. (1977): Aging and ethanol metabolism. *Clin. Pharmacol. Ther.*, 21(3):343–354.
65. Weber, L. D., Nashel, D. J., and Mellow, M. H. (1981): Pharyngeal dysphagia in alcoholic myopathy. *Ann. Intern. Med.*, 95:189–191.
66. Wyngaarden, J. B., and Kelley, W. N. (1972): Gout. In: *The Metabolic Basis of Inherited Disease*, edited by J. B. Stanbury, J. B. Wyngaarden, and D. S. Fredrickson, p. 889. 3rd ed., McGraw-Hill Book Company, New York.
67. Yano, K., Rhoads, G. G., and Kagan, A. (1977): Coffee, alcohol, and risk of coronary heart disease among Japanese men living in Hawaii. *N. Engl. J. Med.*, 297:405–409.

Alcoholism in the Elderly, edited by
J. T. Hartford and T. Samorajski.
Raven Press, New York © 1984.

Neuropsychological Models of Cerebral Dysfunction in Chronic Alcoholics

Gary A. Flinn, Barry Reisberg, and Steven H. Ferris

Geriatric Study and Treatment Program, Millhauser Laboratories, Department of Psychiatry, New York University Medical Center, New York, New York 10016

Evidence of neuropsychological impairment in chronic alcoholics following detoxification has been reported by a number of different investigators using various neuropsychological test procedures. Often there is no difference in overall intelligence between alcoholics and matched controls on testing. There is, however, evidence of more circumscribed impairment in many of these same alcoholics. Often they are mildly to moderately impaired on tasks of short-term memory, nonverbal abstracting, complex memory tasks, and visual-spatial relationships. The ability of the chronic alcoholic to process new information appears to be particularly impaired. However, relative sparing of overrehearsed, overlearned verbal skills and preservation of long-term memory is often reported (1,4,5).

The scientific and pragmatic challenge for the present is to attempt to describe a neuropsychological model that can adequately explain the peculiar set of cognitive deficits observed in chronic alcoholics. In recent years, a number of such neuropsychological models have, in fact, been proposed. Four deserve special attention and will be examined here.

One model contends that excessive, habitual alcohol use causes a premature aging of the brain. Another suggests that the right hemisphere is particularly susceptible to the toxic effects of alcohol. The third argues that prolonged alcohol abuse leads to a diffuse, global state of cerebral dysfunction. The last model to be considered proposes that chronic alcohol abuse selectively disrupts the frontal-limbic-diencephalic system of interconnecting fibers.

PREMATURE AGING MODEL

The premature aging hypothesis is based on the observation that older, nonalcoholic control subjects and detoxified alcoholics 10 to 20 years younger than the controls appear to share a number of specific cognitive deficits. Both groups have difficulty in tasks requiring problem-solving, short-term memory, organization of new information, and visuoperceptual skills (6,15). Thus, Kleinknecht and Goldstein (29) have suggested that habitual abuse of alcohol may result in premature senescence.

Evidence consistent with this model has been provided by Ryan and Butters (39) who demonstrated similar learning and forgetting curves between 34- to 49-year-old alcoholics and 50- to 59-year-old controls. The learning and forgetting curves of the older alcoholics (aged 50–59) and the still older controls (aged 60–65) were likewise similar.

Further evidence of "premature aging" was provided by Blusewicz et al. (4,5). They tested three groups of 20 males each with the Wechsler Adult Intelligence Scale (WAIS) and part of the Halstead-Reitan Neuropsychological Battery. The first group was comprised of young nonalcoholic controls with a mean age of 31. The second group were young alcoholics with a mean age of 33. The third group was comprised of elderly nonalcoholics with a mean age of 71 years. They found that the young alcoholics performed significantly worse than the young controls on most of the tests, but significantly better than the elderly controls.

Jones and Parsons (27) used the Halstead-Category Test to rate the abstraction ability of detoxified, long-term alcoholics. Three groups of 40 each were tested. The first group were detoxified alcoholics, the second group were nonalcoholic brain-damaged patients, and the third group were nonalcoholic, neurologically intact, medical patients who served as controls. These groups were further subdivided according to age: a younger group (25–42 years of age, with a mean age of 36.2) and an older group (43–60 years of age, with a mean age of 50.6).

The older alcoholic and brain-damaged patients performed at a significantly lower level than their younger counterparts. There was, however, no significant difference between the younger and the older nonalcoholic control groups. The younger alcoholic group performed at the level of the younger control group, while the older alcoholics performed significantly worse than the older controls. The authors suggested that an interaction between age and drinking history could help explain the unimpaired performance of the younger alcoholics and the impaired performance of the older alcoholics. Thus, the older alcoholics with the longest history of drinking were rated as the most impaired on the tests, while the younger alcoholics, with a briefer history of drinking scored among the most proficient on the tests.

The authors further speculated that the brain becomes increasingly susceptible to the toxic effects of alcohol as it ages and that the age of the patient, more than the duration of alcohol abuse, will dictate the severity of the neuropsychological impairment. Other studies have supported this hypothesis of age rather than drinking history being of primary importance in the development of cognitive deficits in alcoholics (3,30).

As with the other hypotheses to be presented, there appears to be some evidence that does not entirely support the premature aging hypothesis. For example, Blusewicz and Dustman et al. (4) found elderly and alcoholic groups to perform similarly on only two tests of the Halstead-Reitan Battery. In another survey, even the most severe alcoholics performed at a higher level on the WAIS performance subtests than the aged control subjects (5).

RIGHT-HEMISPHERE DYSFUNCTION MODEL

The right-hemisphere hypothesis contends that the cognitive dysfunction found in alcoholics is lateralized primarily to the right hemisphere (28). Numerous investigators (1,4,5,45) have observed that for chronic alcoholics, the WAIS verbal subtests tend to remain more intact whereas the performance subtests tend to show greater impairment. Vega and Parsons (44) have demonstrated an association between impaired performance-scale scores and right-hemisphere dysfunction. These findings suggest to some that the toxic effects of alcohol disrupt right-hemisphere functions more severely than left-hemisphere functions. Based on this model, it may be predicted that the well-rehearsed, practiced, and repetitive verbal skills for which the left hemisphere is responsible would be less affected than the nonverbal, visual-spatial, visual-motor functions of the right hemisphere.

A number of studies provide data consistent with this prediction. In 18 of 26 patients, Cala et al. (10) found evidence for visual-spatial and visual-motor function impairment, but a preservation of verbal skills. Miglioli et al. (36) retested 30 alcoholics several months after they had originally given evidence of diffuse cerebral dysfunction upon testing during their second week of abstinence. They reported that significant improvement had occurred in verbal memory functions, but none in either short- or long-term visual-spatial memory. Spatial deficits are associated with patients who have right hemisphere lesions.

Poorer performance in the contralaterally controlled left hand has also been advanced as evidence of right-hemisphere dysfunction. It has been noted that on manual tasks, there tends to be a differentially greater degree of impairment in the left hand of alcoholics as compared with the right hand. Jenkins and Parsons (25) described poorer performance in alcoholics with their left hand than in controls using the Tactual Performance Test of the Halstead-Reitan Neuropsychological Battery. Though still exhibiting poorer performance, the difference was not as great between alcoholics and controls on right-hand performance.

There is other evidence, however, that does not support the concept of selective right-hemisphere dysfunction. Løberg (34) found no evidence of a greater deficit in the left-hand, as compared with right-hand performance in alcoholics compared with controls when he analyzed bilateral measures of grip strength, maze coordination, finger dexterity, and tactual-spatial performance. Studies using tachiscopic presentation have likewise failed to support the notion of greater right-hemisphere versus left-hemisphere impairment in chronic alcoholics.

GENERALIZED DYSFUNCTION MODEL

The generalized dysfunction model holds that the toxic effects of alcohol lead to a generalized, diffuse state of cerebral dysfunction. In the past, the relatively intact verbal performance of alcoholics on the WAIS and other tests had cast doubt on this hypothesis. More recently, however, as tests of verbal abilities have become more sophisticated and specific, the verbal performance of alcoholics has been shown to be less intact than previously thought.

Ryan and Butters (40,41) found significant impairment in alcoholics by making the list of paired-associates more difficult. In another study, these same investigators used a four-word delayed recall test and a paired-associate verbal learning task to compare both young and old alcoholics with controls (39). The scores for both young and old alcoholics were significantly lower than those of the controls. Guthrie and Elliot (21) also found alcoholics to be impaired on paired-associate verbal learning tasks. Gudeman et al. (20) demonstrated impaired verbal problem-solving abilities in the alcoholics they studied.

Thus, an examination of the available clinical evidence leads to the conclusion that alcoholics do, in fact, demonstrate deficits in verbal learning, verbal problem-solving, and verbal memory. These deficits, when added to the deficits already described in nonverbal abstracting, problem-solving, perceptual-spatial, and motor tasks appear to support the concept of a generalized, diffuse dysfunction in the brains of detoxified chronic alcoholics.

Evidence from biological studies also appears to support the generalized dysfunction model. Studies using computerized tomography (CT) scans have consistently demonstrated sulcal and ventricular enlargement in the brains of chronic alcoholics. This sulcal and ventricular enlargement is commonly interpreted as atrophy. Figures vary from study to study, but most have reported CT scan findings of cerebral atrophy in at least half the alcoholics studied. Gall et al. (19) reported an incidence of atrophy in 75% of their subjects. In a survey of 240 alcoholics, Cala and Martaglia (9) found 95% to demonstrate CT scan findings consistent with cerebral atrophy. Because brain atrophy is a normal manifestation of aging (11,35), attempts to separate any age changes also present in an age-matched, nonalcoholic control group would be of obvious interest.

FRONTAL-LIMBIC-DIENCEPHALIC DISRUPTION MODEL

The frontal-limbic-diencephalic disruption model also has been proposed to explain the cognitive deficits found in chronic alcoholics. The structural and functional integration of these structures has been well demonstrated (8,12,13). This model emphasizes the similarities between chronic alcoholics and patients with frontal-lobe damage or limbic disorders as revealed by neuropsychological testing. Tarter (43) contends that alcohol selectively disrupts frontal-lobe and limbic functioning. He points to behavioral studies that show that chronic alcohol abusers have deficits in the ability to organize behavior, in the maintenance of a cognitive set, in their ability to incorporate new information to improve performance, and in motor regulation. These deficits have been previously demonstrated in frontal-lobe-damaged patients.

Jenkins and Parsons (26) found that alcoholics continued to exhibit perseveration errors on the Wisconsin Card Sorting Test (WCST) up to after 3 months of abstinence. Perseveration on this particular test has also been demonstrated in nonalcoholic frontal-lobe-damaged patients (37). Tarter (42) found that the degree of impaired performance by alcoholics on the WCST was related to the number of years they had abused alcohol. Alcoholics also manifest deficits in spatial scanning in maze tests (17,18). Such deficits have likewise been demonstrated in patients with well-documented frontal-lobe lesions (37,38).

Brewer and Perrett (7) examined 33 patients whose drinking histories classified them as either heavy social drinkers or alcoholics. Pneumoencephalograms were done to assess the degree of cerebral atrophy. Of the 33 patients, 30 showed evidence of cerebral atrophy and 24 had enlarged ventricles. The cerebral atrophy was rated as severe in more than half of the cases. Frontal lobe atrophy was present in 28 of the 30 patients with cerebral atrophy.

Haug (22) compared the pneumoencephalograms of a group of schizophrenics to a group of alcoholics. Cerebral atrophy was present in 8% of the schizophrenics, but in 74% of the alcoholics. The severity of the cerebral atrophy and the duration of alcohol abuse were positively correlated. The cerebral atrophy was more severe in those patients who had suffered delirium tremens. Cerebral atrophy was present in 20 of 21 patients who demonstrated personality deterioration as evidenced by moral and social inappropriateness, but with relative sparing of intellectual functioning. Haug speculates that as the cerebral pathology in alcoholics increases, they suffer a corresponding decrease in their ability to control their consumption of alcohol. Lemere (32) suggests that some of the features associated with chronic alcoholism, such as the inability to exercise control over consumption, may be partly explained by frontal-lobe damage.

A number of studies using CT scans have likewise demonstrated atrophic changes in the frontal lobes. Cala and Mastaglia (9) noted marked frontal-lobe and interhemispheric fissure atrophy in the alcoholics they studied. Lee et al. (31) also described frontal lobe atrophy, particularly at the interhemispheric fissure. Courville (14) studied the brains of chronic alcoholics at autopsy. He found the anterior frontal lobes to be the most atrophic.

Cerebral blood flow studies of alcoholics have demonstrated decreased blood flow to the frontal regions. Heiss et al. (23,24) studied 35 alcoholics from 20 to 59 years old. They found decreased blood flow in 19 of the 35 patients, mainly in the frontal and parietal regions. Berglund and Ingvar (2), in their study of 54 alcoholics, reported a relative reduction of the blood flow in the inferior frontal and anterior temporal regions in the brains of the older alcoholics, as compared with the younger alcoholics. Though decreased blood flow has been demonstrated in the frontal lobes of alcoholics, they have also been found in the parietal and anterior temporal regions. This weakens the argument for the frontal lobes being selectively affected.

DeObaldia et al. (16) tested 30 alcoholics and 15 controls with the Luria Nebraska Neuropsychological Battery. They compared the pattern of scores for alcoholics with the pattern for frontal-lobe-damaged patients tested by Lewis et al. (33) using the same battery. The frontal-limbic-diencephalic disruption model would be strengthened if similarities could be drawn between the pattern of scores of the alcoholics and the frontal-lobe-damaged patients. However, no such analogous patterns of deficit were noted between either the alcoholics and frontal lobe patients, or between the alcoholics and a group of control subjects.

CONCLUSION

This review suggests that some experimental evidence exists for each of the neuropsychological models presented. The contrary is also true, however; evidence that appears to contradict each of these models also exists. Although the generalized dysfunction and premature aging hypotheses have generated the most interest recently, it is difficult to conclude which of the four models presented best explains the biological, neuropsychological, and behavioral data with any great degree of certainty.

Of particular interest to clinicians involved with the elderly, however, is the suggestion by some that the brain becomes increasingly susceptible to the toxic effects of alcohol as it ages. This would suggest a more serious prognosis in elderly alcoholics than in their younger counterparts and that the curtailment of further alcohol abuse in this age group be of primary importance.

REFERENCES

1. Albert, M. S., Butters, N., and Brandt, J. (1980): Memory for remote events in alcoholics. *J. Stud. Alcohol*, 41:1071–1081.
2. Berglund, M., and Ingvar, D. H. (1976): Cerebral blood flow and its regional distribution in alcoholism and Korsakoffs patients. *J. Stud. Alcohol*, 37:586–597.
3. Bertera, J. H., and Parsons, O. A. (1978): Impaired visual search in alcoholics. *Alcoholism*, 2:9–14.
4. Blusewicz, M. J., Dustman, R. E., Schenkenberg, T., and Beck, E. C. (1977): Neuropsychological correlates of chronic alcoholism and aging. *J. Nerv. Ment. Dis.*, 165:348–355.
5. Blusewicz, M. J., Schenkenberg, T., Dustman, R. E., and Beck, E. C. (1977): Alcoholic and elderly normal groups: An evaluation of organicity and mental aging indices. *J. Clin. Psychol.*, 33:1149–1153.
6. Botwinick, J. (1977): Intellectual abilities. In: *Handbook of the Psychology of Aging*, edited by J. E. Birren and K. W. Shaie, p. 580. Van Nostrand Reinhold, NY.
7. Brewer, C., and Perrett, L. (1971): Brain damage due to alcohol consumption: An air-encephalographic, psychometric and electroencephalographic study. *Br. J. Addict.*, 66:170–182.
8. Brutkowski, S. (1965): Functions of prefrontal cortex in animals. *Physiol. Rev.*, 45:721–746.
9. Cala, L. A., and Mastaglia, F. L. (1980): Computerized axial tomography in the detection of brain damage. *Med. J. Aust.*, 2:193–198.
10. Cala, L. A., Jones, B., Mastaglia, F. L., and Wiley, B. (1978): Brain atrophy and intellectual impairment in heavy drinkers—a clinical, psychometric and computerized tomography study. *Aust. NZ J. Med.*, 8(2):147–153.
11. Cala, L. A., Thickbroom, G. W., Black, J. L., Collins, D. W., and Mastaglia, F. L. (1981): Brain density and cerebrospinal fluid spaces on the cranial CT scan in normal volunteers. *Am. J. Neuroradiol.*, 2:41–47.
12. Clark, W. L. G. (1948): The connections of the frontal lobes of the brain. *Lancet*, 254:353–356.
13. Clark, W. L. G., and Meyer, M. (1950): Anatomical relationships between the cerebral cortex and the hypothalamus. *Br. Med. Bull.*, 6:341–345.
14. Courville, C. (1955): *Effects of Alcohol on the Central Nervous System*. San Lucas Press, Los Angeles.
15. Craik, F. I. M. (1977): Age differences in human memory. In: *Handbook of the Psychology of Aging*, edited by J. E. Birren and K. W. Shaie, p. 384. Van Nostrand Reinhold, NY.
16. DeObaldia, R., Parsons, O. A., and Leber, W. R. (1981): Assessment of neuropsychological

functions in chronic alcoholics using a standardized version of Luria's Neuropsychological Technique. *Int. J. Neurosci.*, 14(1–2):85–93.

17. Fitzhugh, L., Fitzhugh, K., and Reitan, E. (1960): Adaptive abilities and intellectual functioning in hospitalized alcoholics. *Q. J. Stud. Alcohol*, 21:414–423.

18. Fitzhugh, L., Fitzhugh, K., and Reitan, E. (1965): Adaptive abilities and intellectual functioning in hospitalized alcoholics: Further considerations. *Q. J. Stud. Alcohol*, 26:402–411.

19. Gall, von M., Becker, H., Artmann, H., Lerch, G., and Nemeth, N. (1978): Results of computer tomography on chronic alcoholics. *Neuroradiology*, 16:329–331.

20. Gudeman, H. E., Craine, J. F., Golden, C. J., and McLaughlin, D. (1977): Higher cortical dysfunction associated with long term alcoholism. *Int. J. Neurosci.*, 8(1):33–40.

21. Guthrie, A., and Elliott, W. A. (1980): The nature and reversibility of cerebral impairment in alcoholism: Treatment implications. *J. Stud. Alcohol*, 41:147–155.

22. Haug, J. O. (1968): Pneumoencephalographic evidence of brain damage in chronic alcoholics. *Acta Psychiatr. Scand.*, 203:135–143.

23. Heiss, W. D., Kuffer, B., and Demel, I. (1974): Störungen der Hirndurchblutung bei chronischen Alkoholikern in Abhangigkeit vom Klinischen Bild. *Psychiatr. Clin. (Basel)*, 7:181–191.

24. Heiss, W. D., Kufferle, B., Demel, I., Reisner, T., and Roszverky, A. (1976): Cerebral blood flow and severity of mental dysfunction in chronic alcoholism. In: *Cerebral Vascular Disease, 7th International Conference, Salzburg, 1974*, edited by J. S. Meyer, H. Lechner, and M. Reivich, pp. 89–93. Georg Thieme, Stuttgart.

25. Jenkins, R. L., and Parsons, O. A. (1979): Lateralized patterns of tactual performance in alcoholics. In: *Currents in Alcoholism*, Vol. 5, edited by M. Galanter, pp. 285–296. Grune and Stratton, NY.

26. Jenkins, R. L., and Parsons, O. A. (1980): Recovery of cognitive abilities in male alcoholics. In: *Currents in Alcoholism*, Vol. 7, edited by M. Galanter, pp. 229–237. Grune and Stratton, NY.

27. Jones, B., and Parsons, O. A. (1971): Impaired abstracting ability in chronic alcoholics. *Arch. Gen. Psychiatry*, 24:71–75.

28. Jones, B., and Parsons, O. A. (1972): Specific vs. generalized deficits of abstracting ability in chronic alcoholics. *Arch. Gen. Psychiatry*, 26:380–384.

29. Kleinknecht, R. A., and Goldstein, S. C. (1972): Neuropsychological deficits associated with alcoholism: A review and discussion. *Q. J. Stud. Alcohol*, 33:999–1019.

30. Klisz, D., and Parsons, O. A. (1977): Hypothesis testing in younger and older alcoholics. *J. Stud. Alcohol*, 38:1718–1729.

31. Lee, K., Moller, L., Hardt, F., Haubek, A., and Jansen, E. (1979): Alcohol-induced brain damage and liver damage in young males. *Lancet*, 2:759–761.

32. Lemere, F. (1956): The nature and significance of brain damage from alcoholism. *Am. J. Psychiatry*, 113:361–362.

33. Lewis, G. P., Golden, C. J., Moses, J. A., Osmon, D. C., Purisch, A. D., and Hammeke, T. A. (1979): Localization of cerebral dysfunction with a standard version of Luria's neuropsychological battery. *J. Consult. Clin. Psychol.*, 47:1003–1019.

34. Løberg, T. (1980): Dimensions of alcohol abuse in relation to neurophysiological deficits. *J. Stud. Alcohol*, 41:119–128.

35. Meese, W., Kluge, W., Grumme, T., and Hopfenmuller, W. (1980): CT evaluation of the CSF spaces of healthy persons. *Neuroradiology*, 19(3):131–136.

36. Migliolo, M., Buchtel, H. A., Campanini, T., and De Risio, C. (1979): Cerebral hemispheric lateralization of cognitive deficits due to alcoholism. *J. Nerv. Ment. Dis.*, 167(4):212–217.

37. Milner, B. (1963): Effects of different brain lesions on card sorting. *Arch. Neurol.*, 9:90–100.

38. Porteus, S. (1959): *The Maze Test and Clinical Psychology*. Pacific Books, Palo Alto, CA.

39. Ryan, C., and Butters, N. (1980): Learning and memory impairment in young and old alcoholics: Evidence for the premature aging hypothesis. *Alcoholics*, 4:288–293.

40. Ryan, C., and Butters, N. (1980): Further evidence of a continuum-of-impairment encompassing alcoholic Korsakoff patients and chronic alcoholics. *Alcoholism*, 4:190–198.

41. Ryan, C., Butters, N., Montgomery, K., Adinolfi, A., and Didario, B. (1980): Memory deficits in chronic alcoholics: continuities between the "intact" alcoholic and the alcoholic Korsakoff patient. In: *Alcohol Intoxification and Withdrawal*, edited by H. Begleiter and B. Kissin. Plenum Press, NY.

42. Tarter, R. (1971): A Neuropsychological Examination of Cognition and Perceptual Capacities in Chronic Alcoholics. (Unpublished Doctoral Dissertation) University of Oklahoma.

43. Tarter, R. E. (1976): Empirical investigations of psychological deficits. In: *Alcoholism: Interdisciplinary Approaches to an Enduring Problem*, edited by R. S. Tarter and A. A. Sugerman, pp. 359–394. Addison-Wesley, Reading, MA.
44. Vega, A., and Parsons, O. (1969): Relationships between sensory–motor deficits and WAIS verbal and performance scores in unilateral brain damage. *Cortex*, 5:220–241.
45. Wechsler, D. (1941): The effect of alcohol on mental activity. *Q. J. Stud. Alcohol*, 2:479–485.

Alcoholism in the Elderly, edited by
J. T. Hartford and T. Samorajski.
Raven Press, New York © 1984.

Alcoholism and Aging: Electrophysiological Parallels

Robert E. Dustman

*Neuropsychology Laboratory, Veterans Administration Medical Center,
Salt Lake City, Utah 84148*

There are many parallels between data gathered from individuals who have been alcoholic for a substantial portion of their lives and from individuals who are undergoing normal processes of aging. For example, similarities between the two groups have been reported for behavior, test performance, brain pathology, sleep, electroencephalographic tracings, and evoked brain potentials. The parallels have been so striking, in some instances, that it has been hypothesized that alcoholic behavior contributes to a hastening of the aging process (25,26,45,60,67,139). Others (96,126) question a cause-and-effect relationship between alcoholism and aging. Likely, the truth lies somewhere between.

This chapter will examine electrophysiological measures obtained from alcoholics while in an abstinent period and from normally aging humans. Material covered includes EEG, sleep, and evoked potentials (EPs). The reader will note that there have been few studies in which an experimental design included both alcoholics and aging individuals. Most studies focus on alcoholism or aging, but not on both. Conclusions have been drawn regarding similarities or differences between the two populations by comparing recently acquired results from one group with published data for the other. Thus, inferences regarding parallels between aging and alcoholism have not been as clean and clear as they might have been because of differences in experimental procedures. The necessity for including alcoholics and oldsters within a single experimental design, maintaining identical parameters and test procedures for both, will become apparent. One should also keep in mind that it is difficult to study aging independent of the health problems that often accompany approaching senescence. Since poor health may amplify abnormalities associated with normal aging, rigorous health-screening procedures should be employed. This is often not done. When studying alcoholics, one must realize that recovery of cortical function may occur following abstention from drinking (69,88,95, 114,125,126). The rate, duration, and extent of recovery are not yet well defined, further clouding meaningful comparisons between oldsters and alcoholics.

It is not surprising that investigators have studied aging and alcoholism using electrophysiological techniques. The EEG and EP provide a reasonably quick means of measuring the functioning brain. The techniques are noninvasive, are not particularly disquieting, and can yield information that is indicative of "cortical health."

ELECTROENCEPHALOGRAM

The electroencephalogram (EEG) reflects the spontaneous electrical activity of the brain, most likely from dendritic processes in upper cortical layers (66). The EEG was first recorded from humans by Hans Berger (21) in the late 1920s. He observed that the EEG was often characterized by a dominant, relatively slow, high amplitude 8- to 13-Hz frequency, which he termed alpha. Since alpha waves are more easily studied than other brain patterns and since they reflect, to an extent, the conscious state of the organism, they have been responsible for the generation of considerable research. Other EEG rhythms that have been studied frequently are beta (13–40 Hz), delta (0.5–3.5 Hz), and theta (4–7 Hz).

Aging

Many individuals younger than 70 years have no EEG abnormalities; their EEGs are not different from those of normal young adults (134). However, approximately 50% of average adults aged 60 to 70 years do show EEG abnormalities (134). These are often minimal for oldsters who enjoy relatively good health.

Four types of abnormalities have been observed in the EEGs of healthy oldsters (104,110): (a) alpha slowing, (b) changes in beta activity, (c) focal slow waves, and (d) diffuse slow activity. The most common of these is a slowing of alpha, which occurs as a function of both age and health status. Alpha slowing may begin in the mid 40s (101), with an acceleration of slowing after the seventh decade of life (63). For healthy oldsters, decline of alpha frequency may be no more than 1.0 to 1.5 Hz (110,112), and alpha frequency may not be *abnormally* slow even by the age of 100 years (79).

Beta waves, found predominantly over anterior brain regions, occupy a frequency range between 13 and 40 Hz (104,110) and are generally much smaller than alpha waves (110). Increased amounts of low-voltage fast beta activity occur in EEGs of elderly subjects and may comprise 25% of a total record (104). The percentage of beta decreases during extreme old age, after about age 80.

Focal slow-wave activity (1–7 Hz), sometimes accompanied by sharp waves and amplitude asymmetries, is seen in the EEGs of 30% to 40% of the normal elderly (34,104,110). Slow-wave foci usually appear on the left side of the brain and tend to be localized to the anterior temporal area (34). These temporal lobe abnormalities rarely occur before the age of 40 but become more frequent in the fifth and sixth decades when the incidence levels off (110). They likely derive from localized degenerative changes and from cerebral ischemia (110).

Diffuse slow-wave activity is uncommon in the EEGs of normal adults during early senescence. Obrist and Busse (111) reported an incidence of 7% for healthy oldsters younger than 75 years, an incidence not unlike that of healthy young adults. However, the rate increased to 20% for healthy oldsters over 75 years of age, possibly because of reduced cerebral blood flow and metabolic changes due to arteriosclerosis and/or other cardiovascular disease (104,110).

Alcoholism

EEG tracings from abstinent alcoholics have not been particularly useful in delineating brain dysfunction that is assumed to occur as a consequence of heavy drinking (15). For simple or uncomplicated alcoholism, the incidence of EEG abnormalities is not different from the incidence for normal controls (55,65,71,98,107) even in the presence of cortical atrophy documented by brain scan (108). EEG abnormalities that may occur during acute alcoholic states tend to revert to normal with abstention (15,161,168).

There is evidence, however, that alpha production in abstinent alcoholics is reduced below that of normal controls (15,98,107), and, as with normal aging, there is an accentuation of fast EEG activity (19,43,161,168). The importance of these findings is not clear. However, there is a marked improvement in alpha production and a reduction of beta activity after a 4 to 6 week period of abstinence (168), suggesting that these EEG abnormalities may relate to an extended toxic state rather than to chronic cerebral dysfunction.

Summary

There appear to be few parallels between the EEGs of healthy oldsters and the EEGs of abstinent alcoholics. Normal aging is often, but not always, accompanied by alpha slowing, slow-wave foci, and changes in low-voltage fast activity. The incidence of these EEG characteristics correlates with age, disease state, and decreased cognitive function, suggesting a deteriorating CNS. The EEGs of alcoholics without complications are generally not different from those of age-matched normals, particularly if the alcoholics have been abstinent for a period of a few weeks.

Routine recordings of waking EEG may be insensitive to subtle changes in brain function. It may be fruitful to analyze EEG activity of elderly normals and alcoholics using computerized techniques such as "power spectral analysis" (49), which measures amplitude and abundance of brain waves of different frequencies, and "cortical coupling assessment" (36,167). The latter provides simultaneous measures of phase relationships among EEG tracings from several areas of the brain. Both techniques can be used to evaluate the brain while at rest and while working, i.e., reading, solving problems, etc. Procedures such as these may provide new information regarding changes in electrophysiological function resulting from advanced age and excessive drinking.

SLEEP

We spend about one-third of our lives in sleep. Rather than being a passive state, sleep is a complex succession of psychophysiological events that are qualitatively different from those that occur during an awake state (166). Like other complex behavioral phenomena, optimum sleep is dependent upon relatively intact CNS functioning (56,130,131). Thus, factors such as aging and alcoholism, which are believed to degrade cortical function, might be expected to interfere with sleep.

Precise measures of sleep patterns are determined from EEG tracings obtained from subjects during nocturnal recordings. A typical night of sleep includes about five 90-min sleep cycles, each cycle being composed of four levels, or stages, of sleep plus rapid eye movement (REM) sleep. Sleep progresses from light sleep, stages 1 and 2, through deep or slow-wave sleep, stages 3 and 4, which are characterized by high amplitude 1- to 4-Hz delta waves (166). It has been hypothesized that slow-wave sleep, which occupies about 20% of normal sleep recordings, is related to restoring or renewing brain tissue (72). A final level of sleep, REM, also occupies about 20% of normal sleep time. REM is often referred to as being paradoxical sleep since the EEG is characterized by fast, low-voltage brain activity similar to that seen in an awake state.

Aging

Of major concern to normally aging individuals is the decreasing quality of sleep which they experience (106). Although total sleep time of oldsters is not reduced significantly (56), sleep is not as restful because of increased number of awakenings, which increases with age in an almost linear fashion (56,106,164). Deep sleep, associated with EEG slow-wave activity, is particularly disrupted (56,57,106,130).

Oldsters experience less REM sleep than young adults (56,86); this deficit is substantially greater for extremely old subjects (85,106). Reduction of REM sleep is indicative of brain dysfunction and parallels reductions in two other physiological variables that typically decrease with age: alpha frequency and cerebral blood flow (131,133).

What kinds of CNS changes might be implicated in diminished sleep efficiency? Since sleep is a complex behavior dependent on the interplay of cortical and subcortical systems and their chemical substrates, deterioration of some or all of these might interfere with normal sleep. Prinz (130) emphasized that sleep variables follow trends that are similar to life-span curves for brain weight, neuronal population density, brain metabolic rate, and cerebral blood flow. It is known that aging is associated with substantial cell loss in brainstem structures known to be implicated in the neurochemical regulation of sleep; levels of associated neurotransmitters, e.g., serotonin and norepinephrine and the enzyme monoamine oxidase, may be abnormal as well (106,132). Significant cell loss also occurs with advanced age in frontal and other cortical association areas (28,31), which are thought to provide inhibitory control over the alerting effects of the ascending reticular formation (32,37,44), and in horizontal dendritic processes, which have been suggested to provide subtle, modulating influences for complex cortical activities (106,142).

Alcoholism

Parallels between sleep characteristics of normal oldsters and of abstinent alcoholics are fairly striking. Johnson et al. (83) observed that the sleep of 40-year-old alcoholics more closely approximated the sleep of elderly normal individuals than the sleep of age-matched controls. Similar to the sleep of oldsters, the sleep of recently abstinent alcoholics is characterized by reduced amounts of slow-wave sleep, sleep interruptions, and reduced amounts of REM or interrupted REM periods (1,3,4,83,138,166).

Severity of sleep disorder is apparently a function of both age and number of years of excessive drinking; the latter is thought to be more closely related to impaired sleep than the former (138). Quality of sleep does improve with abstinence, however (3,4,83,138), although slow-wave sleep may not reach normal values even after 4 years of abstinence (162). Normal amounts of REM can occur after a few days or weeks of sobriety, but they tend to be fragmented by awakenings or by light sleep (1,3,83). Similar to reports for normal oldsters (58), decreased amounts of REM sleep by abstinent alcoholics are related to impaired cognitive function (20).

Summary

The sleep of alcoholics and of oldsters is similar in several respects: reduced time in deep sleep, excessive sleep interruptions, and impaired REM sleep. Although sleep disorders become more severe with increased age, they apparently become less severe with prolonged abstinence from alcohol abuse. It seems likely that the similarities in sleep dysfunction stem from a commonality of CNS abnormalities: cell loss in brainstem and cortical areas and reduced function of neurotransmitter systems believed to be essential for normal sleep.

CORTICAL EVOKED POTENTIALS

Cortical EPs comprise a family of electrical potentials elicited from the brain by short-duration repetitive stimuli. Because of the versatility inherent in EP techniques, EPs have proved to be a powerful tool for investigating the nervous system. For example, the different sensory systems can be independently probed with a variety of stimuli, brainstem as well as cortical function can be assessed, and the effects of cognition on the brain's electrical activity can be measured.

The present discussion covers those types of EPs for which studies have been done employing abstinent alcoholic and/or normally aging subjects and includes sensory cortical EPs elicited by brief auditory (AEP), somatosensory (SEP), and visual (VEP) stimuli; brainstem auditory EPs (BAEPs); pattern reversal EPs (PREPs); and the long latency EPs that are referred to as P300s or P3s. In addition, studies of changes in EP amplitude as a function of stimulus intensity will be described.

Sensory Cortical Evoked Potentials: AEPs, SEPs, and VEPs

The study of averaged EPs was dependent on technological advances that enabled investigators to extract EPs from the larger background EEG activity. Dawson (46), using a photographic superimposition technique, was one of the first to report a method for obtaining a composite EP waveform. His findings generated interest that resulted in the design and manufacture of specialized computers for EP averaging and in the development of EP software for general-purpose computer systems so that EPs are now studied in laboratories and clinics around the world.

Sensory cortical EPs, which span a time frame of about 250 msec, are thought to encompass two basic brain functions: "sensory receiving," reflected in early components occurring within the first 50 to 60 msec following stimulation, and "information processing," associated with EP components occurring after 60 msec (10,104).

Aging

While no amplitude or latency changes have been reported to occur for AEP waves as a function of adult aging (104,143,144), age effects have been found for SEPs and VEPs. Interestingly, the amplitude of SEP and VEP early waves tends to increase in size with increasing age (50,51,99,144,146,158), perhaps because of decreased central inhibitory function (145). Figure 1, a portrayal of VEPs from 425 normal subjects aged 4 to 86 years, illustrates the enhanced early waves, which are first clearly visible in the evoked potentials of subjects in their forties.

In general, studies of SEPs and VEPs of oldsters have revealed signs of slowing since component latencies of elderly subjects, in comparison with latencies of younger subjects, were delayed [(51,99,144,146,158); see also (89,104,150)]. However, a substantial portion of the delays in VEP waves may have resulted from age-related changes in the visual system that reduce the amount of illumination reaching the retina (23,163). In a recent study of 220 healthy males aged 4 to 90 years, we measured the visual threshold of each subject and adjusted light intensities accordingly before recording VEPs. With adjustment for visual threshold, component latency differences among adult groups were minimal (52,53).

Evaluations were also made of age-related changes in late VEP wave amplitudes elicited by three intensities of flash adjusted for visual threshold. Results for 120 males aged 21 to 90 years highlight the complexity of age-amplitude interactions (24). There were no age-related changes in amplitude for occipital VEPs regardless of intensity (Fig. 2). For frontal and central areas, however, amplitude did change reliably as a function of age, but the presence and magnitude of the age effect was dependent upon stimulus intensity (Fig. 3). For the lowest intensity, VEP amplitude did not differ across age. For the middle intensity, a significant age effect was observed ($p<0.05$); mean amplitudes of the 55- and 66-year-old subjects were significantly larger than the mean for the youngest adult group. Age effects on amplitude were most pronounced for the brightest flash condition ($p<0.001$). Amplitudes for the three oldest groups of subjects were reliably larger than those for the three younger groups.

Alcoholism

Concern must be given to the length of time alcoholics have been abstinent when EPs are recorded, since immediately after cessation of drinking the cortex is hy-

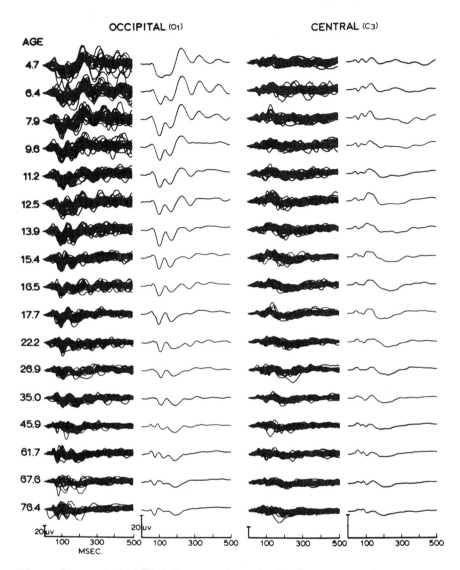

OCCIPITAL (O₁)   **CENTRAL** (C₃)

FIG. 1. Changes in the VEP during maturation and aging. Portrayed are VEPs of 425 individuals aged 4 to 86 years. Each of the 17 age groups, designated by mean age at the left of the figure, is composed of 25 subjects (rather equally divided, male and female). Note the early waves, which are first clearly seen in occipital VEPs of the group aged 45.9 years and are observable thereafter. A downward deflection is positive. (Reproduced from Beck, E. C., and Dustman, R. E., ref. 10a, with permission.)

perexcitable, as evidenced by increased EP voltages (22,125). At least 3 weeks of sobriety are required before the hyperexcitability has dissipated (125). In addition, investigators must be aware that disulfiram (Antabuse®), commonly administered to alcoholics, is associated with enhanced EP amplitudes (117,125).

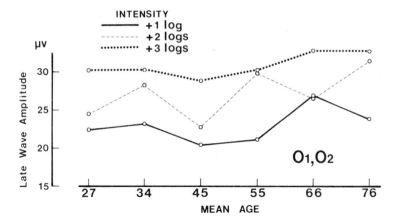

FIG. 2. VEP amplitudes to three intensities of flash. The amplitude measure represents the sum of the amplitudes of three late waves. VEPs were recorded from occipital scalp of 120 males; 20 in each group. (Reproduced from Blusewicz, M. J., et al., ref. 24, with permission. ©The Chemical Rubber Co., CRC Press, Inc.)

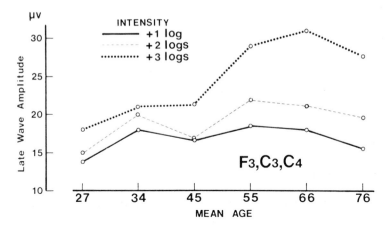

FIG. 3. VEP amplitudes to three intensities of flash. The amplitude measure represents the sum of the amplitudes of three late waves. VEPs were recorded from frontal and central scalp of 120 males; 20 in each group. (Reproduced from Blusewicz, M. J., et al., ref. 24, with permission. ©The Chemical Rubber Co., CRC Press, Inc.)

Porjesz and Begleiter (124) recorded VEPs from 14 alcoholics who had been abstinent for a minimum of 3 weeks and from 14 age-matched controls during three levels of task relevance. EPs were from left and right frontal and parietal scalp. The amplitude of a late VEP component was significantly reduced for alcoholics at all electrode sites. For the controls, amplitude varied with task relevance; this relationship did not exist for the alcoholic individuals, suggesting that they have deficits in selectively attending to relevant stimuli (124).

Salamy et al. (140) recorded AEPs from 11 control subjects and from 11 alcoholic patients after the patients had been sober for 1 and 3 weeks. Again, electrodes were sited bilaterally over frontal and parietal scalp areas. Similar to the findings of Porjesz and Begleiter (124), Salamy et al. (140) reported that the amplitude of a frontally derived EP late wave was significantly smaller for alcoholics than for normals at both the 1- and 3-week recordings. EPs from parietal scalp were reliably smaller for the alcoholics at 1 week but had achieved control levels by 3 weeks.

To investigate alcoholism-aging relationships, Cannon [(38); see also (11,24,54)] compared VEPs and SEPs from 20 young alcoholics who had been abstinent for an average of 6 weeks with VEPs and SEPs from 20 age-matched controls and from 20 healthy elderly subjects whose mean age was 71 years. EPs of the young alcoholics and normal oldsters were alike on some measures. The two groups were similar with respect to amplitudes and latencies of two occipital waves, P100 and N140, and one centrally derived wave, N140. When compared with VEPs from the young controls, these waves were smaller and were delayed (see Fig. 4). However, these late-wave similarities may have resulted from reduced retinal illumination of the elderly subjects. If flash intensity had been adjusted for visual threshold, the oldsters would have received brighter flashes (23,53) and their VEPs might have been similar to those of the young nonalcoholic individuals, since increased flash intensity produces shorter latencies and larger amplitudes (52,53).

For both VEPs and SEPs, early waves were larger and appeared later in responses of the elderly as compared with responses of the two young adult groups, corroborating previous reports of enhanced early-wave amplitude for EPs from normal oldsters (50,51,144,145).

Brainstem Auditory Evoked Potentials

Although BAEPs, also called far field potentials, are generated in brainstem structures, they are recorded from scalp locations. BAEPs typically consist of seven components occurring within about 10 msec following stimulation by rapidly presented clicks (116,122,150). The components are associated with neural activity in the different nuclei and pathways of the auditory system (10,78,154,156).

Aging

Those who have investigated relationships between BAEP characteristics and adult aging have generally reported that BAEP components are delayed in old age (82,87,116,137,150,165). Beagley and Sheldrake (8), however, examined 70 healthy subjects aged 14 to 79 years and did not find increased BAEP latencies in older subjects. It has been suggested that when prolonged latencies are observed for healthy oldsters, the delays are due to cochlear dysfunction (presbycusis) rather than to slowed conduction through brainstem structures (76–78). Recent reports indicate, however, that speed of conduction through auditory (87,116) and somatosensory (80) brainstem structures of older subjects is slowed, suggesting that transmission properties within the brainstem may change with age (116).

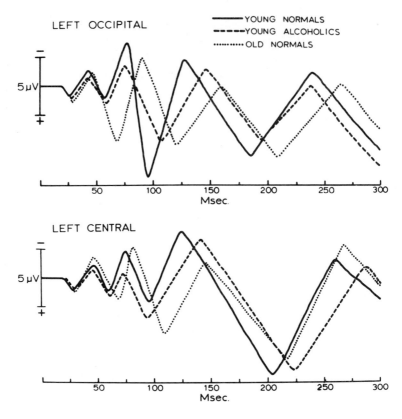

FIG. 4. VEPs from occipital and central scalp of 20 young normal subjects, 20 young alcoholics, and 20 elderly normal subjects. The tracings were constructed by plotting the mean latency and amplitude values of the various VEP waves and drawing interconnecting lines between the mean values. (Reproduced from Dustman, R. E., et al., ref. 54, with permission.)

Alcoholism

BAEP latencies and brainstem transmission time for alcoholics are slowed (17,41,136) when compared with normal values. Begleiter et al. (17) contrasted BAEPs from 17 alcoholics, abstinent for 3 weeks, with BAEPs from 17 age-matched normals. With the exception of wave I, which was slightly earlier for alcoholics, BAEP components for the alcoholic subjects were significantly delayed beyond those of the control group, indicating a slowing of conduction times. Begleiter et al. (17) suggested the slowing may have resulted from alcohol-induced demyelination of brainstem auditory tracts. It is known that brainstem transmission times are prolonged as a result of demyelinating diseases (5,40,157).

Pattern Reversal Evoked Potentials

PREPs are elicited by stimulating the visual system with a display of black and white checks that reverse, i.e., black squares change to white and white squares to black. The alternating checkerboard elicits a simple but stable pattern of potential changes that is restricted to scalp areas overlying the primary visual centers and adjoining visual association areas. PREPs are composed of five measurable waves (148) that extend over a time base of about 200 msec. Following pioneering studies by Halliday et al. (73,74), PREPs have been extensively used in the diagnosis of multiple sclerosis and other demyelinating diseases. PREPs have also been used to determine visual acuity of infants (153) and to monitor CNS changes during the course of treatment for Parkinson's disease (27).

Aging

Studies of age changes in PREPs have usually focused on latency of P100. Most agree that in comparison with younger subjects, P100 occurs later in the PREPs of subjects over 60 years (7,39,147,148,155).

Figure 5 illustrates life-span alterations in P100 latency of PREPs recorded in our laboratory from 137 healthy subjects aged 4 to 90 years (148,151). We found that adult aging was accompanied by increasingly longer latencies for P100 and for two earlier components, P50 and N65, and that the rate of slowing increased after the age of 60 years (148).

Shearer and Dustman (148) estimated that about half of the increased P100 delay that occurred after age 20 years could be attributed to a reduced level of visual stimulation at the retina because of structural changes within the aging eye that restrict the amount of light reaching the retina, i.e., reduced pupillary diameter and

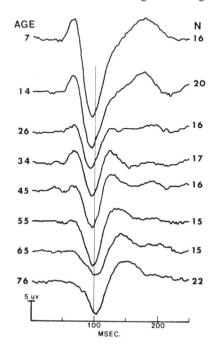

FIG. 5. Group averaged PREPs from an occipital central-frontal central (Oz-Fz) derivation. The mean age of each group is shown at the start of each tracing and the number of subjects at the end. A downward deflection is positive. (Reproduced from Shearer, D. E., and Dustman, R. E., ref. 148, with permission.)

yellowing of the crystalline lens (163). The remaining latency loss was thought to derive from other debilitating processes that are associated with advancing age (148).

Alcoholism

There have been two studies of PREPs of abstinent alcoholics. Porjesz and Begleiter (125,126) reported that P100 was abnormally delayed in alcoholics who had been abstinent for 1 month. Partial latency recovery was observed after an additional 3-month period of abstinence. Posthuma and Visser (129) recorded PREPs from 20 alcoholics who had been medication-free for at least 1 week and from 20 age-matched controls. In comparison to the control group, P100s from the alcoholic subjects were slowed about 8 msec. Although mean P100 latencies for the two groups were not significantly different, between-subject variance of P100 latency for the alcoholics was over 20 times that for the control subjects, indicating that P100s were extremely delayed for some alcoholics and very early for others.

Since delayed PREP waves have been frequently observed in patients with demyelinating diseases (73–75), Porjesz and Begleiter (125) suggested that the prolonged PREP latencies of alcoholics may indicate demyelination in visual system tracts. This is a lead well worth pursuing, since they earlier reported suggestive evidence of demyelination within the auditory system of alcoholics (see BAEPs above).

Late Positive or P300 Component

Unlike the EPs discussed earlier, the P300 component (also called P3) is not tightly coupled to the physical characteristics of the evoking stimuli. The P300, a positive component with a latency usually between 300 and 500 msec, depending on task difficulty (see Fig. 6), appears to be related to stimulus evaluation and

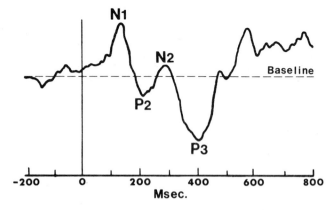

FIG. 6. A typical P300 EP. (Reproduced from Beck, E. C., et al., ref. 12, with permission of the editors and authors, *Exp. Aging Res.*, ©Beech Hill Enterprises, Inc., 1980.)

perhaps is a measure of "central processing time" (48). As such, the P3 has been widely employed by those interested in a better understanding of cognitive processing and in the timing of cognitive events. P3s are best elicited by stimuli that are relatively rare, unexpected, and task-relevant (48).

Aging

Most studies of age effects on P3 latency have reported that P3 latency lengthens as a function of adult aging (12,61,62,68,103,119,120,152), suggesting that the elderly require a longer period of time to process information. For example, Swanson (12,159) recorded P300s from 50 healthy males aged 21 to 86 years. They were presented with eight blocks of 50 visual stimuli of three types: (a) "background," which comprised 80% of the stimuli and were to be ignored; (b) "targets," which were to be counted; and (c) "novel" or unexpected stimuli. The targets and novels each comprised 10% of the total. For half of the blocks, the letter X was background and the letter O target. For the remaining blocks, background and target letters were reversed. As can be seen in Fig. 7, advancing age was associated with longer P3 latencies and P3 slowing was accentuated after age 60 years. The amplitude of P3 did not change as a function of age.

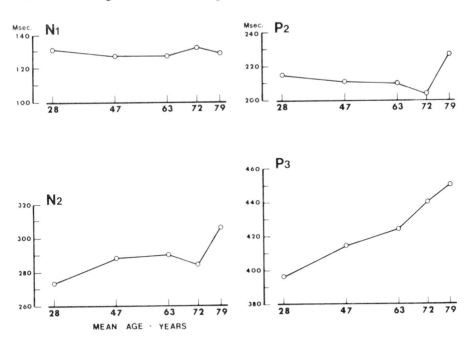

FIG. 7. Comparisons of mean peak latencies of N1, P2, N2, and P3 components of 10 subjects within each of five age groups. Note the distinct age-latency trend for the P3 component. (Reproduced from Beck, E. C., et al., ref. 12, with permission of the editors and authors, *Exp. Aging Res.,* © Beech Hill Enterprises, Inc., 1980.)

Not all studies of P3 latency-age relationships have demonstrated slowing (102,123). Podlesny and Dustman (123) studied interrelationships among signaled reaction time and P3 in three groups of 16 healthy adults (mean ages were 24, 45, and 71 years) using equal probability visual stimuli, X's and O's. P3 latency was constant across age, but P3 amplitude was significantly reduced for older subjects.

With respect to age effects on P3 latency and amplitude, the two studies cited above (12,123), both conducted in the same laboratory, arrived at opposite conclusions, emphasizing again the importance of using identical experimental procedures when comparing alcoholics and normal oldsters.

Alcoholism

The effects of alcoholism on P3 latency and amplitude are difficult to interpret. As for aging, changes in P3 latencies and amplitudes appear to be task-dependent. Some investigators have reported abnormally delayed P3 latencies for alcoholics (6,84,121); others report P3 latencies for alcoholics which are within normal limits (14,126,128). Pfefferbaum et al. (121) recorded P3s from abstinent alcoholics and from age-matched controls using infrequent and frequent tones as stimuli. P3 latency for both target and nontarget stimuli was delayed in responses from the alcoholic subjects. P3 amplitude did not differentiate the two groups for either type of stimulus. Johnson et al. (84) reported prolonged P3 latency for alcoholics in response to visually presented words for difficult task conditions, but not for easy task conditions.

In a series of studies, Begleiter and Porjesz (18,126,127) employed a square, a triangle, and irregular shapes as stimuli. The square and triangle alternated as target and nontarget stimuli. P3 latency for abstinent alcoholics was not reliably different from that for age-matched normal controls, regardless of stimulus type, but was significantly earlier than the latency of P3 for 10 geriatric subjects (mean age of 72 years). However, the alcoholics could be differentiated from age-matched controls and healthy geriatrics on the basis of P3 amplitude. For the young and elderly controls, the target and novel stimuli elicited P3s that were significantly larger than those elicited by background stimuli. This was not the case for the alcoholics; P3 amplitudes for target and novel stimuli were no larger than the amplitude for background stimuli, again suggesting that alcoholics may have an impairment of sensory filtering mechanisms and are unable to attend appropriately (18,126,127). In addition, P3 amplitudes (target and novel stimuli) for the control groups were larger than those for the alcoholic subjects. The amplitude differential may be related to cortical integrity. Begleiter et al. (18) compared P3 responses from controls with P3s from two groups of alcoholic subjects who differed with respect to documented presence or absence of cortical atrophy by computerized tomography (CT) scan. Again, P3 amplitudes for the alcoholics were smaller than those for the age-matched controls. However, P3 amplitudes for those alcoholics with positive signs of atrophy were significantly smaller than amplitudes for alcoholics whose CT scans were negative.

Amplitude/Intensity Slope

For many individuals (augmenters), increased stimulus intensity is paralleled by increased EP amplitude; for others (reducers), amplitudes may become smaller. It has been hypothesized that the augmenting/reducing phenomena are centrally determined and reflect underlying neurophysiological mechanisms that regulate the level of incoming sensory stimulation (33,92,100,118,169). Theoretically, sensory afferent stimulation activates corticofugal impulses, which have inhibitory influence on sensory afferent relays and on the ascending reticular activating system. The cortical excitability levels are thus modulated with resultant alterations in EP amplitudes (33,92,169). It has been suggested that the predisposition to "augment" or "reduce" in response to increased stimulus intensity may be related to levels of inhibitory neurotransmitters, since augmentation was associated with reduced turnover of monoamines, particularly of serotonin and dopamine (70,91,93,94).

Aging

Normal aging appears to be accompanied by deficits in central inhibitory function (9,64,81,105), perhaps related to reduced monoamine availability and utilization (9,105) and to deterioration of anterior cortical areas believed to exert inhibitory control over the ascending reticular formation (32,37,44,141,149).

As part of our studies of 220 healthy males aged 4 to 90 years, we recorded VEPs from frontal, central, and occipital scalp areas. Three intensities of patterned flash (22' checks) were employed: 1, 2, and 3 logs above threshold. Amplitude/intensity (A/I) slope functions were computed for each subject. Positive and negative slope values reflected augmentation and reduction of amplitude, respectively; slope magnitude reflected the size of amplitude change.

Figure 8 illustrates slope values for VEPs recorded from frontal and central scalp locations. The U-shaped age-slope curve reflected highly significant age differences ($F = 7.07$; 10/200 df; $p<0.001$). Slope values for the two youngest and the three oldest groups (see Fig. 8) were reliably larger than slope values for most of the intermediate groups. Thus the young and the old showed a greater electrical responsivity from anterior cortical areas to brighter flashes than subjects of adolescent and young adult ages. The fact that frontal and central scalp slope values were large for youngsters as well as for oldsters adds credence to the notion that A/I slope may reflect underlying CNS excitatory/inhibitory balance. Central inhibitory deficits have been reported for normal children (37,47,59), perhaps owing to low monoamine levels (2,53,109,135) and to late development (myelination) of anterior cortical areas.

A very different age-slope relationship was found for VEPs from occipital scalp (see Fig. 9). Most adults were augmenters, and there were no significant age changes across adult groups. Young children were strong reducers (negative slope). The reduction of occipital VEP amplitude by children to increased intensity may reflect a postulated mechanism within sensory systems (33,91,169) which protects the immature nervous system from overstimulation (29,30,160). The tendency to "re-

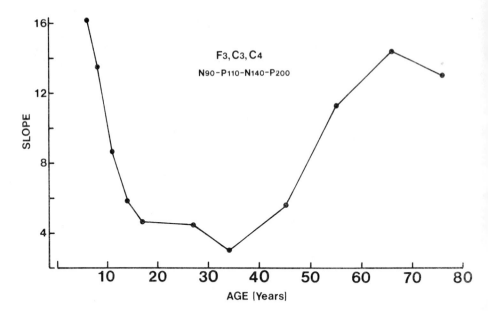

FIG. 8. A/I slope values for three late waves recorded from frontal and central scalp. Amplitude for each subject was summed across waves N90-P110, P110-N140, N140-P200 and across left frontal and left and right central scalp areas. Each age group included 20 males.

duce" VEP amplitude decreased steadily until adolescent years, suggesting that modulation of sensory input levels is developmentally controlled.

Alcoholism

In common with healthy oldsters, abstinent alcoholics reportedly have weak inhibitory systems (90,113,115), decreased monoamine turnover (90,93,94), and damage to anterior cortical areas (35,45,97). And like normal elderly subjects, and children, alcoholics tend to augment VEP amplitudes (42,90,93), presumably because of reduced inhibitory function (90,93,94).

It is not clear, however, that the mechanisms underlying VEP augmentation in normal oldsters and abstinent alcoholics are entirely similar. We reported that VEP augmentation by healthy elderly individuals was restricted to frontal and central cortical areas and did not occur in occipital areas overlying primary visual and visual association areas (52,53). Our recordings were unipolar with electrical activity underlying individual scalp areas being referenced to linked ears. Those reporting VEP A/I augmentation by alcoholics used bipolar recordings from two adjacent occipital areas (90–94) or from occipital and central sites linked together (42), making it difficult to evaluate electrical changes specific to cortical areas.

The enhanced VEP amplitudes of alcoholics associated with increases in flash intensity may reflect CNS hyperexcitability described by Begleiter and Porjesz for animals (13,14,16) and man (18) following cessation of chronic alcohol ingestion.

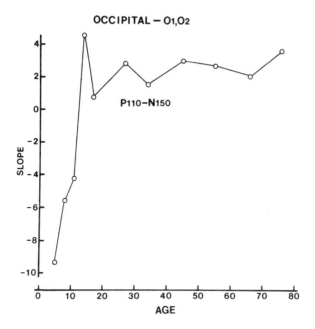

FIG. 9. A/I slope values for VEP component P110-N150 recorded from occipital scalp (O₁ and O₂ combined). Note that mean slope values for children were negative whereas those for most older subjects were positive. Each age group included 20 males. (Reproduced from Dustman, R. E., et al., ref. 52, with permission.)

The hyperexcitability decayed rather rapidly, over a period of weeks, and was observed to occur in a variety of cortical and lower brain structures. Future studies, in which stimulating and recording procedures are similar for the two groups, should provide information as to whether the increased A/I slope of alcoholics reflects relatively short-term hyperexcitability effects or lasting effects resulting from chronic changes in cortical function similar to those known to occur during normal aging.

Summary

With some EP measures, alcoholics and normal oldsters were quite different. For example, on the basis of VEP and P300 studies, it appears that alcoholics have difficulty distinguishing task-relevant stimuli from those that are not; healthy old subjects did not differ from young controls in this respect. Sensory EP studies have typically demonstrated that latencies and amplitudes of early EP waves (sensory receiving) occur later and are larger in responses of normal oldsters as compared with alcoholics and young adult controls.

There were some EP similarities between abstinent alcoholic and elderly subjects. Late waves of sensory EPs for both groups, in comparison to those of control subjects, have been reported to be delayed and reduced in amplitude. These EP characteristics for the elderly, however, may have resulted from sensory dysfunction, e.g., reduced retinal illumination. Results of BAEP and PREP studies suggest that information transmitted through at least some portions of the nervous system is slowed as a result of alcoholism and normal aging. Subjects in both groups tend to be augmenters in visually evoked response studies. This is a particularly interesting parallel since VEP augmentation has been related to inhibitory deficits, and there is anatomical, neurochemical, and behavioral evidence to suggest that inhibitory function of alcoholics and normal oldsters is reduced. But inferences regarding similarity of mechanisms must await further investigation, since procedures for recording from the alcoholics and the oldsters were substantially different.

CONCLUSION

The electrophysiological studies reviewed neither clearly support nor clearly refute the hypothesis that "alcoholism causes premature aging." Brain electrical activity recorded during sleep of abstinent alcoholics and of healthy oldsters rather strongly suggests some commonality of brain dysfunction for the two groups. Resting EEG recorded during periods of wakefulness, however, appears to be relatively insensitive to changes in brain function induced by a history of excessive drinking or by normal aging. While EP procedures offer a versatile approach toward furthering our understanding of brain dysfunction resulting from alcoholism and normal aging, definitive studies have not been done. The variety and complexity of EP procedures dictate that the two populations be studied within one experimental design and with identical procedures, a practice infrequently followed.

Rigorous experimental design, which allows for careful study of healthy oldsters and abstinent alcoholics with a battery of EP and other electrophysiological measures, can lead to meaningful inferences regarding similarities and differences in function of the two groups. To establish the presence or absence of parallels in brain function between alcoholics and the elderly, such studies need to be done.

ACKNOWLEDGMENTS

Thanks are extended to Dr. Don Creel, Dr. Nancy Cohn, and Don Shearer for their helpful comments. This chapter was supported by the Medical Research Service of the Veterans Administration.

REFERENCES

1. Adamson, J., and Burdick, J. A. (1973): Sleep of dry alcoholics. *Arch. Gen. Psychiatry*, 28:146–149.
2. Agrawal, H. C., and Himwich, W. A. (1970): Amino acids, proteins and monoamines of developing brain. In: *Developmental Neurobiology*, edited by W. A. Himwich, pp. 287–310. C. C Thomas, Springfield, IL.
3. Allen, R. P., Wagman, A., Faillace, L. A., and McIntosh, M. (1971): Electroencephalographic (EEG) sleep recovery following prolonged alcohol intoxication in alcoholics. *J. Nerv. Ment. Dis.*, 153:424–433.
4. Allen, R. P., Wagman, A. M. I., and Funderburk, F. R. (1977): Slow wave sleep changes: Alcohol tolerance and treatment implications. In: *Alcohol Intoxication and Withdrawal*, edited by M. M. Gross, pp. 629–640. Plenum Press, NY.

5. Amochaev, A., Johnson, R. C., Salamy, A., and Shah, S. N. (1979): Brain stem auditory evoked potentials and myelin changes in triethyltin-induced edema in young adult rats. *Exper. Neurol.*, 66:629–635.
6. Arzumanov, I. U. L., and Shostakovich, G. S. (1981): Interhemispheric functional relationships in chronic alcoholism. *Zh. Nevropatol. Psikhiatr.*, 81:1367–1371.
7. Asselman, P., Chadwick, D. W., and Marsden, C. D. (1975): Visual evoked responses in the diagnosis and management of patients suspected of multiple sclerosis. *Brain*, 98:261–282.
8. Beagley, H. A., and Sheldrake, M. B. (1978): Differences in brainstem response latency with age and sex. *Br. J. Audiol.*, 12:69–77.
9. Beck, C. H. M. (1978): Functional implications of changes in the senescent brain: A review. *Can. J. Neurol. Sci.*, 5:417–424.
10. Beck, E. C. (1975): Electrophysiology and behavior. *Annu. Rev. Psychol.*, 26:233–262.
10a. Beck, E. C., and Dustman, R. E. (1975): Changes in evoked responses during maturation and aging in man and macaque. In: *Behavior and Brain Electrical Activity*, edited by N. Burch and H. L. Altshuler, pp. 431–472. Plenum Press, NY.
11. Beck, E. C., Dustman, R. E., Blusewicz, M. J., and Cannon, G. W. (1979): Cerebral evoked potentials and correlated neuropsychological changes in the human brain during aging: A comparison of alcoholism and aging. In: *Aging, Vol. 10, Sensory Systems and Communication in the Elderly*, edited by J. M. Ordy and K. Brizzee, pp. 203–226. Raven Press, NY.
12. Beck, E. C., Swanson, C., and Dustman, R. E. (1980): Long latency components of the visually evoked potential in man: Effects of aging. *Exp. Aging Res.*, 6:523–545.
13. Begleiter, H., and Coltrera, M. (1975): Evoked potential changes during ethanol withdrawal in rats. *Am. J. Drug Alcohol Abuse*, 2:263–268.
14. Begleiter, H., DeNoble, V., and Porjesz, B. (1980): Protracted brain dysfunction after alcohol withdrawal in monkeys. In: *Biological Effects of Alcohol*, edited by H. Begleiter, pp. 231–249. Plenum Press, NY.
15. Begleiter, H., and Platz, A. (1972): The effects of alcohol on the central nervous system in humans. In: *The Biology of Alcoholism*, Vol. 2, edited by B. Kissin and H. Begleiter, pp. 293–343. Plenum Press, NY.
16. Begleiter, H. and Porjesz, B. (1977): Persistence of brain hyperexcitability following chronic alcohol exposure in rats. In: *Alcohol Intoxication and Withdrawal*, edited by M. M. Gross, pp. 209–222. Plenum Press, NY.
17. Begleiter, H., Porjesz, B., and Chou, C. L. (1981): Auditory brainstem potentials in chronic alcoholics. *Science*, 211:1064–1066.
18. Begleiter, H., Porjesz, B., and Tenner, M. (1980): Neuroradiological and neurophysiological evidence of brain deficits in chronic alcoholics. *Acta Psychiatr. Scand.*, (Suppl. 286), 62:3–13.
19. Bennett, A. E., Doi, L. T., and Mowery, G. L. (1956): The value of electroencephalography in alcoholism. *J. Nerv. Ment. Dis.*, 124:27–32.
20. Benson, K., Cohen, M., and Zarcone, V. (1978): REM sleep time and digit span impairment in alcoholics. *J. Stud. Alcohol*, 39:1488–1498.
21. Berger, H. (1929): Uber das Elektrenkephalogram des Menschen. *Arch. Psychiat. Nervenkr.*, 87:527–570.
22. Bierley, R. A., Cannon, D. A., Wehl, C. K., and Dustman, R. E. (1980): Effects of alcohol on visually evoked responses in rats during addiction and withdrawal. *Pharmac. Biochem. Behav.*, 12:909–915.
23. Birren, J. E., Casperson, R. C., and Botwinick, J. (1950): Age changes in pupil size. *J. Gerontol.*, 5:216–221.
24. Blusewicz, M. J., Cannon, W. G., and Dustman, R. E. (1982): Alcoholism and aging: Similarities and differences in neuropsychological performance. In: *Alcoholism and Aging: Advances in Research*, edited by W. G. Wood and M. F. Elias, pp. 47–60. CRC Press, Boca Raton, FL.
25. Blusewicz, M. J., Dustman, R. E., Schenkenberg, T., and Beck, E. C. (1977): Neuropsychological correlates of chronic alcoholism and aging. *J. Nerv. Ment. Dis.*, 165:348–355.
26. Blusewicz, M. J., Schenkenberg, T., Dustman, R. E., and Beck, E. C. (1977): WAIS performance in young normal, young alcoholic, and elderly normal groups: an evaluation of organicity and mental aging indices. *J. Clin. Psychol.*, 33:1149–1153.
27. Bodis-Wollner, I., and Yahr, M. D. (1978): Measurements of visual evoked potentials in Parkinson's disease. *Brain*, 101:661–671.

28. Bondareff, W. (1977): The neural basis of aging. In: *Handbook of the Psychology of Aging*, edited by J. E. Birren and K. W. Schaie, pp. 157–176. Van Nostrand Reinhold, NY.

29. Brazelton, T. B. (1973): *Neonatal Behavior Assessment Scale*. Lippincott, Philadelphia, PA.

30. Brazelton, T. B. (1977): Newborn behavior. In: *Scientific Foundations of Obstetrics and Gynecology*, edited by E. E. Philipp, J. H. Barnes, and M. Newton, pp. 550–564. Year Book Medical Publishers, Chicago, IL.

31. Brody, H. (1973): Aging of the vertebrate brain. In: *Development and Aging in the Nervous System*, edited by M. Rockstein, pp. 121–133. Academic Press, NY.

32. Bronson, G. (1965): The hierarchical organization of the central nervous system: implications for learning processes and critical periods in development. *Behav. Sci.*, 10:7–25.

33. Buchsbaum, M. (1976): Self regulation of stimulus intensity: Augmenting/reducing and the average evoked response. In: *Consciousness and Self-Regulation*, Vol. 1, edited by G. E. Schwartz and D. Shapiro, pp. 101–135. Plenum Press, NY.

34. Busse, E. W., and Obrist, W. D. (1963): Significance of focal electroencephalographic changes in the elderly. *Postgrad. Med.*, 34:179–182.

35. Cala, L. A., Jones, B., Wiley, B., and Mastaglia, F. L. (1980): A computerized axial tomography (C.A.T.) study of alcohol induced cerebral atrophy—in conjunction with other correlates. *Acta Psychiatr. Scand.*, (Suppl. 286), 62:31–40.

36. Callaway, E., and Harris, P. R. (1974): Coupling between cortical potentials from different areas. *Science*, 183:873–875.

37. Campbell, B. A., Lytle, L. D., and Fibiger, G. C. (1969): Ontogeny of adrenergic arousal and cholinergic inhibitory mechanisms in the rat. *Science*, 166:635–637.

38. Cannon, W. G. (1974): Cortical evoked responses of young normal, young alcoholic and elderly normal individuals. (Unpublished doctoral dissertation) *Brigham Young University*.

39. Celesia, G. G., and Daly, R. F. (1977): Effects of aging on visual evoked responses. *Arch. Neurol.*, 34:403–407.

40. Chiappa, K. H., Harrison, J. L., Brooks, E. B., and Young, R. R. (1980): Brainstem auditory evoked responses in 200 patients with multiple sclerosis. *Ann. Neurol.*, 7:135–143.

41. Chu, N., and Squires, K. C. (1980): Auditory brainstem response study of alcoholic patients. *Pharmacol. Biochem. Behav.*, 13:241–244.

42. Coger, R. W., Dymond, A. M., Serafetinides, E. A., Lowenstam, I., and Pearson, D. (1976): Alcoholism: Averaged visual evoked response amplitude-intensity slope and symmetry in withdrawal. *Biol. Psychiatry*, 11:435–443.

43. Coger, R. W., Dymond, A. M., Serafetinides, E. A., Lowenstam, I., and Pearson, D. (1978): EEG signs of brain impairment in alcoholism. *Biol. Psychiatry*, 13:729–739.

44. Como, P. G., Joseph, R., Fiducia, J. D., Siegel, J., and Lukas, J. (1979): Visually evoked potentials and after-discharge as a function of arousal and frontal lesion in rats. *Soc. Neurosci. Abstr.*, 5:202.

45. Courville, C. B. (1955): *Effects of Alcohol on the Nervous System of Man*. San Lucas, Los Angeles.

46. Dawson, G. D. (1954): A multiple scalp electrode for plotting evoked potentials. *Electroencephalogr. Clin. Neurophysiol.*, 6:153–154.

47. Diamond, S., Balvin, R. S., and Diamond, F. R. (1963): *Inhibition and Choice*, Harper and Row, NY.

48. Donchin, E., Ritter, W., McCallum, W. C. (1978): Cognitive psychophysiology: The endogenous components of the ERP. In: *Event-Related Brain Potentials in Man*, edited by E. Callaway, P. Tueting, and S. H. Koslow, pp. 349–411. Academic Press, NY.

49. Drechsler, F. (1978): Quantitative analysis of neurophysiological processes of the aging CNS. *J. Neurol.*, 218:197–213.

50. Dustman, R. E., and Beck, E. C. (1966): Visually evoked potentials: Amplitude changes with age. *Science*, 151:1013–1015.

51. Dustman, R. E., and Beck, E. C. (1969): The effects of maturation and aging on the waveform of visually evoked potentials. *Electroencephalogr. Clin. Neurophysiol.*, 26:2–11.

52. Dustman, R. E., Shearer, D. E., and Snyder, E. W. (1982): Age differences in augmenting/reducing of occipital visually evoked potentials. *Electroencephalogr. Clin. Neurophysiol.*, 54:99–110.

53. Dustman, R. E., and Snyder, E. W. (1981): Life-span changes in visually evoked potentials at central scalp. *Neurobiol. Aging*, 2:303–308.

54. Dustman, R. E., Synder, E. W., Callner, D. A., and Beck, E. C. (1979): The evoked response

as a measure of cerebral dysfunction. In: *Evoked Brain Potentials and Behavior*, edited by H. Begleiter, pp. 321–363. Plenum Press, NY.

55. Dyken, M., Grant, P., and White, P. (1961): Evaluation of electroencephalographic changes associated with chronic alcoholism. *Dis. Nerv. Syst.*, 22:284–286.

56. Feinberg, I. (1978): Sleep patterns in dementia: issues, evidence and strategies. In: *Senile Dementia: A Biomedical Approach*, edited by K. Nandy, pp. 155–167. Elsevier/North-Holland Biomedical Press, NY.

57. Feinberg, I., Hibi, S., and Carlson, V. R. (1977): Changes in EEG amplitude during sleep with age. In: *The Aging Brain and Senile Dementia*, edited by K. Nandy and I. Sherwin, pp. 85–98. Plenum Press, NY.

58. Feinberg, I., Koresko, R. L., and Heller, N. (1967): EEG sleep patterns as a function of normal and pathological aging in man. *J. Psychiatr. Res.*, 5:107–144.

59. Fishbein, H. D. (1976): *Evolution, Development and Children's Learning.* Goodyear Publishing, Pacific Palisades, CA.

60. Fitzhugh, L. C., Fitzhugh, K. B., and Reitan, R. M. (1965): Adaptive abilities and intellectual functioning of hospitalized alcoholics: Further considerations. *Q. J. Stud. Alcohol*, 26:402–411.

61. Ford, J. M., Hink, R. F., Hopkins, W. F., Roth, W. T., Pfefferbaum, A., and Kopell, B. S. (1979): Age effects on event-related potentials in a selective attention task. *J. Gerontol.*, 34:388–395.

62. Ford, J. M., Roth, W. T., Mohs, R. C., Hopkins, W. F., and Kopell, B. S. (1979): Event-related potentials recorded from young and old adults during a memory retrieval task. *Electroencephalogr. Clin. Neurophysiol.*, 47:450–459.

63. Friedlander, W. J. (1958): Electroencephalographic alpha rate in adults as a function of age. *Geriatrics*, 13:29–31.

64. Frolkis, V. V., and Bezrukov, V. V. (1979): *Aging of the Central Nervous System.* Karger, NY.

65. Gerson, I. M., and Karabell, S. (1979): The use of the electroencephalogram in patients admitted for alcohol abuse with seizures. *Clin. Electroencephalogr.*, 10:40–48.

66. Glaser, G. H. (1963): The normal electroencephalogram and its reactivity. In: *EEG and Behavior*, edited by G. H. Glaser, pp. 3–23. Basic Books, NY.

67. Goldstein, G., and Shelly, C. (1982): A multivariate neuropsychological approach to brain lesion localization in alcoholism. *Addict. Behav.*, 7:165–175.

68. Goodin, D. S., Squires, K. C., Henderson, B. H., and Starr, A. (1978): Age-related variations in evoked potentials to auditory stimuli in normal human subjects. *Electroencephalogr. Clin. Neurophysiol.*, 44:447–458.

69. Goodwin, D. W., and Hill, S. Y. (1975): Chronic effects of alcohol and other psychoactive drugs on intellect, learning and memory. In: *Alcohol, Drugs and Brain Damage*, edited by G. Rankin, pp. 55–69. Addiction Research Foundation, Toronto.

70. Gottfries, C. G., Knorring, L. von, and Perris, C. (1976): Neurophysiological measures related to levels of 5-hydroxyindoleacetic acid, homovanillic acid and tryptophan in cerebrospinal fluid of psychiatric patients. *Neuropsychobiology*, 2:1–8.

71. Greenblatt, M., Levin, S., and Ferruccio, Di C. (1944): The electroencephalogram associated with chronic alcoholism, alcoholic psychosis and alcoholic convulsions. *Arch. Neurol. Psychiat.*, 52:290–295.

72. Groves, P., and Schlesinger, K. (1979): *Biological Psychology.* Wm. C. Brown, Dubuque, IA.

73. Halliday, A. M., McDonald, W. I., and Mushin, J. (1972): Delayed visual evoked response in optic neuritis. *Lancet*, May 6, 982–985.

74. Halliday, A. M., McDonald, W. I., and Mushin, J. (1973): Visual evoked response in diagnosis of multiple sclerosis. *Br. Med. J.*, 4:661–664.

75. Halliday, A. M., McDonald, W. I., and Mushin, J. (1974): Delayed visual evoked responses in progressive spastic paraplegia. *Electroencephalogr. Clin. Neurophysiol.*, 37:328.

76. Harkins, S. W. (1981): Effects of age and interstimulus interval on brainstem auditory evoked potential. *Int. J. Neurosci.*, 15:107–118.

77. Harkins, S. W. (1981): Effects of presenile dementia of the Alzheimer's type on brainstem transmission time. *Int. J. Neurosci.*, 15:165–170.

78. Harkins, S. W., and Lenhardt, M. (1980): Brainstem auditory evoked potentials in the elderly. In: *Aging in the 1980's*, edited by L. W. Poon, pp. 101–114. American Psychological Association, Washington DC.

79. Hubbard, O., Sunde, D., and Goldensohn, E. S. (1976): The EEG in centenarians. *Electroencephalogr. Clin. Neurophysiol.*, 40:407–417.

80. Hume, A. L., Cant, B. R., Shaw, N. A., and Cowan, J. C. (1982): Central somatosensory conduction time from 10 to 79 years. *Electroencephalogr. Clin. Neurophysiol.*, 54:49–54.

81. Jakubczak, L. F. (1973): Age and animal behavior. In: *The Psychology of Adult Development and Aging*, edited by C. Eisdorfer and M. P. Lawton, pp. 98–111. American Psychological Association, Washington DC.

82. Jerger, J., and Hall, J. (1980): Effects of age and sex on auditory brainstem response. *Arch. Otolaryngol.*, 106:387–391.

83. Johnson, L. C., Burdick, J. A., and Smith, J. (1970): Sleep during alcohol intake and withdrawal in the chronic alcoholic. *Arch. Gen. Psychiatry*, 22:406–418.

84. Johnson, R., Pfefferbaum, A., Hart, T., and Kopell, B. S. (1982): Cognitive changes in long-term alcoholics. *Psychophysiology*, 19:327–328.

85. Kahn, E., and Fisher, C. (1969): Some correlates of rapid eye movement sleep in the normal aged male. *J. Nerv. Ment. Dis.*, 148:495–505.

86. Kales, A., Wilson, T., Kales, J. D., Jacobson, A., Paulson, M. J., Kollar, E., and Walter, R. D. (1967): Measurements of all-night sleep in normal elderly persons: Effects of aging. *J. Am. Geriatr. Soc.*, 15:405–414.

87. Kjaer, M. (1980): Recognizability of brain stem auditory evoked potential components. *Acta Neurol. Scand.*, 62:20–33.

88. Kish, G. B., Hagen, J. M., Woody, M. M., and Harvey, H. L. (1980): Alcoholics' recovery from cerebral impairment as a function of duration of abstinence. *J. Clin. Psychol.*, 36:584–589.

89. Klorman, R., Thompson, L. W., and Ellingson, R. J. (1978): Event related brain potentials across the life span. In: *Event-Related Brain Potentials in Man*, edited by E. Callaway, P. Tueting, and S. H. Koslow, pp. 511–570. Academic Press, NY.

90. Knorring, L. von (1976): Visual averaged evoked responses in patients suffering from alcoholism. *Neuropsychobiology*, 2:233–238.

91. Knorring, L. von (1978): Visual averaged evoked responses in patients with bipolar affective disorders. *Neuropsychobiology*, 4:314–320.

92. Knorring, L. von, Monakhov, K., and Perris, C. (1978): Augmenting/reducing: an adaptive switch mechanism to cope with incoming signals in healthy subjects and psychiatric patients. *Neuropsychobiology*, 4:150–179.

93. Knorring, L. von and Oreland, L. (1978): Visual averaged evoked responses and platelet monoamine oxidase activity as an aid to identify a risk group for alcoholic abuse. A preliminary study. *Prog. Neuropsychopharmacol.*, 2:385–392.

94. Knorring, L. von, and Perris, C. (1981): Biochemistry of the augmenting-reducing response in visual evoked potentials. *Neuropsychobiology*, 7:1–8.

95. Leber, W. R., Jenkins, R. L., and Parsons, O. A. (1981): Recovery of visual-spatial learning and memory in chronic alcoholics. *J. Clin. Psychol.*, 37:192–197.

96. Leber, W. R., and Parsons, O. A. (1982): Premature aging and alcoholism. *Int. J. Addict.*, 17:61–88.

97. Lezak, M. D. (1976): *Neuropsychological Assessment*. Oxford University Press, NY.

98. Little, S. C., and McAvoy, M. (1952): Electroencephalographic studies in alcoholism. *Q. J. Stud. Alcohol*, 13:9–15.

99. Luders, H. (1970): The effects of aging on the wave form of the somatosensory cortical evoked potential. *Electroencephalogr. Clin. Neurophysiol.*, 29:450–460.

100. Lukas, J. H., and Siegel, J. (1977): Cortical mechanisms that augment or reduce evoked potentials in cats. *Science*, 198:73–75.

101. Mankovsky, N. B., and Belonog, R. P. (1971): Aging of the human nervous system in the electroencephalographic aspect. *Geriatrics*, 26:100–116.

102. Marsh, G. R. (1975): Age differences in evoked potential correlates of a memory scanning process. *Exp. Aging Res.*, 1:3–16.

103. Marsh, G. R., and Thompson, L. W. (1972): Age differences in evoked potentials during an auditory discrimination task. *Gerontologist*, 12:44.

104. Marsh, G. R., and Thompson, L. W. (1977): Psychophysiology of aging. In: *The Psychology of Aging*, edited by J. E. Birren and K. W. Schaie, pp. 219–248. Van Nostrand Reinhold, NY.

105. McGeer, P. L., and McGeer, E. G. (1980): Chemistry of mood and emotion. *Annu. Rev. Psychol.*, 31:273–307.

106. Miles, L. E., and Dement, W. C. (1980): Sleep and aging. *Sleep*, 3:119–220.
107. Naitoh, P. (1973): The value of electroencephalography in alcoholism. 3. *Ann. N.Y. Acad. Sci.*, 215:303–320.
108. Newman, S. D. (1978): The EEG manifestations of chronic ethanol abuse: relation to cerebral cortical atrophy. *Ann. Neurol.*, 3:299–304.
109. Nies, A., Robinson, D. S., Davis, J. M., and Ravaris, C. L. (1973): Changes in monoamine oxidase with aging. In: *Psychopharmacology and Aging*, edited by C. Eisdorfer and W. E. Fann, pp. 41–54. Plenum Press, NY.
110. Obrist, W. D. (1976): Problems of aging. In: *Handbook of Electroencephalography and Clinical Neurophysiology*, Vol. 6, Part A, edited by G. E. Chatrian and G. C. Lairy, pp. 275–292. Elsevier, Amsterdam.
111. Obrist, W. D., and Busse, E. W. (1965): The electroencephalogram in old age. In: *Application of Electroencephalography in Psychiatry*, edited by W. P. Wilson, pp. 185–205. Duke University Press, Durham, NC.
112. Otomo, E., and Tsubaki, T. (1966): Electroencephalography in subjects 60 years and over. *Electroencephalogr. Clin. Neurophysiol.*, 20:77–82.
113. Parsons, O. A. (1975): Brain damage in alcoholics: altered states of unconsciousness. In: *Alcohol Intoxication and Withdrawal*, edited by M. M. Gross, pp. 569–584. Plenum Press, NY.
114. Parsons, O. A., and Farr, S. P. (1981): The neuropsychology of alcohol and drug use. In: *Handbook of Clinical Neuropsychology*, edited by S. B. Filskov and T. T. Boll, pp. 320–365. John Wiley, NY.
115. Parsons, O. A., and Tarter, R. E. (1972): Altered motor control in chronic alcoholics. *J. Abnorm. Psychol.*, 80:308–314.
116. Patterson, J. V., Michalewski, H. J., Thompson, L. W., Bowman, T. E., and Litzelman, D. K. (1981): Age and sex differences in the human auditory brainstem response. *J. Gerontol.*, 36:455–462.
117. Peeke, S. C., Prael, A. R., Herning, R. I., Rogers, W. Benowitz, N. L., and Jones, R. T. (1979): Effect of disulfiram on cognition, subjective response, and cortical-event-related potentials in nonalcoholic subjects. *Alcoholism*, 3:223–229.
118. Petrie, A., Holland, T., and Wolk, I. (1963): Sensory stimulation causing subdued experience: Audio-analgesia and perceptual augmentation and reduction. *J. Nerv. Ment. Dis.*, 137:312–321.
119. Pfefferbaum, A., Ford, J. M., Roth, W. T., and Kopell, B. S. (1980): Age differences in P3-reaction time associations. *Electroencephalogr. Clin. Neurophysiol.*, 49:257–265.
120. Pfefferbaum, A., Ford, J. M., Roth, W. T., and Kopell, B. S. (1980): Age-related changes in auditory event-related potentials. *Electroencephalogr. Clin. Neurophysiol.*, 49:266–276.
121. Pfefferbaum, A., Horvath, T. B., Roth, W. T., and Kopell, B. S. (1979): Event-related potential changes in chronic alcoholics. *Electroencephalogr. Clin. Neurophysiol.*, 47:637–647.
122. Picton, T. W., Hillyard, S. A., Krausz, H. I., and Galambos, R. (1974): Human auditory evoked potentials. I: Evaluation of components. *Electroencephalogr. Clin. Neurophysiol.*, 36:179–190.
123. Podlesny, J. A., and Dustman, R. E. (1982): Age effects on heart rate, sustained potential, and P3 responses during reaction-time tasks. *Neurobiol. Aging*, 3:1–9.
124. Porjesz, B., and Begleiter, H. (1979): Visual evoked potentials and brain dysfunction in chronic alcoholics. In: *Evoked Brain Potentials and Behavior*, edited by H. Begleiter, pp. 277–302. Plenum Press, NY.
125. Porjesz, B., and Begleiter, H. (1981): Human evoked brain potentials and alcohol. *Alcohol: Clin. Exper. Res.*, 5:304–317.
126. Porjesz, B., and Begleiter, H. (1982): Evoked brain potential deficits in alcoholism and aging. *Alcohol: Clin. Exper. Res.*, 6:53–63.
127. Porjesz, B., Begleiter, H., and Garozzo, R. (1980): Visual evoked potential correlates of information processing deficits in chronic alcoholics. In: *Biological Effects of Alcohol*, edited by H. Begleiter, pp. 603–623. Plenum Press, NY.
128. Porjesz, B., Begleiter, H., and Samuelly, I. (1980): Cognitive deficits in chronic alcoholics and elderly subjects assessed by evoked brain potentials. *Acta Psychiatr. Scand.*, (Suppl. 286), 62:15–29.
129. Posthuma, J., and Visser, S. L. (1982): Visual evoked potentials and alcohol-induced brain damage. In: *Clinical Applications of Evoked Potentials in Neurology*, edited by J. Courjon, F. Mauguiere, and M. Revol, pp. 149–155. Raven Press, NY.

130. Prinz, P. N. (1976): EEG during sleep and waking states. In: *Experimental Aging Research*, edited by M. F. Elias, B. E. Eleftheriou and P. K. Elias, pp. 135–163. EAR, Inc., Bar Harbor, ME.
131. Prinz, P. N. (1977): Sleep patterns in the healthy aged: Relationship with intellectual function. *J. Gerontol.*, 32:179–186.
132. Prinz, P. N., Halter, J., Benedetti, C., and Raskind, M. (1979): Circadian variation of plasma catecholamines in young and old men: Relation to rapid eye movement and slow wave sleep. *J. Clin. Endocrinol. Metab.*, 49:300–304.
133. Prinz, P. N., Obrist, W. D., and Wang, H. S. (1975): Sleep patterns in healthy elderly subjects: Individual differences as related to other neurobiological variables. *Sleep Res.*, 4:132.
134. Rizvi, C. A. (1978): EEG changes in old age: Normal and pathological. *Va. Med.*, 105:637–639.
135. Robinson, D. S., Nies, A., Davis, J. N., Bunney, W. E., Davis, J. M., Colburn, R. W., Bourne, H. R., Shaw, D. M., and Coppen, A. J. (1972): Ageing, monoamines, and monoamine-oxidase levels. *Lancet*, 1:290–291.
136. Rosenhamer, H. J., and Silfverskiold, B. P. (1980): Slow tremor and delayed brainstem auditory evoked responses in alcoholics. *Arch. Neurol.*, 37:293–296.
137. Rowe, M. J. (1978): Normal variability of the brain-stem auditory evoked response in young and old adult subjects. *Electroencephalogr. Clin. Neurophysiol.*, 44:459–470.
138. Rundell, O. H., Williams, H. L., and Lester, B. K. (1977): Sleep in alcoholic patients: Longitudinal findings. In: *Alcohol Intoxication and Withdrawal*, edited by M. M. Gross, pp. 389–402. Plenum Press, NY.
139. Ryan, C., and Butters, N. (1980): Learning and memory impairments in young and old alcoholics: evidence for the premature-aging hypothesis. *Alcohol: Clin. Exper. Res.*, 4:288–293.
140. Salamy, J. G., Wright, J. R., and Faillace, L. A. (1980): Changes in average evoked responses during abstention in chronic alcoholics. *J. Nerv. Ment. Dis.*, 168:19–25.
141. Scheibel, M. E., and Scheibel, A. B. (1966): The organization of the nucleus reticularis thalami: A Golgi study. *Brain Res.*, 1:43–62.
142. Scheibel, M. E., and Scheibel, A. B. (1975): Structural changes in the aging brain. In: *Aging*, Vol. 1, edited by H. Brody, D. Harman, and J. M. Ordy, pp. 11–37. Raven Press, NY.
143. Schenkenberg, T. (1970): Visual, auditory, and somatosensory evoked responses of normal subjects from childhood to senescence. (Unpublished doctoral dissertation) University of Utah.
144. Schenkenberg, T., and Dustman, R. E. (1970): Visual, auditory, and somatosensory evoked response changes related to age, hemisphere, and sex. *Proc. Am. Psychol. Assoc.*, 183–184.
145. Shagass, C. (1972): *Evoked Brain Potentials in Psychiatry*. Plenum Press, NY.
146. Shagass, C., and Schwartz, M. (1965): Age, personality and somatosensory evoked responses. *Science*, 148:1359–1361.
147. Shaw, N. A., and Cant, B. R. (1980): Age-dependent changes in the latency of the pattern visual evoked potential. *Electroencephalogr. Clin. Neurophysiol.*, 48:237–241.
148. Shearer, D. E., and Dustman, R. E. (1980): The pattern reversal evoked potential: The need for laboratory norms. *Am. J. EEG Technol.*, 20:185–200.
149. Skinner, J. E., and Yingling, C. D. (1977): Central gating mechanisms that regulate event-related potentials and behavior. A neural model for attention. In: *Progress in Clinical Neurophysiology*, edited by J. E. Desmedt, pp. 28–68. Karger, Basel.
150. Smith, D. B. D., Thompson, L. W., and Michalewski, H. J. (1980): Averaged evoked potential research in adult aging—status and prospects. In: *Aging in the 1980's*, edited by L. W. Poon, pp. 135–151. American Psychological Association, Washington, DC.
151. Snyder, E. W., Dustman, R. E., and Shearer, D. E. (1981): Pattern reversal evoked potential amplitudes: Life span changes. *Electroencephalogr. Clin. Neurophysiol.*, 52:429–434.
152. Synder, E., and Hillyard, S. (1977): Effects of age on event-related potentials. *Soc. Neurosci. Abstr.*, 3:120.
153. Sokol, S. (1978): Measurement of infant visual acuity from pattern reversal evoked potentials. *Vision Res.*, 18:33–39.
154. Starr, A., and Achor, L. J. (1979): Anatomical and physiological origins of auditory brain stem responses (ABR). In: *Human Evoked Potentials*, edited by D. Lehman and E. Callaway, pp. 415–429. Plenum Press, NY.
155. Stockard, J. J., Hughes, J. F., and Sharbrough, F. W. (1979): Visually evoked potentials to electronic pattern reversal: Latency variations with gender, age, and technical factors. *Am. J. EEG Technol.*, 19:171–204.

156. Stockard, M. M., and Rossiter, V. S. (1977): Clinical and pathologic correlates of brain stem auditory response abnormalities. *Neurology*, 27:316–325.
157. Stockard, J. J., Rossiter, V. S., Wiederholt, W. C., and Kobayashi, R. M. (1976): Brain stem auditory-evoked responses in suspected central pontine myelinolysis. *Arch. Neurol.*, 33:726–728.
158. Straumanis, J. J., Shagass, C., and Schwartz, M. (1965): Visually evoked cerebral response changes associated with chronic brain syndrome and aging. *J. Gerontol.*, 20:498–506.
159. Swanson, C. I. H. (1979): Age differences in evoked responses to three types of visual stimuli. (Unpublished doctoral dissertation) University of Utah.
160. Tronick, E., Als, H., and Brazelton, T. B. (1979): Early development of neonatal and infant behavior. In: *Human Growth, Vol. 3, Neurobiology and Nutrition*, edited by F. Falkner and J. M. Tanner, pp. 305–328. Plenum Press, NY.
161. Varga, B., and Nagy, T. (1960): Analysis of alpha-rhythm in the EEG of alcoholics. *Electroencephalogr. Clin. Neurophysiol.*, 12:933.
162. Wagman, A. M. I., and Allen, R. P. (1975): Effects of alcohol ingestion and abstinence on slow wave sleep of alcoholics. In: *Alcohol Intoxication and Withdrawal*, edited by M. M. Gross, pp. 453–466. Plenum Press, NY.
163. Weale, R. A. (1965): On the eye. In: *Behavior, Aging and the Nervous System*, edited by A. T. Welford and J. E. Birren, pp. 307–325. Thomas, Springfield, IL.
164. Webb, W. B., and Swinburne, H. (1971): An observational study of sleep of the aged. *Percept. Mot. Skills*, 32:895–898.
165. Wedel, H. von (1979): Differences in brainstem response with age and sex. In: *Models of the Auditory System and Related Signal Processing Techniques*, Scand. Audiol. Suppl. 9, edited by M. Hoke and E. deBoer, pp. 205–209.
166. Williams, H. L., and Salamy, A. (1972): Alcohol and sleep. In: *The Biology of Alcoholism*, Vol. 2, edited by B. Kissin and H. Begleiter, pp. 435–483. Plenum Press, NY.
167. Yingling, C. D. (1977): Lateralization of cortical coupling during complex verbal and spatial behaviors. In: *Language and Hemispheric Specialization in Man: Cerebral ERPs*, edited by J. E. Desmedt, pp. 151–160. Karger, Basel.
168. Zilm, D. H., Huszar, L., Carlen, P. L., Kaplan, H. L., and Wilkinson, D. A. (1980): EEG correlates of the alcohol-induced organic brain syndrome in man. *Clin. Toxicol.*, 16:345–358.
169. Zuckerman, M., Murtaugh, T., and Siegel, J. (1974): Sensation seeking and cortical augmenting-reducing. *Psychophysiology*, 11:535–542.

Alcoholism in the Elderly, edited by
J. T. Hartford and T. Samorajski.
Raven Press, New York © 1984.

Interactions of Normal Aging, Senile Dementia, Multi-Infarct Dementia, and Alcoholism in the Elderly

*†John Stirling Meyer, **John W. Largen, Jr., †Terry Shaw,
*Karl F. Mortel, and *Robert Rogers

*Cerebrovascular Research and †Cerebral Blood Flow Laboratory, Veterans
Administration Medical Center, Houston, Texas 77211; **Cerebral Blood Flow
Laboratory, Texas Research Institute of Mental Sciences, Texas Medical Center,
Houston, Texas 77030*

Associated with normal aging, there is progressive loss of nerve cells of the brain with cerebral atrophy measurable at necropsy, together with a decline in neurotransmitter levels measured at autopsy, which appear to precede the neuronal loss. During life, age-related brain atrophy is measurable as progressive enlargement of the ventricles by computerized tomography (CT) scanning with narrowing of gyri and poor discrimination of gray and white matter. Neurophysiological measures such as the electroencephalogram (EEG) and evoked potentials (EPs) show slowing and attenuation. Decreased cerebral metabolic demand with advancing age results in progressive decreases of cerebral blood flow (CBF) as the metabolism of gray and white matter becomes reduced. This is particularly evident as an age-related decrease in gray matter flow. Cognitive and neurological functioning, including memory, ability to abstract, motor speed, and other measures of neuropsychological functions, exhibit progressive declines with age. Debilitating effects of premorbid and morbid disease states, particularly risk factors for stroke and cerebrovascular disease, exacerbate age-related declines in neurophysiological, neuropsychological, and cerebral metabolic functioning.

The main focus of this chapter is to describe and correlate declines in brain functioning measured in normal aging, dementia, and alcoholism as reflected by decreases in regional cerebral blood flow (rCBF). The primary emphasis is devoted to recent cross-sectional and longitudinal (prospective) studies of rCBF, measured by the ^{133}Xe inhalation technique and carried out in this laboratory among large cohorts of patients and normal healthy volunteers over the past 7 years. CBF represents an indirect measure of brain function since normally there is tight coupling between CBF, neurotransmitter activity, cerebral metabolism, and neuronal functioning. Debilitating effects of excessive neuronal abiotrophy, arch-typified by the dementia of the Alzheimer's type (DAT), result in gross enhancement of age-related declines in rCBF and metabolism in a diffuse manner but most strikingly in the cerebral cortex and basal ganglia. Likewise, repeated and bilateral strokes enhance the likelihood of dementia (multi-infarct dementia, MID) with advancing age. Such insults to the aging brain not only result in functional impairment but are associated with reduced potential for recovery.

Excessive and chronic alcohol ingestion is, by itself, associated with atrophy of the brain, neurotransmitter dysfunction, neuropsychological impairment, and decreased CBF. This is partially or completely reversible in early stages of the disease, particularly in the young. However, chronic alcohol intake may, of itself, lead to Wernicke-Korsakoff's dementia. In the elderly, effects of alcohol are superimposed upon an aging and atrophic brain with an already decreased functional reserve. The present communication will discuss possible relationships between chronic and excessive alcohol intake as a risk factor for hastening normal age-related plus disease-related declines in rCBF. Such rCBF declines with aging are not observed to the same degree in nondrinking individuals and ultimately may lead to dementia. Several of these interacting factors are preventable or remediable. Optimal health measures with continued neural activity (mental exercise) appear to delay rCBF declines of normal aging and the dementing processes.

NEUROPATHOLOGICAL, STRUCTURAL, AND NEUROTRANSMITTER CHANGES ASSOCIATED WITH NORMAL AGING, DEMENTIA, AND ALCOHOLISM

Normal Aging

Effects of alcoholism in the elderly must be considered against a background of normal age-related changes. In normal aging, there are significant age-related declines in the integrative action of the entire nervous system. With advancing age, virtually all tests of motor performance show significant and progressive declines with age, including reaction time, fine coordination, agility, motor strength, and speed of repetitive voluntary movements. Similarly, tests of olfactory, auditory, visual, and tactile sensory functioning exhibit age-related attenuation of functioning. Measurements of peripheral motor nerve, sensory nerve, and central spinal cord conduction velocities also decrease sharply after age 60 (38).

These declines in neurological performance with age correlate with neuropathological changes of the aging nervous system. Brain weight shows progressive declines beginning in the fourth and fifth decades owing to neuronal degeneration and replacement gliosis. Lipofuscin granules accumulate in neurons with aging, especially in thalamic nuclei, cortical pyramidal cells, and olivary and dentate nuclei. Age-related changes in the dendritic architecture of the cortical neurons have been described (124). Considerable reductions in neuronal populations of the neocortex are present by the seventh decade (23,62). There are losses of up to 35% of small glial cells and up to 60% of large neurons in the cortex (62). The locus ceruleus loses up to 35% of its neurons; however, the brainstem nuclei, including the vestibular and inferior olivary nuclei, remain relatively spared. In normal aging, localized senile plaques, neurofibrillary tangles, and granulovacuolar degeneration are observed but not to the degree and widespread nature seen in DAT.

In keeping with the above review of the pathology of normal aging, CT estimates of brain volume based on pixel counts have shown progressive age-related decreases in brain volume which decline more rapidly after 50 years of age (151). Likewise, age-related quantitated increases in ventricular volume and widening of cortical sulci have been reported (7,57). Significant correlations have been reported between measures of ventricular enlargement and/or cortical atrophy with various measures of cognitive and intellectual functioning. However, others report (41,98) only weak relationships between CT measures of atrophy and cognitive performance if effects of advancing age are statistically controlled.

Dementia

The term "dementia" generally refers to organic, diffuse disorders of the brain in adult life manifested by deterioration of measured cognitive functioning relative to previous normal levels (141,142). Wells (142) emphasized the evolving and progressive nature of symptoms and character of dementia, which frequently represent wide spectrums of cognitive and behavioral dysfunction. Estimates of prevalence rates of dementia within general populations vary widely owing to methodological differences in sampling techniques and to the severity of the dementia. Best estimates range from 1.6 to 9.1% for severe dementia and from 2.6 to 24.7% for mild dementia in elderly populations (140). Retrospective analyses of autopsied brains report that DAT accounts for 50% of dementing disorders while 12% are accounted for by MID (140). Other estimates rank MID to be responsible for about 20% of dementias, with mixed DAT and MID (MIX) for another 12%. In any event, DAT, MID, and MIX account for approximately 80% of chronic dementing disorders.

DAT is a primary degenerative disorder of the central nervous system with insidious onset and steady, progressive, and diffuse deterioration involving bilateral regions of the brain and including cortex and subcortical structures (144). Memory loss, particularly for recent events, is among the earliest and most salient features. Other clinical features include impaired abstract thinking, reduced capacity for logical reasoning and concept formation, and impaired judgement. There are also changes in personality, and in later stages there may be widespread manifestations of cerebral disease. The rapidity of the degenerative process varies from case to case, with 3 to 5 years as the mean interval before severe incapacitation occurs. Grasp, sucking, and glabellar reflexes are regularly elicited as signs of cortical release, even in mild-to-moderate cases, although similar signs are sometimes observed in cognitively well-preserved "normal" aged. Later signs may include dysphasia, dyslexia, dyspraxia, and dysgraphia with eventually the appearance of gross dementia including disorientation, incontinence, and total inability for self-care followed by death usually due to intercurrent infection (142).

Classic MID can usually be differentiated from DAT after evaluation by neuropsychological tests plus a detailed history of symptom presentation, of risk factors for stroke, and neurological and cardiovascular evaluations. Considerations in the diagnosis of MID have been summarized by Hachinski and associates (58). The Ischemic Index modified after Mayer-Gross by Hachinski et al. (59) has been shown to have high diagnostic accuracy in differentiating MID from DAT, and its validity as a diagnostic predictor has been confirmed by neuropathological verification (121). The Ischemic Index assigns scores on the basis of history and symptoms suggestive of dementia due to cerebrovascular disease such as history of hypertension, abrupt onset, step-wise deterioration, fluctuating course, and the presence of focal neurological signs and symptoms. In addition, documented risk factors for cerebrovascular disease (hypertension, arteriosclerotic heart disease, diabetes mellitus, and hyperlipidemia) are frequently associated with MID (146). As will be discussed later, even nondemented aging subjects with one or more risk factors for stroke may experience mild-to-moderate disorders of EEG, neuropsychological functioning, and CBF.

In the present discussion, so-called presenile and senile forms of Alzheimer's disease are considered as a single nosological entity since recent clinical, morphological, and genetic studies indicate that no difference exists between the two forms except age of onset before 65 years for the presenile form (32).

Gross morphological changes relevant to DAT include reductions in brain size and weight, diffuse atrophy of the brain characterized by narrowing of gyri, widening of sulci, and progressive enlargement of the lateral and third ventricles. Frequent atrophic involvement of the medial temporal, parietal, parahippocampal, and hippocampal gyri have been particularly emphasized (135).

The most significant histological features include the presence of senile plaques, neurofibrillary tangles, granulovacuolar degeneration, and neuronal loss particularly in the *nucleus basalis* of Meynert (18,34). Compared with brains obtained from normals of similar age, neuronal loss is significantly greater in DAT and may be marked throughout the cortex and to a lesser extent in the subcortical structures. Similarly, quantitatively greater differences have been demonstrated in the number of senile plaques, neurofibrillary tangles, and amount of granulovacuolar degeneration in DAT compared with aged normals. The possibility of a neuropathological volumetric "threshold" has been considered, beyond which additional quantitative neuropathological degeneration of the brain inevitably results in dementia (33,137).

In MID, autopsy studies reveal patterns of multiple foci of ischemic destruction, often including lacunar or small infarcts throughout both hemispheres. Extensive ischemic softening of multiple zones of cortical tissue are usually found in widely varying patterns of distribution. The quantitative element is significant since apparently well-preserved older individuals have been shown to have multiple areas of ischemic softening (136). In addition, studies have confirmed the quantitative relationship between volumetric quantity of cerebral softenings and the severity of dementia during life (137). It has also been well established that in many demented patients, significant cerebral softenings coexist with characteristic changes of Alzheimer type (MIX) (33).

CT studies carried out on elderly patients with dementing disorders have reported that 50 to 60% exhibit mild-to-moderate ventricular enlargement with 34% showing sulci enlargement on the CT scan (22,65). Again there are exceptions as the CT scan may appear to be within normal limits in earlier cases with well-documented dementia, and there is considerable overlap between CT evidence of atrophy in early dementia and in elderly controls. However, age of patient, etiology, and severity of the dementia influence the results of these measures. Even in cases of dementia with normal CT scans, density measures may be decreased (98). However, neither ventricular enlargement nor cortical atrophy by CT scan may be considered pathognomonic for dementia, nor does dementia necessarily predict atrophy on the CT scan.

Patients with MID more predictably differ from nondemented controls by CT scanning, since they exhibit multifocal and asymmetrical changes not present in patients with DAT (129), although, once again, there may be overlap with CT scans of elderly nondemented controls.

Alcoholism

Evidence of cerebral atrophy has frequently been reported at necropsy of brains of patients with a history of alcoholism (34,86). Histological examinations reveal widespread neuronal loss, particularly in the frontal regions. Such changes cannot be attributed to secondary factors such as nutritional status (54,86). Long-term maintenance of rats on an ethanol-containing diet resulted in significant neuronal loss of hippocampal pyramidal and dentate gyrus granule cells in the absence of malnutrition (139). Likewise, in a similar paradigm, 50 to 60% loss of dendritic spines of hippocampal pyramidal cells and dentate gyrus granule cells have been reported in mice (119). Pneumoencephalography of alcoholics during life has shown considerable cortical and ventricular atrophy and, to a lesser extent, atrophy of the cerebellar vermis (30,60). Cerebral atrophy was reported to be more enhanced in patients with history of delirium tremens, alcoholic hallucinosis, and Wernicke-Korsakoff's dementia. However, alcoholic patients without dementia or neurological symptoms may likewise exhibit such atrophy (60). Similarly, malnutrition appears to predispose alcoholics to cerebral atrophy, but the latter also occurs in patients with adequate nutrition presumably owing to the direct toxic effects of alcohol (60,111). In well-controlled CT scan studies, cerebral atrophy has been found in 52 to 73% and cerebellar atrophy in 62% of alcoholics under age 55 (27,28,75,83). These atrophic changes could not be explained on the basis of normal age-related changes and occurred in heavy drinkers with good nutrition, without history of delirium tremens, alcoholic seizures, hepatic disease, or head trauma. Evidence of partial reversibility of cerebral atrophy in some abstinent young alcoholics has been reported by serial CT scanning (29).

Carlen and associates (28) reported that if the degree of brain atrophy was plotted against age, alcoholics showed significantly more rapid rates of development of cerebral atrophy than controls, suggesting that alcohol enhances the rate of cerebral atrophy associated with aging and places the alcoholic at greater risk for development of functional impairment compared with age-matched, nonalcoholic controls.

Several alcohol-related variables have direct relevance for both morphological and behavioral cerebral disorders. These include duration of alcoholism, average intake, type of beverage, pattern of drinking (binge versus steady), and period of time between abstinence and measurement (110). Secondary medical complications such as multiple head trauma, liver disease, and nutritional status also significantly affect the level and pattern of atrophy and neuropsychological functioning. Although it is well established that alcoholic Wernicke-Korsakoff's disease is caused by thiamine deficiency, secondary to nutritional deficiency, there is also considerable evidence for direct toxic effects of alcohol on brain tissues (49). In animals given chronic ethanol-containing diets, there is direct evidence for neuronal impairment and behavioral deficiencies independent of nutritional status (49). In addition, human studies report significant morphological and neuropsychological impairment in chronic alcoholics specifically selected for history of adequate nutrition, absence of liver disease, head injury, delirium tremens, and alcoholic hallucinosis. Evidence of partial reversibility of cerebral atrophy and neuropsychological impairment following prolonged abstinence similarly argues for direct toxic effects of alcohol on the cerebrum (122).

In recent years, research has implicated a deficit in the cholinergic system in normal aging and in Alzheimer's disease. Activity of choline acetyltransferase (CAT), the synthesizing enzyme of acetylcholine, has been shown in postmortem studies to be reduced in both the cortex and the hippocampus during normal aging (6,89), which becomes excessively reduced in DAT (6,37). On the other hand, postmortem examinations have also revealed comparable declines in cholinergic muscarinic receptor sites in the cortex of normal senescent individuals and of patients with DAT (143), implicating some presynaptic impairment. Recent data indicate that in DAT there is a selective degeneration of the nucleus basalis of Meynert, a major source of cholinergic innervation projecting to the cerebral cortex (143). The dramatic and selective deficit in cholinergic function in normal aging, which is exaggerated in DAT, is particularly significant in light of the well-established association between cholinergic functioning and memory (8,39).

There is evidence for declines of other neurotransmitter systems as well. With normal advancing age there is evidence for reduced activity in dopamine, noradrenaline, serotonin, and gamma-aminobutyric acid (GABA) systems (123).

NEUROPSYCHOLOGICAL STUDIES OF NORMAL AGING VERSUS DAT, MID, ALCOHOLIC DEMENTIA, AND WERNICKE-KORSAKOFF'S DISEASE

Normal Aging

The patterns of psychological decline in normal aging are well documented in several reviews (16,21,97). In the early literature, declines in general intelligence were frequently reported. The conclusions were, however, based on cross-sectional analysis of data, which is subject to error from cohort effects and may exaggerate age-related deterioration. More recent longitudinal studies indicate that, in fact, intellectual functions tend to remain relatively preserved until late in adulthood, but there is considerable between-subject variability in rate of decline of intellectual functioning with advancing age (21,97). General intelligence, however, is a multivariate construct of diverse integrated abilities that have been shown to vary at disproportionate rates with aging. Subtests requiring psychomotor speed, perceptual integrative ability, recent memory, flexibility, and assimilation ability tend to show faster declines than verbal abilities, remote memory, and tasks requiring utilization of previously acquired information.

Extensive reviews of learning and memory in the aged have indicated attenuated performance on verbal memory tasks such as paired-associates learning, supraspan tasks, and memory for paragraphs as well as tasks of nonverbal memory (21,35). However, more recent analytic studies have shown that such declines may be accentuated or minimized by alterations of a number of parameters influencing learning and memory in the elderly, such as rate of stimulus presentation, learning times, task meaningfulness, word familiarity, and organizability of the information to be tested.

A generalized slowing in psychomotor performance (tapping speed, reaction time) and slowing of cognitive task-completion time have been consistently reported among the elderly (17,21).

In studies incorporating neuropsychological test batteries, age-related declines in performance have been documented (5,117,118). Relative to younger groups, elderly subjects show greatest performance decrements on tests highly weighted in "immediate adaptive ability" and equal or superior performance on tests most heavily dependent on "prior experience and stored information" (116). Neuropsychological tests most sensitive to the effects of aging are also sensitive to the effects of brain damage (116). However, it should be noted that cutoff points for many neuropsychological test variables have not been standardized for different ages.

One of the more significant variables affecting test performance in the elderly is that of physical health. Approximately 75 to 80% of individuals over the age of 65 years have at least one chronic disabling condition, and it has been extensively documented that health factors, particularly disease of the cardiovascular system, may be instrumental in contributing to psychological performance deficits (21). Eisdorfer and Wilkie (43) summarized research indicating that cardiovascular and cardiopulmonary functional status directly influence intellectual functioning, reaction times, and speed of information processing. Similarly, uncontrolled hypertension has been shown to adversely influence response speed, intellectual functioning, and neuropsychological performance. Furthermore, elevated serum cholesterol levels have been shown to relate to neuropsychological test performance and brain atrophy (88,117,118).

The foregoing discussion is similar to the findings of EEG research in relation to aging as summarized by Obrist (102), which underscored the malignant influence of institutionalization and poor health, particularly the effects of chronic cardio-vascular and cerebrovascular disease. Healthy, active individuals living in the community manifested minimal EEG changes compared with young adult norms, with the possible exception of extreme senescence (87,101). In contrast, institutionalization of subjects and those with chronic circulatory disease were associated with accentuated abnormalities of EEG records, particularly in regard to loss of alpha frequency, changes in amplitude, and the appearance of diffuse slow-wave activity (101,104). Uncontrolled fluctuation in blood pressure, either alone or in combination with vascular disease, has been shown to be associated with diffuse slow-wave activity in elderly psychiatric patients (105). The theoretical mechanisms have been addressed by Obrist (102), who proposed a model based upon relationships of EEG to CBF and cerebral metabolism, the latter thought to be the ultimate rate-limiting step responsible for EEG changes. Reduced cerebral metabolism was thought to be due to by-hypoxic and ischemic conditions secondary to arteriosclerotic-based cerebrovascular insufficiency.

DAT

Progressive deterioration of intellect and memory are characteristic neuropsychological deficits consistently reported in DAT (97). Review of the literature shows that dementia patients predictably show lowered intelligence quotients compared with normal age-matched subjects (97). There is a selective impairment in recent memory characterized by a reduction in ability to learn new material or register ongoing events. The nature of the memory deficits has been systematically explored by Inglis and co-workers (66) and Miller and associates (97). Deficits in both figural and semantic memory have been found (84), and patients with pathologically verified DAT displayed high rates of intrusions compared with other categories of dementia (51). In measures of verbal and nonverbal remote memory, patients with senile dementia evidence significant difficulty compared with normal elderly volunteers (78,145).

Increased psychomotor slowing has been reported in dementia patients on simple pegboard tasks (96) as well as in oculomotor reaction (115) and choice reaction times (116). Language deficits may occur within the context of overall impairment of higher cortical functioning. While naming dysfunction, perseveration, poverty of speech, and verbal fluency impairment are commonly reported features, deficits in the linguistic character of spoken language also evolve with progressive deterioration (9,120). Studies incorporating neuropsychological test batteries have reported significant declines in tests of concept formation, reasoning, and organizational ability (131).

MID

Unfortunately, there are few studies that have attempted to differentiate MID from DAT based on neuropsychological testing, although there are some indications that different etiologies of dementia may produce different profiles of test scores

(50,52,112,113). Perez and associates (112,113) utilized intellectual and memory subtests to differentiate DAT from MID and from vertebrobasilar insufficiency (VBI). Striking variability was noted in test performance of the MID group, and the degree and pattern of performance varied with each patient, depending upon the localization, severity, and number of infarcts.

Alcoholic Dementia

Numerous reviews report that chronic alcoholism is associated with a variety of cognitive and neuropsychological deficits (53,74,110,134). In general, there was a wide degree of intellectual impairment found in alcoholics, ranging from little difference from normal, to levels of impairment resembling that of established brain damage. Several studies demonstrate that the severity of functional deficits correlates with the duration of alcoholism (42,71,133) and average quantity of alcohol ingested (or with estimated lifetime consumption). Of particular relevance to the level of impairment was the period of time between sobriety and testing.

Chronic alcoholism has been found not to disrupt cognitive and neuropsychological functioning in a diffuse or generalized fashion. Rather, specific clusters of functions are affected while others remain spared. The majority of studies agree that general intelligence remains relatively unaffected in chronic alcoholism (48,74,133). However, a fairly consistent pattern of intact verbal abilities with slightly lowered performance abilities has frequently emerged (110,134). In a review by Parsons (110), it was concluded that the patterns of neuropsychological deficits most frequently evidenced in alcoholics were relatively impaired performance on tasks involving visual spatial analysis, tactual spatial analysis, nonverbal abstraction, and set flexibility. The pattern of neuropsychological impairment is not specific to alcoholics, but many of these measures are sensitive to aging effects as well as to brain damage in general. Other research suggests that basic lower-order processes remain intact, but more complex behaviors involving synthesis and integration among different modalities tend to become impaired (31).

Memory deficits as assessed via standard clinical instruments tend not to be seriously affected in chronic alcoholics. However, research summarized by Butters and Cermak (26) demonstrates that subtle memory and information processing deficits can be elicited in chronic alcoholics. It was further demonstrated that these deficits are qualitatively similar to impairment in patients with Wernicke-Korsakoff's disease. These data are consistent with a "continuity of impairment" hypothesis (109) ranging from subtle impairment in nonalcoholic heavy drinkers (109) through progressively greater impairment in short-term alcoholics, long-term alcoholics, and ultimately Wernicke-Korsakoff's disease (26).

There is ample evidence for recovery of function with abstinence from alcohol (53), but despite considerable recovery, the level of improvement often remains below normal, and certain functions do not appear to improve, suggesting some permanent residual impairment (85).

Age adversely affects the degree of impairment as well as degree of recovery in chronic alcoholics. It is suggested that cognitive and neuropsychological decline associated with chronic alcohol ingestion parallels the effects of normal aging (19,20,48,74,132,138). Several studies demonstrate similarities between young alcoholics and elderly normals on a variety of neuropsychological tests (20,64). Recovery of function has also been shown to vary with age. Alcoholics under the age of 40 years tended to recover from memory impairment following sobriety whereas those over age 40 maintained impairment over the time period examined (45). In animal research, senescent mice show greater toxicity to chronic alcohol ingestion with enhanced behavioral impairment compared with younger animals (46,147).

Wernicke-Korsakoff's Disease

The chronic stage of Wernicke-Korsakoff's disease is best characterized by relatively intact intellectual functioning with severe anterograde and retrograde amnesia (25,26). Intelligence measured by standard instruments does not significantly differ from age- and education-matched normal controls. A key psychometric indication of Wernicke-Korsakoff's disease is a relatively well-preserved IQ with a Wechsler Memory Quotient 20 to 30 points below normal (26). New learning and memory are severely impaired, resulting in an anterograde amnesia since the onset of illness. A retrograde amnesia for remote events has been experimentally shown by the administration of historical questions and famous faces representing prior decades (2). Alcoholic Korsakoff patients also share with chronic alcoholics impairment in visuoperceptual ability (26).

CBF IN NORMAL AGING, DAT AND MID, ALCOHOLISM, AND WERNICKE-KORSAKOFF'S DISEASE

Normal Aging

Until recently there was controversy regarding the extent to which changes in CBF reflect normal consequences of aging. In 1956, Kety (72) summarized 16 studies on aging where CBF was measured utilizing the nitrous oxide method, an invasive procedure that yields blood flow and oxygen consumption for the entire brain with an error exceeding $\pm 10\%$. Combined results from these studies showed that there was a rapid fall in cerebral circulation and metabolism between puberty and adolescence, followed by gradual, but progressive declines from the third decade through senescence with an accompanying progressive increase in cerebrovascular resistance.

Later studies with the nitrous oxide method reported no significant declines with advancing age when a highly selected small group of healthy aged volunteers were examined (36,130). These volunteers were highly selected community-resident, senescent persons in excellent health and without evidence of gross mental decline, having a mean age of 71 years. In such a group where physical illness, institutionalization, and social adversity had been selectively eliminated, no statistically significant differences were found in average total CBF or cerebral oxygen consumption compared with a group of normal young subjects. Reductions in CBF in individual cases, when found, were thought to be associated with arteriosclerotic disease. These findings were taken to suggest that if CBF reductions were observed in normal elderly subjects, they were associated with either degenerative or vascular pathology.

Recent studies have been carried out in larger groups of healthy normal volunteers using noninvasive methods and measuring gray matter flow rather than total CBF (107,108). These studies consistently report steady, progressive declines in gray matter flow with advancing age as measured by the ^{133}Xe inhalation method.

Melamed et al. (90) selected forty-four normal subjects with an age range between 19 to 79 years and excluded any subjects with cerebral pathology, including dementia or focal neurologic deficits, hypertension, coronary and peripheral vascular disease, or pulmonary abnormalities. Advancing age was associated with significant reductions in bihemispheric blood flow from all regions measured. These data support a progressive age-related decline in CBF continuing from youth through old age.

Meyer, Shaw, and co-workers (91,94,99,125–127) have systematically analyzed rCBF in gray matter flow of normal volunteers by cross-sectional and longitudinal studies and have demonstrated significant age-related declines in healthy normal volunteers as well as more rapid declines in normal subjects with risk factors for stroke. A group of normal, right-handed volunteers were studied, ranging in age from 30 to 98 years and specifically selected for optimal health (medically and neurologically normal, without risk factors for atherosclerotic disease, and socially active). Cross-sectional studies indicated that there were progressive declines in mean hemispheric gray matter flow with advancing age (127,128). Significant correlations were found between resting gray flow and age, with a mean yearly decline of 0.53 ml per 100 g of brain tissue per minute (91,94).

Regional flow did not decline homogeneously with age. Mean left hemispheric gray matter values were initially higher than that of the right hemisphere but tended to decline with advancing age at a more rapid pace. The prefrontal regions of the brain exhibited the most rapid age-related declines whereas regions exhibiting the least decline were those surrounding both Sylvian fissures, precentral areas of the left hemisphere, and the parietal areas of the right. Thus, age-related declines in rCBF were found in normal, optimally healthy volunteers, which could not be explained by disease factors. Reasons for the decline were attributed to normal atrophy of the brain with advancing age and progressive rigidity of the cerebral vessels.

A second group of neurologically normal, asymptomatic, and otherwise healthy volunteers were examined for flow changes with advancing age. However, the second group possessed one or more risk factors for cerebral atherosclerosis and stroke (hypertension, diabetes mellitus, hyperlipidemia, heart disease). Given the high rate of chronic diseases in the population over 65 (75 to 80%), this latter group more typically represents the elderly population at large. These volunteers with risk factors showed a more rapid decline of rCBF values with advancing age (99,127,150), resulting in a uniform shift of their CBF values below resting values of their nonrisk-factored counterparts. Regional declines resembled those of the normal nonrisk-factored group. The mechanism for enhanced rate of decline was presumed to be due to an increase in the rate of cerebral atherosclerosis, which was later confirmed in tests of cerebral vasodilator and vasoconstrictor responses, which likewise decline with age.

Risk-factored and nonrisk-factored, healthy, aged volunteers have recently been studied longitudinally over a course of 42 months (92,126) and more recently up to 48 months. In addition, other groups of patients with transient ischemic attacks (TIA), stroke, and MID were similarly studied prospectively over the same period. The longitudinal data confirmed that healthy, nonrisk-factored, elderly subjects showed reductions in resting CBF with the passage of time. Normal volunteers with risk factors showed similar but more rapid rates of decline and their gray flow values were consistently lower. The rate of CBF decline was even more rapid in patients with TIA, and most severe declines occurred in those with completed strokes and MID. In summary, the normal decline of rCBF with advancing age is accelerated in a stepwise fashion by successive stages of severity of cerebrovascular disease.

CBF Measurements and Alcoholism

CBF has been measured in alcoholic patients during withdrawal from acute excess and following delirium tremens using the nitrous oxide method (44) and was found to be decreased together with cerebral utilization of oxygen and glucose. Following abstinence, CBF tended to become more restored to normal levels while cerebral utilization of oxygen and glucose also increased but remained reduced.

Berglund and associates (11,13) examined serial rCBF measures in chronic alcoholics during various withdrawal periods from alcohol. During the first two days of withdrawal, a mean global rCBF reduction of 19% was found, followed by rapid return toward normal levels during the following week of abstinence. The degree of rCBF reduction correlated significantly with a measure of confusion. Patients with the longest preceding drinking period demonstrated the most pronounced initial decreases in CBF, which was symmetrical over both hemispheres.

Recovery of function was examined in a small group of chronic alcoholics who were followed over a 7-week period of abstinence (15) using serial measures of the ^{133}Xe inhalation technique. Results indicated that after the first week of abstinence, there were no further increases in mean CBF. One patient with alcoholic hallucinosis who actively experienced auditory hallucinations during rCBF measurement showed elevations in the left Sylvian fissure while another with both visual and auditory hallucinations manifested higher occipital and temporal-parietal flows (14).

Heiss and associates (61) compared chronic alcoholic patients with a group of control subjects utilizing the ^{133}Xe intracarotid bolus injection method and the gamma camera. Mean CBF, gray matter flow, and weight of gray matter were significantly reduced in chronic alcoholics. The reductions in CBF were proportional to the severity of the alcoholic encephalopathy.

Regional cerebral blood flow in 60 alcoholic patients was found to be significantly reduced relative to healthy controls and to patients with Wernicke-Korsakoff's disease (12). Flow values demonstrated significant declines with age, though young alcoholics showed similar flow values to young healthy controls and alcoholics over age 50 exhibited flow values commensurate with presenile dementia. In his review of the literature, Berglund (11) concluded that age-related declines in CBF were more pronounced in alcoholics, which suggested accelerated effects of normal aging.

Wernicke-Korsakoff's Disease

Using the nitrous oxide method, Shimojho and co-workers (128) examined patients with Wernicke-Korsakoff's disease within 5 to 28 days following initial hospital admission. CBF, cerebral oxygen consumption, and glucose metabolism were found to be strikingly reduced below normal levels and remained reduced for several weeks after treatment. In contrast, Berglund and Ingvar (12) measured rCBF values in patients with treated Korsakoff's disease of long-standing nature utilizing the ^{133}Xe intracarotid technique. rCBF was found comparable to that of normal healthy controls and significantly higher than that of alcoholics without Wernicke-Korsakoff's disease, suggesting some improvement with treatment despite chronicity of symptoms.

Activation Studies of CBF

Cerebrovascular capacitance has been tested by measuring rCBF before and during hypocapnia induced by hyperventilation, hypercarbia induced by 5% carbon dioxide (CO_2), and hyperoxia by inhalation of 100% oxygen. CO_2 is a cerebral vasodilator and oxygen, a cerebral vasoconstrictor.

Cerebral vasodilator responses to hypercarbia were measured in a group of normal healthy volunteers without risk factors for cerebrovascular disease (150). The CO_2 response exhibited a linear and progressive decline with advancing age. The vasodilator response to hypercarbia was diffuse and symmetrical in normal subjects and in patients with DAT, whereas in patients with MID, multifocal reduced responses were found.

In normal volunteers with risk factors, cerebral vasodilator responses to CO_2 were reduced to a greater extent than in healthy normals without risk factors. Patients with chronic infarction, ischemia with TIA, and VBI showed even greater reductions in CO_2 responsiveness.

Vasoconstrictive responsiveness in aging has been measured both by inhalation of 100% oxygen (3) and by hyperventilation-induced hypocapnia (91,147). Cerebral vasoconstriction responses were found to be progressively decreased with advancing age from the second through ninth decades.

DAT and MID

Numerous studies have documented reductions of both CBF and of cerebral oxygen consumption in aged subjects with dementia that exceed those seen in age-matched controls (59,80,81,106,128). However, in early or mild DAT, rCBF may present as relatively normal. Obrist (103) compared CBF values in a group of patients with dementia with a normal elderly group and a group of normal young subjects. The normal elderly group demonstrated a 28% reduction in gray matter flow values compared with the young normals. However, the dementia group, who were an average of 20 years younger than the elderly normals, showed a 38% reduction relative to young controls.

In DAT, rCBF values are diffusely reduced but most marked in both frontal (67,70,149) and frontotemporal regions (106) and occasionally in bilateral temporo-occipital parietal regions (67,68,70). The reduction of rCBF in DAT has been found to correlate with clinical symptomology as well as with the distribution of Alzheimer changes and atrophy reported at autopsy (56).

In DAT, rCBF reductions are symmetrical and diffuse (59,100,114,149), which is attributed to the diffuse decline in neuronal function and metabolism in DAT with a secondary readjustment in rCBF in response to decreased demand. In MID, there are patchy multifocal reductions corresponding to infarcted regions with relatively normal flow in nonischemic portions of the brain (59,100,114,149). Such variable and asymmetrical patterns of CBF reflect the basic character of the disease (55,149).

The cerebrovascular capacitance response to hypercapnia in DAT and MID has been investigated in earlier CBF studies with mixed results, but, in general, CO_2 responsiveness was found to be reduced in vascular dementia and relatively preserved in DAT (148–150). Yamaguchi et al. (149) tested the responsiveness to CO_2 inhalation (5%) in DAT and MID patients. The CO_2 response was well preserved and symmetrical in the DAT group, in contrast to the MID group, which displayed significantly decreased responsiveness in a patchy distribution analogous to the areas affected by vascular damage due to infarction.

Cerebral vasoconstrictor responsiveness during 100% oxygen inhalation was tested in dementia by Amano et al. (3). In DAT, the response was normal, showing no difference from age-matched controls. Regional responses were diffuse and symmetrical without differences between hemispheres. On the other hand, responsiveness in the MID group was again patchy and nonhomogenous. Responses were asymmetrical between hemispheres and also differed within the hemispheres in a distribution that correlated with zones of multiple cerebral infarctions. In some cases, there were paradoxical vasodilatory responses.

Results with inhalation of 100% oxygen suggest that this test is a safe, reliable technique for differentiation of DAT and MID. The normal CBF responsiveness of DAT during CO_2 and oxygen inhalation confirms the pathological nature of the disorder, which is a primary neuronal degenerative disorder with little or no vascular pathology.

Behavioral Activation

Meyer and associates tested cerebrovascular functional reserve in demented patients using a standard procedure for psychophysiological activation (91,149). DAT and MID patients as well as alcoholic patients with Wernicke-Korsakoff's disease showed an absence of significant CBF increases during the activation procedure, unlike those consistently found in normal controls of all ages. The data were interpreted as indicating a failure of local activation of the regional cortical neurons as well as diminished activation of the reticular activating system in these late forms of organic dementia.

In other studies of moderately impaired DAT patients, Ingvar et al. (69) examined rCBF changes measured before and during presentation of a more complex activation procedure, the Raven's Progressive Matrices. In the activation run, only minimal generalized increases were noted in hemispheric CBF with marked individual variability in regional pattern, direction, and extent of change. However, there was evidence for reduced responses to mental activation in association areas. In the Largen et al. (79) study also employing the Raven's Progressive Matrices, patients with mild or early DAT showed excessive CBF increases bilaterally. The data were interpreted as indicating greater "brain work" and/or arousal during attempts to solve the nonverbal reasoning tasks.

Stable Xenon-Enhanced CT in Aging and Dementia

The CT CBF technique is a recent technical development that permits quantitative measurement of local cerebral blood flow (LCBF) in three dimensions with excellent resolution (40,93,95). In addition, local blood-brain partition coefficients ($L\lambda$) may be measured for each region of interest rather than assigning assumed normal values.

In normal healthy volunteers, gray matter of the cortex as well as subcortical structures including basal ganglia and thalamus showed significant age-related declines of LCBF with normal $L\lambda$ values up to the ninth decade (4,95). There were also significant declines in white matter flow with advancing age, but these were not as marked as those seen in gray matter. Patients with TIA showed reduced LCBF but normal $L\lambda$ values. However, patients with stroke showed areas of zero flow and bordering areas of reduced LCBF and $L\lambda$ values. In DAT, LCBF values were diffusely and severely reduced in the cortex and thalamus compared with age-matched controls, and the severity of LCBF reduction correlated with severity of dementia. In addition, basal ganglia and white matter flow were not significantly different from age-matched normals (4,95). In MID patients there were multiple focal zones of reduced LCBF, often with reduced $L\lambda$ values.

Positron Emission Tomography in Aging and Dementia

Regional cerebral glucose and oxygen metabolism have now been measured by cross-sectional analysis in normal aging and dementia using positron emission tomography (PET) scanning. These methods involve labeling of the substrates to be measured by short-lived, positron-emitting radionuclides. Utilizing the (^{18}F) fluorodeoxyglucose (FDG) method, Kuhl and associates (77) reported a gradual decrease in mean local cerebral glucose metabolism with advancing age, which was symmetrical and relatively homogeneous throughout the cerebral cortex, cau-

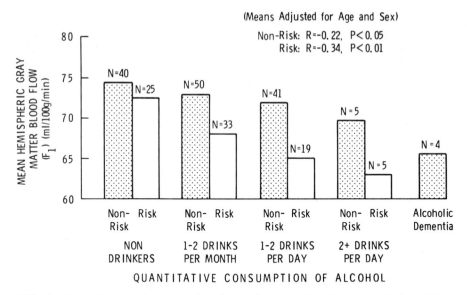

FIG. 1. Comparisons between quantity of alcohol consumed and mean hemispheric blood flow of gray matter in normal volunteers without other risk factors, normal volunteers with risk factors, and alcoholics with Wernicke-Korsakoff dementia. Enhanced reduction of gray matter blood flow is illustrated (which was measured by the ^{133}Xe inhalation method) when plotted against the amount of habitual consumption of alcohol among drinkers and compared with nondrinkers. The nonrisk group consisted of subjects without any risk factors for stroke whereas the risk group consisted of subjects with hypertension, hyperlipidemia, heart disease, and/or diabetes. The alcohol dementia group (who suffered from chronic Wernicke - Korsakoff dementia) show further reductions of CBF associated with their irreversible alcoholic encephalopathy.

date nucleus, and thalamus. Furthermore, age-related declines were maximal in frontal regions similar to the previously described rCBF declines. The declines in regional cerebral glucose consumption with advancing age have been confirmed in other laboratories (1). In addition, there is an accompanying decline in regional oxygen consumption with advancing age.

Regional glucose metabolism has also been measured in DAT (1,10,47) where there was a bilateral and diffuse reduction of glucose metabolism, particularly in the frontal and parietal cortex and thalamus (10). Such changes have been found to correlate with performance on cognitive tests (47). These metabolic data are consistent with the rCBF data reported earlier.

RECENT STUDIES CORRELATING CBF WITH ALCOHOL CONSUMPTION IN AGING POPULATIONS

A large pool of normal aged volunteers has been studied prospectively in order to correlate ^{133}Xe inhalation measurements of rCBF with multiple risk factors for cerebral vasular disease and stroke, including alcohol consumption (92,125). These nonalcoholic neurologically intact subjects were classified into groups according to their alcohol consumption. Figure 1 illustrates data on group differences in rCBF values (gray flow) measured in this laboratory and compares them with similar measurements in Wernicke-Korsakoff's disease. The nonrisk-factored group represented optimally healthy volunteers, ranging in age from 43 to 98 years (mean age of 60 years), without risk factors for cerebrovascular disease. These histograms reveal significant declines in resting rCBF, which correlates with the quantity of alcohol consumed on a regular basis. These declines cannot be explained on the basis of age or sex, which were statistically controlled. Particularly noteworthy was the observation that in aged patients, even relatively mild consumption of alcohol appears to be associated with slight CBF declines, and the greater the mean consumption of alcohol, the lower the resting rCBF. The majority of subjects in the "2 or more drinks per day" group consumed considerably more alcohol than indicated by the histogram label. The group showing lowest mean rCBF values were patients under treatment with well-established, chronic Wernicke-Korsakoff's disease due to severe alcoholism. These findings were cross-validated by comparison with a second group of elderly volunteers of similar age but with risk factors for atherosclerosis. The same pattern of significantly enhanced decline in rCBF values was evidenced, which correlates with the volume of alcohol consumed on a regular basis. As reported from this laboratory previously, rCBF findings among normal volunteers with risk factors displayed rCBF levels below that of their nonrisk-factored counterparts, and these reductions were enhanced by a history of chronic alcohol ingestion.

SUMMARY AND CONCLUSIONS

Evidence has been summarized indicating that with advancing age, there are significant and progressive age-related declines in brain morphology, histology, neurotransmitter functioning, neuropsychological functioning, and rCBF and metabolism. The morphological declines result in progressive loss of neuronal reserve, and the potential redundancy of function is lost, eventually leading to functional decline, which fosters the development of dementia (10). Direct toxic and secondary effects of prolonged ingestion of alcohol are likewise associated with cerebral atrophy, neuronal loss, and disruption of neurotransmitter functioning. In chronic alcoholism, these changes may occur prior to brain atrophy due to age-related effects, although CT data have indeed confirmed that alcoholics develop cerebral atrophy at an enhanced rate, placing them at greater risk for functional impairment. Combined effects of chronic alcoholism and advancing age are additive in nature, exacerbating the effects of either alone.

Normal aging is also associated with progressive declines in neuropsychological functioning, especially those abilities of an integrative nature and immediate adaptive ability. Neuropsychological functioning, like EEG, has been shown to be adversely affected by disease factors, particularly cerebrovascular and cardiovascular disease, conditions common in the elderly. Neuropsychological functions most sensitive to normal aging are also the most sensitive to the toxic effects of chronic alcoholism, and severity of dysfunction tends to be correlated with the duration of alcoholism as well as with daily average consumption. Patterns of neuropsychological deficits in young alcoholics resemble the patterns of elderly nonalcoholics. Furthermore, advancing age adversely affects both the degree of neuropsychological dysfunction as well as the potential for recovery in alcoholics. In summary, chronic alcoholism in the young results in a pattern of premature or accelerated aging. The aging brain is much more susceptible to the ill-effects of chronic alcoholism later in life.

Cross-sectional and longitudinal studies have systematically demonstrated that with normal aging, there are significant declines in CBF and metabolism not attributable to disease factors. [133]Xenon inhalation studies of optimally healthy volunteers demonstrate that gray matter blood flow shows a significant decline with advancing age, most rapid decreases occurring in prefrontal regions. Cerebrovascular responsiveness to hypercarbia and hyperoxia likewise exhibits a progressive decline with advancing age. Normal and otherwise healthy volunteers with risk factors for cerebroatherosclerosis manifest lower rCBF values across all ages and demonstrate enhanced age-related rates of rCBF decrease. Progressive declines in rCBF with advancing age are accelerated in a stepwise fashion by successive severities of involvement by cerebrovascular disease. Normal volunteers with risk factors show reduced CO_2 cerebral vasomotor responsiveness compared with their nonrisk-factored counterparts, whereas patients with chronic infarction or TIA show even greater reductions in cerebral vasomotor responsiveness. CBF declines with normal advancing age because of two major factors: (a) abiotrophy of the cerebrum with decline in neuronal population and associated reduction in metabolic demand and (b) progressive rigidity of the cerebral vessels as a function of arteriosclerosis.

Available studies indicate that rCBF is reduced in chronic alcoholism and that age-related declines become more pronounced in alcoholics, suggesting that alcoholism accelerates the normal effects of aging. In this laboratory, measurements indicate significant declines in resting rCBF, correlating with increased consumption of alcohol in otherwise optimally healthy elderly volunteers. These observations were also replicated in independent groups of aged volunteers with risk factors for atherosclerosis when those who drank alcohol were compared with those who did not.

When neuropathological, neuropsychological, CBF, and metabolic dysfunctions are examined in two major forms of dementing disorders with independent etiologies (DAT, a degenerative disorder of the central nervous system, and MID, a cerebrovascular disorder), both types of dementia are characterized by intellectual loss and memory deficits, the specific neuropsychological patterns reflecting the nature and distribution of the respective cerebral pathologies. rCBF is diffusely reduced in DAT whereas MID is characterized by patchy, multifocal reductions corresponding to infarcted regions. Cerebrovascular responsiveness to CO_2 and 100% oxygen is well preserved and symmetrical in DAT but is significantly decreased in a patchy manner in MID. Tests of rCBF responsiveness confirm that the enhanced rate of rCBF decline in risk-factored volunteers is due to an increased rate of cerebral atherosclerosis superimposed on normal age-related brain atrophy.

Further studies are indicated to elucidate complex interactions between chronic alcoholism and normal advancing age. The abiotrophy in aging appears to be enhanced by the toxic effects of alcoholism. Neuropathological changes characteristic of chronic alcoholism combine with those of advancing age in an additive fashion and in some cases culminate in neuronal loss beyond a "neuronal threshold" of loss, which results in premature dementia (134–136). Secondary effects of alcoholism include poor nutrition, head injury, delirium tremens, alcoholic hallucinosis, and epilepsy, which may be expected to exacerbate cerebral functional decline. There are studies suggesting that acute alcohol ingestion and chronic alcoholism may adversely affect cardiac functioning and impair CBF (24,76). Furthermore, there is some evidence that chronic alcohol ingestion may be associated with an increased risk for stroke (63,82), either directly or indirectly (73,110).

ACKNOWLEDGMENTS

This research was supported by the Veterans Administration, Washington, D.C.; United State Public Health Service Grant NSO9287; and the Texas Department of Mental Health and Mental Retardation.

REFERENCES

1. Alavi, A., Ferris, S., Wolf, A., Christman, D., Folwer, J., MacGregor, R., Farkas, T., Greenberg, J., Dann, R., and Reivich, M. (1981): Determination of regional cerebral metabolism in dementia using F-18 deoxyglucose and positron emission tomograph. *Cerebral Vascular Disease 3*, 10th Salzburg Conference, International Congress Series 532, Excerpta Medica: pp. 109–112.
2. Albert, M. S., Butters, N., and Levin, J. (1979): Temporal gradients in the retrograde amnesia of patients with alcoholic Korsakoff's Disease. *Arch. Neurol.*, 36:211–216.
3. Amano, T., Meyer, J. S., Okabe, T., Shaw, T., and Mortel, K. F. (1982): *Cerebral Vasomotor Responses During Oxygen Inhalation: Results in Normal Aging Versus Dementia (in press).*
4. Amano, T., Meyer, J. S., Okabe, T., Shaw, T., and Mortel, K. (1983): Stable xenon CT cerebral blood flow measurements computed by a single compartment-double integration mode in normal aging and dementia. *Comput. Assist. Tomogr.*, 6:923–932.
5. Bak, J. S., and Greene, R. L. (1980): Changes in neuropsychological functioning in an aging population. *J. Consult. Clin. Psychol.*, 48:395–399.
6. Ball, M. J. (1977): Neuronal loss, neurofibrillary tangles and granulovaculor degeneration in the hippocampus with normal aging and dementia: A quantitative study. *Acta Neuropath.*, 37:111–118.
7. Barron, S. A., Jacobs, L., and Kinkel, W. R. (1976): Changes in size of normal lateral ventricles during aging determined by computerized tomography. *Neurology*, 26:1011–1013.
8. Bartus, R. T., Dean, R. L., Beer, B., and Lippa, A. S. (1982): The cholinergic hypothesis of geriatric memory dysfunction. *Science*, 217:408–417.
9. Bayles, K. A. (1982): The use of language tasks in identifying etiologically different dementias. *Int. Neuropsychol. Soc.*, Pittsburgh, PA.
10. Benson, D., Kuhl, D., Phelps, M., Cummings, J., and Tsai, S. (1981): Positron emission computed tomography in the diagnosis of dementia. *Ann. Neurol.*, 10:76.
11. Berglund, M. (1981): Cerebral blood flow in chronic alcoholics. *Alcoholism: Clinical and Experimental Research.* 5:295–303.
12. Berglund, M., and Ingvar, D. H. (1976): Cerebral blood flow and its regional distribution in alcoholism and in Korsakoff's psychosis. *J. Stud. Alcohol*, 37:586–597.
13. Berglund, M., and Risberg, J. (1977): Regional cerebral blood flow during alcohol withdrawal related to consumption and clinical symptomatology, *Acta Neurol. Scand.*, 56(Suppl 64):480–481.

14. Berglund, M., and Risberg, J. (1981): Regional cerebral blood flow during alcohol withdrawal. *Arch. Gen. Psychiatry,* 38:351–355.
15. Berglund, M., Bliding, G., Bliding, A., and Risberg, J. (1980): Reversibility of cerebral dysfunction in alcoholism during the first seven weeks of abstinence—a regional cerebral blood flow study. *Acta Psychiatr. Scand.,* 62(Suppl. 286):119–127.
16. Birren, J. E., and Schaie, K. W. (1977): *Handbook of Psychology of Aging.* Van Nostrand Reinhold, NY.
17. Birren, J. S., Woods, A. M., and Williams, M. V. (1979): Speed of behavior as an indicator of age changes and the integrity of the nervous system. In: *Brain Function in Old Age: Evaluation of Changes and Disorders,* edited by F. Hoffmeister, C. Muller, and H. P. Krause. Springer-Verlag, NY.
18. Blessed, G., Tomlinson, B. E., and Roth, M. (1968): The association between quantitative measures of dementia and of senile change in the cerebral gray matter of elderly subjects. *Br. J. Psychiatry,* 114:797–811.
19. Blusewicz, M. J., Dustman, R. E., Schenkenberg, T., and Beck, E. C. (1977): Neuropsychological correlates of chronic alcoholism and aging. *J. Nerv. Ment. Dis.,* 165:348–355.
20. Blusewicz, M. J., Schenkenberg, T., Dustman, R. E., and Beck, E. C. (1977): WAIS performance in young normal, young alcoholic, and elderly normal groups: An evaluation of organicity and mental aging indices. *J. Clin. Psychol.,* 33:1149–1153.
21. Botwinick, J. (1978): *Aging and Behavior,* Springer-Verlag, New York.
22. Brinkman, S. A., Sarwar, M., Levin, H. S., and Morris, H. H. (1981): Quantitative indexes of computed tomography in dementia and normal aging. *Radiology,* 138:89–92.
23. Brody, H. (1955): Organization of the cerebral cortex (Part 3). *J. Comp. Neurol.,* 102:511–556.
24. Burch, G. H., and Giles, T. D. (1974): Alcoholic cardiomyopathy. In: *The Biology of Alcoholism,* Vol. 3, edited by B. Kissen and H. Begleiter. Plenum Press, NY.
25. Butters, N. (1979): Amnesic disorders. In: *Clinical Neuropsychology,* edited by K. M. Heilman and E. Valenstein. Oxford University Press, New York.
26. Butters, N., and Cermak, L. S. (1980): *Alcoholic Korsakoff's Syndrome.* Academic Press, NY.
27. Cala, L. A., Jones, B., Mastaglia, F. L., and Wiley, B. (1978): Brain atrophy and intellectual impairment in heavy drinkers—a clinical, psychometric and computerized tomography study. *Aust. NZ J. Med.,* 8:147–153.
28. Carlen, P. L., Wilkinson, D. A., Wortzman, G., Holgate, R., Cordingley, J., Lee, M. A., Huszar, L., Moddel, G., Singh, R., Kiraly, L., and Rankin, J. G. (1981): Cerebral atrophy and functional deficits in alcoholics without clinically apparent liver disease. *Neurology,* 31:377–385.
29. Carlen, P. L., Wortzman, G., Holgate, R. C., Wilkinson, D. A., and Rankin, J. G. (1978): Reversible cerebral atrophy in recently abstinent chronic alcoholics measured by computed tomography scans. *Science,* 200:1076–1078.
30. Carlsson, C., Claeson, L. C., Karlsson, K. I., and Pettersson, L. F. (1979): Clinical, psychometric and radiological signs of brain damage in chronic alcoholism. *Acta Neurol. Scand.,* 60:85–92.
31. Chmielewski, C., and Golden, C. J. (1980): Alcoholism and brain damage: An investigation using the Luria-Nebraska neuropsychological battery. *Int. J. Neurosci.,* 10:99–105.
32. Constantinidis, J. (1978): Is Alzheimer's Disease a major form of senile dementia? Clinical, anatomical, and genetic data. In: *Aging, Vol. 7, Alzheimer's Disease: Senile Dementia and Related Disorders,* edited by R. Katzman, R. D. Terry, and K. L. Bick. Raven Press, NY.
33. Corsellis, J. A. N. (1962): *Mental Illness With Aging Brain.* Maudsley Monograph 9, Oxford University Press, London.
34. Courville, C. B. (1955): *Effects of Alcohol in the Nervous System of Man.* San Lucas Press, Los Angeles, CA.
35. Craik, F. I. M. (1977): Age differences in human memory. In: *Handbook of the Psychology of Aging,* edited by J. E. Birren and K. W. Schaie. Van Nostrand Reinhold, NY.
36. Dastur, D. K., Lane, M. H., Hansen, D. B., Kety, S. S., Butler, R. N., Perlin, S., and Sokoloff, L. (1963): In: *Human Aging: A Biological and Behavioral Study,* edited by J. E. Birren, R. N. Butler, S. W. Greenhouse, L. Sokoloff, and M. R. Yarrow, NSPHS Publication No. 986, U.S. Government Printing Office, Washington, DC.
37. Davies, P., and Malone, A. J. F. (1976): Selective loss of cholinergic neurons in Alzheimer's Disease. *Lancet,* 2:1403.
38. Dorfman, L. J., and Bosley, T. M. (1979): Age-related changes in peripheral and central nerve conduction in man. *Neurology,* 29:38–44.

39. Drachman, D. A. (1977): Memory and cognitive function in man: Does the cholinergic system have a specific role? *Neurology*, 27:783–790.
40. Drayer, B. P., Wolfson, S. K., Reinmuth, O. M., Dujovny, M., Boehnke, M., and Cook, T. F. (1978): Xenon enhanced CT for analysis of cerebral integrity, perfusion, and blood flow. *Stroke*, 9:123–130.
41. Earnest, M. P., Heaton, R. K., Wilkinson, W. G., and Manke, W. F. (1979): Cortical atrophy, ventricular enlargement, and intellectual impairment in the aged. *Neurology*, 29:1138–1143.
42. Eckardt, M. J., Parker, E. S., Noble, E. P., Feldman, D. J., and Gottschalk, L. A. (1978): Relationship between neuropsychological performance and alcohol consumption in alcoholics. *Biol. Psychiatry*, 13:551–565.
43. Eisdorfer, C., and Wilkie, F. (1977): Stress, disease, aging and behavior. In: *Handbook of the Psychology of Aging*, edited by J. E. Birren and K. W. Schaie, Van Nostrand Reinhold, NY.
44. Eisenberg, S. (1968): Cerebral blood flow and metabolism in patients with delirium tremens. *Clin. Res.*, 16:71.
45. Ellenberg, L., Rosenbaum, G., Goldman, M. S., and Whitman, R. D.: Recoverability of psychological functioning following alcohol abuse: Lateralization effects. *J. Consult. Clin. Psychol.*, 48:503–510.
46. Ernst, A. J., Dempster, J. P., Yee, R., St. Dennis, C., and Nakand, L. (1976): Alcohol toxicity, blood alcohol concentration and body water in young and adult rats. *J. Stud. Alcohol*, 37:347–356.
47. Ferris, S. H., de Leon, M. J., Wolf, A. P., Farkas, T., Christman, D. R., Reisberg, B., Fowler, J. S., MacGregor, R., Goldman, A., George, A. E., Fowler, J. S., MacGregor, R., Goldman, A., George, A. E., and Rampal, S. (1980): Positron emission tomography in the study of aging and senile dementia. *Neurobiol. Aging*, 1:127–131.
48. Fitzhugh, L., Fitzhugh, K., and Reitan, R. (1965): Adaptive abilities and intellectual functioning of hospitalized alcoholics: Further considerations. *J. Stud. Alcohol*, 26:402–411.
49. Freund, G. (1973): Chronic central nervous system toxicity of alcohol. *Annu. Rev. Pharm.*, 13:217–277.
50. Fuld, P. A. (1978): Psychological testing in the differential diagnosis of the dementias. In: *Aging, Vol. 7, Alzheimer Disease: Senile Dementia and Related Disorders*, edited by R. Katzman, R. D. Terry, and K. L. Bick. Raven Press, NY.
51. Fuld, P. A., Katzman, R., Davies, P., and Terry, R. D. (1982): Intrusions as a sign of Alzheimer dementia: Chemical and pathological verification. *Ann. Neurol.*, 11:155–159.
52. Gianotti, G., Caltagirone, C., Masullo, C., and Miceli, G. (1980): Patterns of neuropsychological impairment in various diagnostic groups of dementia. In: *Aging, Vol. 13, Aging of the Brain and Dementia*, edited by L. Amaducci, A. N. Davison, and P. Antuono, Raven Press, NY.
53. Goodwin, D. W., and Hill, S. Y. (1975): Chronic effects of alcohol and other psychoactive drugs on intellect, learning and memory. In: *Alcohol, Drugs and Brain Damage*, edited by G. Rankin. Addition Research Foundation, Toronto.
54. Grenell, R. G. (1972): Effects of alcohol on the neuron. In: *The Biology of Aging*, Vol. 2, edited by N. Kissen and H. Begleiter. Plenum Press, NY.
55. Gustafson, L., and Risberg, J. (1979): Regional cerebral blood flow measurements by the ^{133}Xe inhalation technique in differential diagnosis of dementia. *Acta Neurol. Scand.*, 60(Suppl 72):546–547.
56. Gustafson, L., Brun, A., and Ingvar, D. H. (1977): Presenile dementia: Clinical symptoms, pathoanatomical findings and cerebral blood flow. In: *Cerebral Vascular Disease*, edited by J. S. Meyer, H. Lechner, M. Reivich. Excerpta Medica, Amsterdam/Oxford.
57. Gyldensted, C. (1977): Measurements of the normal ventricular system and hemispheric sulci of 100 adults with computed tomography. *Neuroradiology*, 14:183–192.
58. Hachinski, V., Lassen, N. A., and Marshall, J. (1974): Multi-infarct dementia. *Lancet*, 2:207–209.
59. Hachinski, V. C., Iliff, L. D., Zilhka, E., Duboulay, G. H., McAllister, V. L., Marshall, J., Russell, R. W. R., and Symon, L. (1975): Cerebral blood flow in dementia. *Arch. Neurol.*, 32:632–637.
60. Haug, J. O. (1968): Pneumoencephalographic evidence of brain damage in chronic alcoholics. *Acta Psychiatr. Scand.*, 44(Suppl 203):135–143.
61. Heiss, W. D., Kufferle, B., Demel, I., Reisnel, T., and Roszuczky, A. (1976): Cerebral blood flow and severity of mental dysfunction in chronic alcoholism. In: *Cerebral Vascular Disease*,

edited by J. S. Meyer, M. Reivich, and H. Lechner. 17th Int. Conf., Salzburg, Georg Thieme, Stuttgart, 89–93.

62. Henderson, G., Tomlinson, B. E., and Gibson, P. H. (1980): Cell counts in human cerebral cortex in normal adults throughout life using an image analyzing computer. *J. Neurol. Sci.*, 46:113–136.

63. Hillbom, M., and Kaste, M. (1978): Does ethanol intoxication promote brain infarction in young adults? *Lancet*, 2:1181–1183.

64. Hochla, N. A. N., and Parsons, O. A. (1982): Premature aging in female alcoholics: A neuropsychological study. *J. Nerv. Ment. Dis.*, 170:241–245.

65. Huckman, M. S., Fox, J., and Topel, J. (1975): The validity of criteria for the evaluation of cerebral atrophy by computed tomography. *Radiology*, 116:85–94.

66. Inglis, J. (1970): Memory disorder. In: *Symptoms of Psychopathology*, edited by C. G. Costello, John Wiley and Sons, NY.

67. Ingvar, D. H., and Lassen, N. A. (1979): Activity Distribution in the Cerebral Cortex in Organic Dementia as Reviewed by Measurements of Cerebral Blood Flow. In: *Brain Function in Old Age*, edited by F. Hoffmeister, C. Muller, and H. P. Krause. Springer-Verlag, NY.

68. Ingvar, D. H., and Gustafson, L. (1970): Regional cerebral blood flow in organic dementia with early onset. *Acta Neurol. Scand.*, 46(Suppl 43):42–73.

69. Ingvar, D. H., Risberg, J., Schwartz, M. S. (1975): Evidence of subcortical function of association cortex in presenile dementia. *Neurology*, 25:964–974.

70. Ingvar, D. H., Brun, A., Hagberg, B., and Gustafson, L. (1978): Regional Cerebral Blood Flow in the Dominent Hemisphere in Confirmed Cases of Alzheimer's Disease, Pick's Disease, and Multi-Infarct Dementia: Relationships to Clinical Symptomatology, and Neuropathological Findings. In: *Alzheimer's Disease*, edited by R. Katzman, R. D. Terry, and K. L. Bick. Raven Press, NY.

71. Jones, B., and Parsons, O. A. (1972): Specific vs generalized deficits of abstracting ability in chronic alcoholics. *Arch. Gen. Psychiatry*, 26:380–384.

72. Kety, S. S. (1956): Human cerebral blood flow and oxygen consumption as related to aging. *Res. Publ. Assoc. Res. Nerv. Ment. Dis.*, 31:31–45.

73. Klatsky, A. L., Friedman, G. D., Siegelaub, A. B., and Gerald, M. J. (1977): Alcohol consumption and blood pressure: Kaiser-Permanente multiphasic health examination data. *N. Engl. J. Med.*, 296:1194–2000.

74. Kleinknect, R. A., and Goldstein, S. G. (1972): Neuropsychological deficits associated with alcoholism. *J. Stud. Alcohol*, 33:999–1019.

75. Kroll, P., Seigel, R., O'Neill, B., and Edwards, R. P. (1980): Cerebral cortical atrophy in alcoholic men. *J. Clin. Psychiatry*, 41:417–421.

76. Knott, D. H., and Beard, J. D. (1972): Changes in cardiovascular activity as a function of alcohol intake. In: *The Biology of Alcoholism*, edited by B. Kissen and H. Begleiter. Plenum Press, NY.

77. Kuhl, D. E., Metter, E. J., Reige, W. H., and Phelps, M. E. (1982): Effects of human aging in patterns of local cerebral glucose utilization determined by the (^{18}F) fluorodeoxyglucose method. *J. Cereb. Blood Flow Metab.*, 2:163–171.

78. Largen, J. W., Sheer, D., and Faibish, G. (1981): Verbal and nonverbal remote memory in early Alzheimer's Disease. *American Psychological Association*, Los Angeles.

79. Largen, J. W., Shaw, T., Weinman, M., and Meyer, J. S. (1981): Order effects and responsiveness of regional cerebral blood flow in early putative Alzheimer's Disease. *J. Cereb. Blood Flow Metab.*, (Suppl), 1:483–484.

80. Lassen, N. A., Feinberg, I., and Lane, M. H. (1960): Bilateral studies of cerebral oxygen uptake in young and normal subjects and in patients with organic dementia. *J. Clin. Invest.*, 39:491–500.

81. Lassen, N. A., Munck, O., and Tottey, E. R. (1957): Mental function and cerebral oxygen consumption in organic dementia. *Arch. Neurol. Psychiatry*, 77:126–133.

82. Lee, K. (1979): Alcoholism and cerebrovascular thrombosis in the young. *Acta Neurol. Scand.*, 59:270–274.

83. Lishman, W. A., Ron, M., and Acker, W. (1980): Computed tomography of the brain and psychometric assessment of alcoholic patients—a British study. In: *Psychopharmacology of Alcohol*, edited by M. Sandur. Raven Press, NY.

84. Logue, P., and Wyrick, L. (1979): Initial validation of Russell's revised Wechsler memory scales: A comparison of normal aging versus dementia. *J. Consult. Clin. Psychol.*, 47:176–178.

85. Long, J. A., and McLachlan, F. C. (1974): Abstract reasoning and perceptual–motor efficiency in alcoholics. *J. Stud. Alcohol*, 35:1220–1229.
86. Lynch, M. J. G. (1960): Brain lesions in chronic alcoholism. *Arch. Path.*, 69:342–353.
87. Marsh, G. R., and Thompson, L. W. (1977): Psychophysiology of aging. In: *Handbook of the Psychology of Aging*, edited by J. E. Birren and K. W. Schaie. Van Nostrand Reinhold, NY.
88. Mathew, N. T. Meyer, J. S., Achari, A. N., Dodson, R. F. (1976): Hyperlipidemia, neuropathy and dementia. *Eur. Neurol.*, 14:370–382.
89. McGeer, P. L., and McGeer, E. G. (1975): Age changes in human for some enzymes associated with metabolism of catecholamines, GABA, and acetylcholine. In: *Neurobiology of Aging*, edited by J. M. Ordy and K. B. Brisse. Plenum Press, NY.
90. Melamed, E., Lavy, S., Bentin, S., Cooper, G., and Rinot, Y. (1980): Reduction in regional cerebral blood flow during normal aging in man. *Stroke*, 11:31–35.
91. Meyer, J. S. (1978): Improved method for noninvasive measurement of regional cerebral blood flow by [133]xenon inhalation (Part II). *Stroke*, 9:205–210.
92. Meyer, J. S., and Shaw, T. (1984): Cerebral blood flow and aging. In: *Clinical Neurology of Aging*, edited by M. L. Albert. Oxford University Press *(in press)*.
93. Meyer, J. S., Hayman, L. A., Yamamoto, M., Sakai, F., and Nakajima, S. (1980): Local cerebral blood flow measured by CT after stable xenon inhalation. *AJNR*, 1:213–225.
94. Meyer, J. S., Ishihara, N., Deshmukh, V. D., Naritomi, H., Sakai, F., Hsu, M. C., and Pollack, P. C. (1978): An improved method for noninvasive measurement of regional cerebral blood flow by [133]xenon inhalation. (Part I). Description of method and normal values obtained in healthy volunteers. *Stroke*, 9:195–204.
95. Meyer, J. S., Hayman, L. A., Amano, T., Nakajima, S., Shaw, T., Lauzon, P., Derman, S., Karacan, I., and Harati, Y. (1981): Mapping local blood flow of the human brain by CT scanning during stable xenon inhalation. *Stroke*, 12:426–436.
96. Miller, E. (1974): Psychomotor performance in presenile dementia. *Psychosom. Med.*, 4:65–68.
97. Miller, E. (1977): *Abnormal Aging*. John Wiley and Sons, New York.
98. Naeser, M. A., Gebhardt, C., and Levine, H. L. (1980): Decreases computerized tomography number in patients with presenile dementia. *Arch. Neurol.*, 37:401–409.
99. Naritomi, H., Meyer, J. S., Sakai, F., Yamaguchi, F., and Shaw, T. (1979): Effects of normal advancing age on regional cerebral blood flow. Studies in normal subjects and subjects with risk factors for atherothrombotic stroke. *Arch. Neurol.*, 36:410–416.
100. Obrien, M. D., and Mallet, B. (1970): Cerebral cortex perfusion rates in dementia. *J. Neurol. Neurosurg. Psychiatry*, 33:497–500.
101. Obrist, W. D. (1963): The electroencephalogram of healthy aged males. In: *Human Aging 5: A Biological and Behavioral Study*, edited by J. G. Birren, R. N. Butler, S. W. Greenhouse, L. Sokoloff, and M. R. Yarrow. USPHS Publication No. 986, US Government Printing Office, Washington, DC.
102. Obrist, W. D. (1975): Cerebral physiology of the aged relation to psychological function. In: *Behavior and Brain Electrical Activity*, edited by N. Burch and H. I. Altshuler. Plenum Press, NY.
103. Obrist, W. D. (1978): Non-invasive studies of cerebral blood flow in aging and dementia. In: *Aging, Vol. 7, Alzheimer's Disease, Senile Dementia and Related Disorders*, edited by R. Katzman, R. D. Terry, and K. L. Bick. Raven Press, NY.
104. Obrist, W. D., and Bissell, L. F. (1955): The electroencephalogram in aged patients with cardiac and cerebral vascular disease. *J. Geront.*, 10:315–330.
105. Obrist, W. D., Busse, E. W., and Henry, C. E. (1961): Relation of electroencephalogram to blood pressure in elderly persons. *Neurology*, 11:151–158.
106. Obrist, W. D., Chivian, E., Cronquist, and Ingvar, D. H. (1970): Regional cerebral blood flow in senile and presenile dementia. *Neurology*, 20:315–322.
107. Obrist, W. D., Thompson, H. K., King, C. H., and Wang, H. S. (1967): Determination of regional cerebral blood flow by inhalation of [133]xenon. *Circ. Res.*, 20:124–135.
108. Obrist, W. D., Thompson, H. K., Wang, H. S., and Wilkinson, W. E. (1975): Regional cerebral blood flow estimated by [133]xenon inhalation. *Stroke*, 6:245–256.
109. Parker, E. S., and Noble, E. P. (1977): Alcohol consumption and cognitive functioning in social drinkers. *J. Stud. Alcohol*, 38:1224–1232.
110. Parsons, O. A., and Far, S. P. (1981): The neuropsychology of alcohol and drug use. In: *Handbook of Clinical Neuropsychology*, edited by S. B. Filskov and T. J. Boll. John Wiley and Sons, NY.

111. Pell, S., and D'Alonzo, C. A. (1968): The prevalence of chronic disease among problem drinkers. *Arch. Environ. Health*, 16:679–684.
112. Perez, F. I., Gay, J. R. A., Taylor, R. L., and Rivera, V. M. (1975): Patterns of memory performances in the neurologically impaired aged. *Can. J. Neurol. Sci.*, 2:347–355.
113. Perez, F. I., Rivera, V. M., and Meyer, J. S. (1975): Analysis of intellectual and cognitive performance in patients with multi-infarct dementia, vertebrobasilar insuffiency with dementia, and Alzheimer's Disease. *J. Neurol. Neurosurg. Psychiatry*, 38:533–540.
114. Perez, F. I., Mathew, N. T., Stump, D. A., and Meyer, J. S. (1977): Regional cerebral blood flow statistical patterns and psychological performance in multi-infarct dementia and Alzheimer's Disease. *J. Can. Neurol.*, :53–61.
115. Pirozzolo, F. J., and Hansch, E. C. (1981): Oculomotor reaction time in dementia reflects degree of cerebral dysfunction. *Science*, 214:349–351.
116. Pirozzolo, F. J., Christensen, K. J., Ogle, K. M., Hausch, E. C., and Thompson, W. G. (1981): Simple and choice reaction time in dementia: Clinical implications. *Neurobiol. Aging*, 2:113–117.
117. Reed, H. B. C., and Reitan, R. M. (1963): Changes in psychological test performance associated with the normal aging process. *J. Gerontol.*, 18:271–274.
118. Reitan, R. M. (1955): The distribution according to age of a psychologic measure dependent upon organic brain functions. *J. Gerontol.*, 10:338–340.
119. Riley, J. N., and Walker, D. W. (1978): Morphological alterations in hippocampus after long-term alcohol consumption in mice. *Science*, 201:640–648.
120. Rosen, W. G. (1980): Verbal fluency in aging and dementia. *J. Clin. Neuropsychol.*, 2:135–146.
121. Rosen, W. G., Terry, R. D., Fuld, P. A., Katzman, R., and Peck, A. (1980): Pathological verification of ischemic score in differentiation of dementias. *Ann. Neurol.*, 7:486–488.
122. Ryan, C., Butters, N., Didario, B., Adinolfi, A. (1980): The relationship between abstinence and recovery of function in male alcoholics. *J. Clin. Psychol.*, 2:125–134.
123. Samorajski, T., and Hartford, J. (1980): Brain physiology of aging. In: *Handbook of Geriatric Psychiatry*, edited by E. W. Busse and D. G. Blazer. Van Nostrand Reinhold, NY.
124. Scheibel, M. F., and Scheibel, A. (1975): Structural changes in the aging brain. In: *Aging, Vol. 1, Clinical, Morphologic, and Neurochemical Aspects in the Aging Central Nervous System*, edited by S. H. Brody and J. M. Ordy. Raven Press, NY.
125. Shaw, T. G., and Meyer, J. S. (1981): Aging and cerebrovascular disease. In: *Diagnosis and Management of Stroke and TIAs*, edited by J. S. Meyer and T. Shaw. Addison-Wesley Publishing Company, Menlo Park, CA.
126. Shaw, T. G., Cutaia, M. M., Mortel, K. F., Meyer, J. S., Nakajima, S., Amano, T. (1981): Prospective measurements of cerebral blood flow in normal and abnormal aging. *Neurology*, (Suppl)31:102, p.104.
127. Shaw, T. G., Meyer, J. S., Sakai, F., Yamaguchi, F., Yamamoto, M., and Mortel, K. (1979): Effects of normal aging versus risk factors for stroke in regional cerebral blood flow (rCBF). *Acta Neurol. Scand.*, :462–463.
128. Simard, D., Olesen, J., Paulson, O. B., Lassen, N. A., and Skinhoj, E. (1971): Regional cerebral blood flow and its regulation in dementia. *Brain*, 94:273–288.
129. Soininen, H., Puranen, M., and Riekkinen, P. J. (1982): Computed tomography findings in senile dementia and normal aging. *J. Neurol. Neurosurg. Psychiatry*, 45:50–54.
130. Sokoloff, L. (1966): Cerebral circulatory and metabolic changes associated with aging. *Res. Publ. Assoc. Res. Nerv. Ment. Dis.*, 41:237–254.
131. Storrie, M. C., and Doerr, H. O. (1979): Characteristics of Alzheimer's type dementia utilizing an abbreviated Halstead-Reitan battery. *J. Clin. Neuropsychol.*, 2:78–82.
132. Sun, A. U., Ordy, J. M., and Samorajski, T. (1975): Effects of alcohol on aging in the nervous system. In: *Neurobiology of Aging: An Interdisciplinary Approach*, edited by J. M. Ordy and K. R. Brizzee. Plenum Press, NY.
133. Tarter, R. E. (1973): An analysis of cognitive deficits in chronic alcoholics. *J. Nerv. Ment. Dis.*, 157:138–147.
134. Tarter, R. E. (1975): Psychological deficit in chronic alcoholics: A review. *Int. J. Addict.*, 10:327–368.
135. Tomlinson, B. C. (1977): The pathology of dementia. In: *Dementia*, 2nd ed., edited by C. E. Wells, F. A. Davis Company, Philadelphia, PA.
136. Tomlinson, B. E., Blessed, G., and Roth, M. (1968): Observations on the brains of nondemented old people. *J. Neurol.*, 7:331–356.

137. Tomlinson, B. E., Blessed, G., and Roth, M. (1970): Observations on the brains of demented old people. *J. Neurol. Sci.*, 11:205–242.
138. Vestal, R. E., McGuire, E. A., Tobin, J. D., Andres, R., Norris, A. H., and Mezey, E. (1977): Aging and ethanol metabolism. *Clin. Pharm. Ther.*, 21:343–354.
139. Walker, D. W., Barnes, D. G., Zornetzer, S. F., Hunter, B. E., and Kubanis, P. (1980): *Science*, 209:711–713.
140. Wang, H. S. (1977): Dementia of old age. In: *Aging and Dementia*, edited by W. C. Smith and M. Kinsbourne. Spectrum Publications, NY.
141. Wells, C. E. (1977): Diagnostic Evaluation and Treatment in Dementia. In: *Dementia*, 2nd ed., edited by C. E. Wells. F. A. Davis Company, Philadelphia, PA.
142. Wells, C. E. (1977): Dementia: definition and description. In: *Dementia*, 2nd ed., edited by C. E. Wells. F. A. Davis Company, Philadelphia, PA.
143. White, P., Hiley, C. R., Goodhardt, M., Carrasco, L. H., Keet, J. P., Williams, I. E. I., and Bowen, D. M. (1977): Neocortical cholinergic neurons in elderly people. *Lancet*, 1:688–631.
144. Whitehouse, P. J., Price, D. L., Struble, R. G., Clark, A. W., Coyle, J. T., and DeLong, M. R. (1982): Alzheimer's Disease and senile dementia. Loss of neurons in the basal forebrain. *Science*, 215:1237–1239.
145. Wilson, R. S., Kaszniak, A. W., and Fox, J. H. (1981): Remote memory in senile dementia. *Cortex*, 17:41–48.
146. Wolf, P., and Kannel, W. (1982): Controllable risk factors for stroke: Preventative implications of trends in stroke mortality. In: *Diagnosis and Management of Stroke and TIAs*, edited by J. S. Meyer and T. Shaw. Addison-Wesley Publishing Company, Menlo Park, CA.
147. Wood, W. G. (1976): Age-associated differences in response to alcohol in rats and mice: A biochemical and behavioral review. *Exp. Aging Res.*, 2:543–562.
148. Yamaguchi, F., Meyer, S., Sakai, F., and Yamamoto, M. (1979): Normal human aging and cerebral vasoconstrictive responses to hypocapnia. *J. Neurol. Sci.*, 44:87–94.
149. Yamaguchi, F., Meyer, J. S., Yamamoto, M., Sakai, F., and Shaw, T. (1980): Non-invasive regional cerebral blood flow measures in dementia. *Arch. Neurol.*, 37:410–418.
150. Yamamoto, M., Meyer, J. S., Sakai, F., and Yamaguchi, F. (1980): Aging and cerebral vasomotor responses to hypercarbia: Responses in normal aging and persons with risk factors for stroke. *Arch. Neurol.*, 37:489–496.
151. Yamagura, H., Ito, M., Kubota, K., Matsuzawa, T. (1980): Brain atrophy during aging: A quantitative study with computed tomography. *J. Gerontol.*, 35:492–498.

Alcoholism in the Elderly, edited by
J.T. Hartford and T. Samorajski.
Raven Press, New York © 1984.

Psychiatric Aspects of Alcoholism in Geriatric Patients

James T. Hartford and Ole J. Thienhaus

*Department of Psychiatry, College of Medicine, University of Cincinnati,
Cincinnati, Ohio 45267*

Alcohol abuse and dependence in the elderly tend to be seriously underestimated as a factor in presenting psychopathology and as a cause of many routine problems seen in emergency rooms and acute care clinics. A general tendency to neglect alcoholism as part of the differential diagnosis is compounded by a lack of knowledge about the effects of alcohol on elderly patients. Behavior that would be identified in younger patients as a problem may be passed off in the elderly as eccentric.

Even when alcoholism is considered in assessing the geriatric patient, making the diagnosis can still be difficult (28). Many of the problems noted in younger patients are not seen in the elderly. Absence from work, difficulties in the family, and problems from driving while intoxicated are often absent in the presentation of the geriatric patient. History from family members that may provide the crucial clues to the diagnosis of the younger alcoholic is frequently not available.

It is not unusual for the problems of alcoholism to blend into pathology that may arise as the sociological consequences of the aging process. The actual incidence of alcoholism in the elderly ranges from 15 to 25%. Even with the knowledge that alcoholism is relatively common, it can be extremely difficult to differentiate the problems of aging and other medical or psychiatric conditions in the elderly person from alcoholism.

The clinician must also bear in mind that elderly patients who are not alcohol-dependent but who drink are more prone to alcohol-related problems than their younger counterparts. Serious falls, difficulties due to memory loss and confusion, and sleep problems are very common in the elderly drinker. Such complications arise from the greater direct impact that alcohol has on mental functioning in the elderly. This higher susceptibility may be due to the effects of aging on ethanol metabolism, or it may be related to the physiological changes and general decrease in size as a result of the aging process (29).

Many geriatric patients have serious medical illnesses and are maintained on multiple medications. This exposes the elderly drinker to a variety of specific hazards. Alcohol tends to interact with many drugs to increase the incidence or severity of side effects, such as confusion, sedation, memory loss, and cardiovascular problems. Patients who are drinking are also at great risk to forget their medication or take an improper dosage. Finally, alcohol may interfere with the metabolism and absorption of many medical drugs, such as chloralhydrate and barbiturates.

In the following discussion, the descriptive symptomatology of alcoholism according to the *Diagnostic and Statistical Manual of Mental Disorders (DSM-III)* published by the American Psychiatric Association (APA) is briefly reviewed (4). The mechanisms by which alcoholism interfaces with other types of psychiatric pathology and its respective causative, concurrent, and reactive nature in relationship to major mental disorders are also discussed. Various treatment modalities will be described and examined with special emphasis on their clinical applicability to elderly patients.

DIAGNOSTIC CONSIDERATIONS

For clinical purposes alcohol-abuse disorder and alcohol dependence (alcoholism) are diagnosed according to operational criteria developed and adopted by the APA.

The *DSM-III* makes the diagnosis of alcohol dependence contingent on the presence of two symptom clusters: (a) a pattern of pathological alcohol use or alcohol-related impairment in social or occupational functioning and (b) signs of either tolerance or withdrawal.

The reference to social and occupational functioning clearly reflects the problems of applying these standard diagnostic criteria to elderly patients. The criteria were standardized on younger patients in whom alcohol dependence would be likely to cause impairment in these areas. In the elderly patient, however, there is often limited opportunity for assessing social or occupational functioning (5).

The clinician may have to focus primarily on the pattern of alcohol use. If daily use of alcohol is a prerequisite for adequate functioning, or there is an inability to cut down or stop drinking, or if there is a history of binge drinking and repeated amnesic periods for events occurring while intoxicated, the presence of the pattern of pathological alcohol use is established. This pattern by itself is the hallmark of an alcohol-abuse disorder. Alcohol dependence (alcoholism) shows the additional feature of tolerance, that is, the need for markedly increased amounts of alcohol to achieve the desired effect, or the development of the withdrawal syndrome after cessation of or even reduction in drinking.

While many elderly males live with family members or have a surviving spouse, many do not, and even more elderly alcoholic females live alone. In either population, signs of tolerance or withdrawal may easily be missed. But they may escape notice even in cases where observation is present; tolerance phenomena may be masked by the aged person's greater susceptibility to the effects of alcohol. Unless the patient's access to alcohol is interfered with, the symptomatology of withdrawal may never occur. Because of the lack of obligation to function either at work or socially, the elderly alcoholic is infrequently motivated to keep abstinent for any prolonged period of time.

PATHOGENETIC CONCEPTS

It is helpful and important to differentiate primary alcoholism from what has been described as secondary alcoholism (24). Primary or early onset alcoholism is probably at least, in part, genetically determined. It is usually present from a relatively young age and qualifies as a disease that follows a fairly predictable course (12). Geriatric patients falling into this category are usually described as "alcoholics grown old."

Secondary alcoholism develops in the context of a preexisting problem. This may be a psychiatric illness, such as depression or stress related to a personality disorder, or it may arise from the sociological changes incurred as part of the aging process. The pressures of growing old may predispose the individual to develop secondary alcoholism (7,24) and there is epidemiological evidence to support this hypothesis, even though intricacies of statistical data gathering cast some doubt on the actual figures for the incidence of reactive alcoholism in the geriatric population (5). It is clear that an aging person with preexisting inadequate personality traits has an increased risk of developing alcohol abuse and secondary alcohol dependency. The term "secondary" suggests the etiology of the alcoholism to be the result of a primary illness. Occasionally, treatment of the primary illness may result in cessation of the alcohol abuse. Usually, however, this is not the case. For this reason, it must be continually borne in mind that alcoholism is a problem that must be focused upon as a separate entity, and the fact that the alcohol abuse developed in response to another problem becomes a secondary issue.

It may be helpful to conceptualize the pathogenesis of secondary alcoholism in a psychodynamic frame of reference: the (drug) alcohol temporarily helps to restore a balance between the mind's coping mechanisms and adverse forces that are experienced as overpowering.

Problems that do not appear extraordinary to others may be experienced as extremely threatening to the self-esteem or motivation for survival of an individual whose internal capacity to deal with stress is inadequately developed or waning. In order to defend against the attendant anxiety and avoid the pain of depression, such an individual will be more likely to turn to drugs that promise relief. Because alcohol is the most available among a number of such substances (which include minor tranquilizers), it is frequently the one chosen (22).

Structural personality defects that predispose individuals to inadequate coping behavior in response to stress are central features of personality disorders. These are characterized by maladaptive behavior that is typical of the individual's current and long-term functioning and are not limited to episodes of illness. Such behavior tends to cause significant impairment in either social or occupational functioning (4). Personality disorders that seem to be especially predisposed to substance-abuse disorders are borderline, passive-aggressive, and, to a lesser degree, compulsive and dependent personality disorders (16).

The ability of the individual to cope with external stress and adapt to continually changing circumstances tends to be a primary issue in the development of secondary alcoholism. In patients with personality disorders, the patients' inner resources are inadequate to respond to the increasing stress of aging.

In another group of patients with reactive alcoholism it is the sheer weight of painful, disturbing external factors that impinge upon an individual who may have been able to withstand less exorbitant stresses in the past. The well-known concomitants of aging combine to generate such stress. There is bereavement from the loss of parents, siblings, friends, and spouse. There are changes in the immediate surrounding social structure such as the leaving of children, retirement from competitive employment, moves into different living quarters. Finally, there may be a decline in physical and mental capacities and often deteriorating health.

The distinction between primary and secondary alcoholism does not in itself provide a solution to the long-standing controversy about whether or not alcohol dependence is a disease in its own right. It does offer the clinician an operational concept to help organize thoughts about the development of the disorder and, especially in the geriatric population, a place to begin in assessment and treatment planning.

ALCOHOLISM AND MENTAL DISORDERS

Some 30% of alcoholics have been diagnosed as having either a schizophrenic or major affective disorder (16). A preexisting major depressive illness was found to be present in 5 to 15% of patients diagnosed as having an alcohol-dependence disorder (25). Occasionally alcoholism and a major mental disorder coexist with only minimal mutual impact. As a general rule, however, alcohol abuse and dependence, in individuals with a primary psychiatric illness, are directly related to the psychiatric illness, and these problems compound one another (14).

The relationship between dementia and alcoholism is of particular importance to the geropsychiatrist. A frequent presenting complaint of the elderly patient is memory impairment. In patients with a primary dementia, very often the problem is first brought to the attention of the clinician by the patient's family. In these cases, the patients typically deny having memory problems or rationalize their loss of memory as "normal at my age." Such patients are equally prone to either minimize or deny the use of alcohol. Elderly patients who are under the influence of alcohol may appear to be confused and manifest poor memory without signs of obvious drunkenness. Because dementia fluctuates from time to time and, in the early stages, may vary widely, the differential may be difficult to make.

Alcohol abuse in patients with dementia feeds into a vicious cycle: alcohol has direct neurotoxic properties (9) that tend to compound the effect of malnutrition, especially vitamin deficiencies. The basal ganglia, hippocampus, reticular activating formation, and neocortex undergo neuronal loss with aging faster than do other regions of the brain. These structures are therefore particularly vulnerable in the elderly person's brain, and toxic damage will result in further cognitive impairment (15). The alcohol that is ingested in order to alleviate some of the distress secondary to deteriorating organic brain syndrome eventually accelerates the debilitating dementing process.

It is not unusual for patients with a primary problem of dementia to develop some degree of alcohol-related problems. The functional losses of dementia pose a serious threat to the individual's self-esteem. This can generate secondary, reactive psychopathological features whose presentation depends on the resilience and nature of defense mechanisms available to the individual. Preexisting obsessive-compulsive traits may become intensified, the patient may, by means of increasing projection, develop paranoid features or hallucinate. The undermining of self-esteem will eventually result in depression, and at any stage during the process, alleviation of subjective distress may be sought through alcohol.

Suicide deserves special attention because it is a serious problem among alcoholics. The general disinhibiting pharmacological action of ethanol has been shown to have a direct impact on the incidence of suicide: Alcohol abuse was found to play a role in 30% of suicides (3). The problem is even greater in individuals with major mental disorders, for they have a significantly greater risk of committing suicide, possibly four times as great as the average (27). The rate of suicides is also increased in the older age groups: 23% of all suicides reported in the United States in 1976 were committed by persons 60 years of age or older (19). On the other hand, only 15% of the entire population belonged to that age group (18).

The elderly alcohol abuser may experience all the major stresses that lead to suicide: increased age, alcohol abuse, social isolation, loneliness, and recent loss. Assessment for suicidal potential and manifest suicidal risk should be a part of every assessment where the possibility of alcohol abuse exists.

TREATMENT

There is no predictable course or cure for alcoholism. This is especially true for the elderly alcoholic. There are, however, many different approaches and therapeutic techniques that can be employed to alleviate complications associated with alcohol abuse and in many cases to effectively and definitively treat the underlying problem. The clinical management of the alcoholic patient combines pharmacological approaches with psychosocial therapies. A primary goal in treatment is to get the patient to stop drinking. In many cases, this is not possible, and the clinician must settle for minimizing the patient's desire or need for alcohol.

Any treatment should relate to the reasons why the patient comes to treatment: either a significant person in the alcoholic's life has brought him for therapy, or some distressing consequence of the alcohol dependence has motivated the patient to actively seek treatment. In either case, this can function as the basis for change, the first step toward effective treatment.

A thorough physical examination is indicated as part of the assessment of an alcoholic of any age, and it is crucial in the elderly alcoholic. Physical assessment should include a complete battery of laboratory tests to monitor the functioning of the pancreas, thyroid, liver, lungs, and cardiovascular system. Any concomitant physical illnesses should be identified and stabilized. It may be necessary to hospitalize the patient for the assessment in order to do an adequate and thorough workup. The time and effort required for the physical workup are significant. This commitment can function as reinforcement of the clinician's investment in the patient. A sense of mutual respect and trust is extremely important in the treatment of the elderly alcoholic: it is this alliance that, perhaps more than any other factor, will determine a successful or unsuccessful outcome.

Pharmacological approaches are threefold. The first type is directed at the underlying contributing or primary illnesses. The second kind of pharmacotherapy aims at correcting sequelae or concomitant features of the alcohol dependence such as anemia, malnutrition, hypertension, or uncontrolled diabetes mellitus. Finally, there is the deconditioning approach with disulfiram (Antabuse®).

Disulfiram should be used in the elderly alcoholic only where careful medical monitoring is possible and preferably by clinicians with experience in the use of the drug. Disulfiram reinforces abstinence by a rather marked toxic response when alcohol-containing substances are ingested. In young patients, the toxic response is an unpleasant experience that can have serious implications. In the elderly patient, these responses could be potentially life-threatening.

It has been described how mental disorders can contribute to alcohol-abuse disorder and alcoholism. If caught early, i.e., before the use of alcohol has gone out of control and grown into an autonomous process, the effective treatment of underlying disorders can have substantial impact on the incipient development of the secondary alcohol dependence. By effectively treating major psychiatric illnesses such as schizophrenia, manic-depressive illness, or major depressive disorders with appropriate psychopharmacological agents, the impact of secondary alcoholism can be significantly minimized or even eliminated. In many cases of alcohol abuse in the elderly, especially where a full-blown alcohol-dependence disorder has already developed, treatment of underlying illnesses will not be curative.

For those patients with dementia due to an identifiable organic cause, medical or surgical therapies may contain or prevent a condition that would otherwise lead to an increased risk of alcohol dependence. In patients whose cognitive impairment is idiopathic, or of the Alzheimer's variety, it is possible to minimize problems with alcohol abuse through careful education of the patient and structuring their environment and access to alcohol.

There is little controversy about the treatment of sequelae or concomitant features of alcoholism. Malnutrition and hypovitaminosis (vitamin-B complex) are widespread, especially among elderly alcoholics with their typically limited natural support systems. A well-balanced diet and additional multivitamins are essential parts of the medical management of alcoholic patients.

The hazards of alcohol withdrawal deserve special attention. These require careful monitoring of the vegetative signs and mental status in an inpatient setting, and prompt therapy, e.g., chlordiazepoxide (Librium®) when prodromal signs of delirium tremens (DTs) occur. It should be kept in mind that the characteristic warning signs of impending DTs may be masked by cardiovascular medications such as propranolol, which are frequently taken by elderly patients (30).

Disulfiram blocks the further degradation of acetaldehyde, a product in the oxidative breakdown of ethanol in the liver. Increased levels of acetaldehyde cause tachycardia, headache, dizziness, dyspnea, nausea, and vomiting. There is additionally an initial rise in blood pressure followed by marked hypotension. All these effects occur some 5 to 15 min after ingestion of alcohol in a patient who took 0.5 g of disulfiram during the preceding 12 hr (23).

The method is based on behavioral concepts of operant conditioning. It can be expected that the desire to drink alcohol will dissipate if the ingestion is regularly followed by intensive unpleasant physical symptoms. Disulfiram in connection with psychotherapy has been shown to be effective in the treatment of alcoholism (11). In an elderly patient, however, disulfiram should only be used in carefully selected cases. Not only is it incompatible with many other medications, i.e., phenytoin, isoniazid, cough syrups, and many lotions (10), but the nature of the unpleasant reactions triggered by alcohol in a person on disulfiram makes it hazardous in the elderly.

Psychosocial therapies include individual psychotherapy, therapy with the patient's family, group therapy, Alcoholics Anonymous (AA), and rehabilitative measures. All these can be started even if the patient is in the hospital and continued in an outpatient facility. Frequently the preferred course of action is to initiate measures aimed at behavioral change in a structured, controlled inpatient setting. However, there is no convincing support in the literature for the view that programs that are outpatient based from the start are less effective (8).

Individual therapy, usually in conjunction with other modalities in the framework of an overall comprehensive case management, will often require behavioral techniques (13,20). These approaches are directed toward teaching the patient alternatives to excessive drinking. The syndrome of alcoholism is broken down into component parts that can then be isolated and studied. Modification of behavior and stabilization of results are achieved by means of the punishment-reward principle of operant conditioning (26).

All individual psychotherapy must address the alcoholic patient's main defense mechanism, denial (21). Denial is also the prevailing defense in the alcoholic's family. Education regarding the nature of alcohol dependency and the fact that it is an illness is indicated for both the alcoholic and those close to him or her.

Group therapy is frequently helpful. Usually the group is comprised of alcoholic patients, and the sharing of experiences by similarly afflicted persons promotes the development of meaningful insight. The interdependence on peers in a group setting replaces the single, intense relationship with an individual therapist (6). In geropsychiatric facilities, therapy is offered in groups consisting entirely of elderly patients. While it is preferable that the group include all alcoholics, this is not always possible. No studies are available to date that would compare the relative benefits for elderly alcoholics in a geriatric group versus a group composed exclusively of alcohol-dependent patients of various ages. It appears, however, that elderly alcoholics do better in geriatric groups (31).

Alcoholics Anonymous employs concepts of group therapy. It provides an escape from the intense feeling of psychosocial isolation and offers, instead, a feeling of belonging and acceptance on the basis of empathic understanding by others who suffer from the same condition (1). AA fosters a sense of mutual responsibility by instituting sponsorships (2). Each member has an individual sponsor and, in turn, sponsors somebody else for monitoring each one's sobriety. The focus of AA is entirely on the drinking; no defensive deviation to possible causative or contributing factors is permitted.

AA is popular with elderly alcoholics: in North America 34% of AA members are 50 years old and older (17). AA is compatible with other therapies. The elderly patient in AA may need the support of a therapist who is in tune with those components of the patient's predicament that are especially related to his/her advanced age.

SUMMARY

Alcoholism is a serious and common problem in the elderly patient. It is difficult to diagnose because of the age-related decrease in socialization and employment. Conventional diagnostic criteria rely heavily on impairment of socialization and work record. These indices are of less value in the elderly population and more easily hidden by the elderly alcohol abuser. Older persons who have decreased social contacts can easily justify this by their circumstances. Because work by the elderly is occasional, tends to be voluntary, and is often totally absent, assessment of work-related stresses or absenteeism is not helpful in the diagnosis. A drinking pattern of daily use of alcohol or an inability to cut down or stop drinking, and/or the occurrence of binge drinking are more useful in establishing a diagnosis of alcoholism or an alcohol-abuse disorder in the elderly.

Once the diagnosis is made, treatment modalities for the elderly are similar to those employed for younger patients. The exception is the use of disulfiram (Antabuse®), which presents greater risk to the elderly because of the side effects associated with its pharmacological action. Treatment of the elderly alcoholic should include a careful and thorough physical examination with attention to any concomitant physical or psychiatric illnesses.

There is empirical evidence that elderly alcoholics do better in geriatric groups than in homogeneous groups of alcoholics of various ages. Currently there are no studies available to document the validity of these clinical experiences adequately. It is hoped that in the near future further research will specifically target problems of the elderly alcohol abuser. Such efforts may be expected to lead to a comprehensive differential evaluation of the various therapeutic approaches as they apply to the geriatric patient.

REFERENCES

1. A.A. (1939): *Alcoholics Anonymous*. Works Publishing, NY.
2. Alibrandi, L. A. (1978): The folk psychotherapy of Alcoholics Anonymous. In: *Practical Approaches to Alcoholism Psychotherapy*. Edited by S. Zimberg, J. Wallace, and S. B. Blume, Plenum Press, NY.
3. American Medical Association (1977): *Manual on Alcoholism*, 3rd ed., AMA, Chicago, IL.
4. American Psychiatric Association (1980): *Diagnostic and Statistical Manual of Mental Disorders*. 3rd ed., APA, Washington, DC.
5. Blazer, D. G., and Pennybacker, M. R. (1983): Epidemiology of alcoholism in the elderly. In: *Alcoholism in the Elderly*, edited by J. T. Hartford and T. Samorajski, Raven Press, NY.
6. Blume, S. B. (1978): Group psychotherapy in the treatment of alcoholism. In: *Practical Approaches to Alcoholism Psychotherapy*, edited by S. Zimberg, J. Wallace, and S. B. Blume, Plenum Press, NY.
7. Droller, H. (1964): Some aspects of alcoholism in the elderly. *Lancet*. 2:137–139.
8. Emerick, C. D. (1975): A review of psychologically oriented treatment of alcoholism. II. The relative effectiveness of different treatment approaches and effectiveness of treatment versus no treatment. *J. Stud. Alcohol*. 36:88–108.
9. Freund, G. (1982): The interaction of chronic alcohol consumption and aging on brain structure and function. *Alcohol. Clin. Exp. Res.*, 6:13–21.
10. Geffner, E. S., editor (1982): *The Psychiatrist's Compendium of Drug Therapy 1982/1983*. Biomedical Information, NY.
11. Gerrein, J. R., Rosenberg, C. M., and Manohar, V. (1973): Disulfiram maintenance in outpatient treatment of alcoholism. *Arch. Gen. Psychiatry*, 28:798–802.
12. Goodwin, D. W., Schulsinger, F., Hermansen, L., et al. (1973): Alcohol problems in adoptees raised apart from alcoholic biologic parents. *Arch. Gen. Psychiatry*, 28:235–244.
13. Hamburg, S. (1975): Behavior therapy in alcoholism. *J. Stud. Alcohol*. 36:69–87.
14. Harrington, L. G., and Price, A. C. (1962): Alcoholism in a geriatric setting. V. Incidence of mental disorders. *J. Am. Geriatr. Soc.*, 10:209–211.
15. Hartford, J. T., and Samorajski, T. (1982): Alcoholism in the geriatric population. *J. Am. Geriatr. Soc.* 30:18–24.
16. Kolb, L. C. (1982): *Modern Clinical Psychiatry*, 10th ed., Saunders, Philadelphia, PA.
17. Leach, B. (1973): Does Alcoholics Anonymous really work? In: *Alcoholism, Progress in Research and Treatment*. Edited by P. G. Bourne, Academic Press, NY.
18. Madden, T. A., Turner, I. R., and Eckenfels, E. J. (1982): *The Health Almanac*. Raven Press, NY.
19. Miller, M. (1979): *Suicide after Sixty*. Springer, New York.
20. Miller, P. M. (1975): A behavioral intervention program for chronic public drunkenness offenders. *Arch. Gen. Psychiatry*. 32:915–918.
21. Moore, R. A., and Murphy, T. C. (1961): Denial of alcoholism as an obstacle to recovery. *Q. J. Stud. Alcohol*. 22:597–609.
22. National Commission on Marijuana and Drug Abuse (1973): *Drug Use in America: Problem in Perspective (2nd report)*. U.S. Government Printing Office, Washington, DC.
23. Ritchie, J. M. (1980): The aliphatic alcohols. In: *The Pharmacological Basis of Therapeutics*. 6th ed., edited by A. G. Gilman, L. S. Goodman and A. Gilman. Macmillan, NY.
24. Rosin, A. J., and Glatt, M. M. (1971): Alcohol excess in the elderly. *J. Stud. Alcohol*. 32:53–59.
25. Schuckit, M. A. (1979): Alcoholism and affective disorder: Diagnostic confusion. In: *Alcoholism and Affective Disorders*, edited by D. W. Goodwin and C. K. Erikson, Spectrum Publications, NY.
26. Selzer, M. L. (1981): Alcoholism and alcoholic psychoses. In: *Comprehensive Textbook of Psychiatry*, Vol. 2, 3rd ed., edited by H. I. Kaplan, A. M. Freedman, and B. J. Sadock, Williams and Wilkins, Baltimore, MD.
27. Stengel, E. (1970): *Suicide and Attempted Suicide*. 2nd ed., Penguin Books, Baltimore, MD.
28. Vaillant, G. E. (1978): Alcoholism and drug dependence. In: *The Harvard Guide to Modern Psychiatry*, edited by A. M. Nicholi, Belknap Press, Cambridge, MA.

29. Vestal, R. E., McGuire, E. A., Tobin, J. D., et al. (1977): Aging and ethanol metabolism. *Clin. Pharmacol. Ther.*, 21:343–354.
30. Zechnich, R. J. (1982): Beta blockers can obscure diagnosis of delirium tremens. Letter to the editor. *Lancet.* 1:1071–1072.
31. Zimberg, S. (1978): Psychosocial treatment of elderly alcoholics. In: *Practical Approaches to Alcoholism Psychotherapy*, edited by S. Zimberg, J. Wallace, and S. B. Blume, Plenum Press, NY.

Alcoholism in the Elderly, edited by
J. T. Hartford and T. Samorajski.
Raven Press, New York © 1984.

Aging, Alcoholism, and Addictive Behavior Change: Diagnostic Treatment Models

*Carlo C. DiClemente and **Jack R. Gordon

*Alcoholism Treatment Center and **Clinical Services Division, Texas Research Institute
of Mental Sciences, Houston, Texas 77030

The dictionary definition of diagnosis is the act or art of identifying a disease from its signs and symptoms or, from another perspective, an analysis of the cause or nature of a condition or problem. The goal of the diagnosis is to develop a systematic taxonomy or classification that will help put the problem in its proper perspective in order to make relevant interventions. Identifying or understanding a particular problem or disease does not, however, always lead to effective intervention. Identifying the symptoms unique to a specific, biologically caused disease enables the diagnostician to search for the biological malfunction or invading agent that causes the disease. Only after the malfunction or agent is identified can an effective cure be found. This approach is less effective for diseases or maladaptive syndromes like addictive behaviors, which have a learned component. In those, the connections between symptom picture and the cause or nature of the illness are less clear and the diagnostic work more complicated.

Several basic approaches have been used to analyze the cause or nature of addictive behaviors. The epidemiologist looks for who is susceptible to or at risk of developing alcohol problems. Epidemiological data may provide a demographic map of the problem, isolate risk factors, and identify groups of people who should be studied more intensively or targeted for intervention. In an etiological approach to alcoholism one looks for the roots of alcoholism or addictive behavior. An etiological model would enable us to understand the development of the problem and the critical factors that distinguish the alcoholic from the social drinker. A categorical approach is often less ambitious. Although some attempts at categorization also include assumptions about etiology, the main task of categorization is to identify separate and separable disorders. Models developed from this approach tend to focus on symptoms that cluster together to form an entity or syndrome. The current third edition of the American Psychiatric Association's *Diagnostic and Statistical Manual of Mental Disorders (DSM-III)* is the best example of categorization, as it defines alcoholism as alcohol dependence, a pattern of pathological use with evidence of tolerance and/or withdrawal.

Although all these approaches are important, useful, and have implications for treatment, they are not treatment models. Treatment of addictive behaviors must focus on behavior change. The statement that alcoholics cannot demonstrate alcohol dependence unless they drink alcohol is at once simplistic and profound. Behavior change in alcohol consumption is the critical dimension in alcoholism treatment, and it is not adequately addressed by the epidemiological, etiological, and categorical models. A comprehensive treatment model must be directed to addictive behavior change.

A variety of models have been proposed to promote more effective treatment of the alcoholic patient. This chapter is not an exhaustive survey but rather a discussion and critique of some issues in developing treatment models.

SUBCLASSIFICATION

Even before Jellinek's descriptive classification of alcoholism, researchers and theoreticians have tried to divide the heterogeneous population of alcoholics according to dimensions relevant for treatment. As Gibbs (12) notes, researchers have proposed some dimensions relevant to treatment: the alcoholic's drinking history and pattern of use (39), behavioral and biological characteristics (17), rehabilitation needs, and personality characteristics (26,35). Many of these attempts have little value for treatment, however, because no link has been found between subclasses and treatment effectiveness.

Attempts to subclassify alcoholic groups deal with patient characteristics and patient problems. Gibbs (12), focusing on patient characteristics, developed classifications based on social stability and intellectual functioning, dividing alcoholics into groups for whom specific treatments would be relevant. The four treatments were (a) outpatient treatment with disulfiram (Antabuse®) and medication, (b) outpatient treatment with group or individual insight-oriented therapy, (c) treatment in a structured residential facility, and (d) inpatient treatment with individual or group counseling. These treatment recommendations were, however, rationally derived and not research-based. Social stability and intellectual functioning are, moreover, very general characteristics containing a heavy socioeconomic bias. The focus on patient characteristics may have some merit for classifying patients, but its utility for planning treatment has yet to be proved. Nevertheless, patient characteristics rather than type of therapy have been related consistently to therapy outcome. Treatment prognosis for persons with higher social status and stability is better than for those lower on the scale regardless of type of intervention (2,36). A patient's drinking history and social environment also have been shown to influence remission rates (1). Currently, treatment factors have been shown to account for a small portion of outcome variance; a patient's background and motivation to seek help seem to be critical factors in recovery (25).

Using a problem-oriented approach, Kissin (16) describes a pathogenetic classification of alcoholics that focuses on three predisposing etiological elements: biological, psychological, and social mechanisms. His three-dimensional model illustrates the interaction of the three factors. Each individual is evaluated for physical dependence, psychological maladjustment, and social maladjustment. Kissin believes that the individual's pattern of pathology, as it is related to these dimensions, should direct the therapist to a rational therapeutic regimen. With regard to intervention, Kissin describes a core and special-therapies model for treating the chronic alcoholic. The model addresses, first, the special problems of withdrawal symptoms, family problems, medical problems, severe psychopathology and indigence, and the interventions appropriate to these problems. Then he recommends a core-therapy approach consisting of Alcoholics Anonymous (AA), individual therapy, group therapy, religious counseling, psychodrama, and behavioral therapy to treat what he considers the basic problem of the alcoholic—psychological dependence.

Although the use of subclassification models to design relevant, effective treatment programs holds some promise, these models are fraught with problems. Well-motivated, intelligent, socially stable alcoholics would probably do well in any treatment program. The task of a treatment model is not to eliminate treatment failures but to design a comprehensive assessment that will facilitate treatment for all alcoholics. Gibbs focuses on patient characteristics; Kissin looks primarily at patient problems. Several questions remain. Are these models sufficiently comprehensive and detailed? Do they focus on characteristics related to changing addictive behaviors? Finally, should types of alcoholics or types of problems be the primary considerations for treatment, or should a new classification system be developed?

DECISION-MAKING

Motivation has already been mentioned as a critical factor in treatment outcome. If, as Kissin (16) states, it is harder to become dry than to stay dry, an important and often overlooked aspect of addictive behavior change is the individual's decision to change. Decision-making is relevant to any change whether the individual enters therapy or not.

Recent studies have shown that 30 to 50% of the individuals who received only minimal treatment for their alcoholism improved (1, 10). Edwards and his colleagues (9) demonstrated that a single counseling session produced an outcome at one year follow-up not significantly different from that of a treatment group. In an exploratory study of what we believe is erroneously called "natural" or "spontaneous" remission, Tuchfield et al. (37) examined factors relevant to what we would call self-change. Many conditions that caused patients to initiate their commitment to changing their drinking behavior were decision-making variables like identification with a negative role model, serious health problem, and personal humiliation. The patient's decision to attempt to modify an addictive behavior is critical to treatment outcome.

Motivation, "hitting bottom," and constructive coercion have been the major ways in which decision-making variables have been addressed in alcoholism treatment. A more sophisticated approach to decision-making is needed. Janis and Mann (15) developed a decision-making model relevant to addictive behaviors. They enumerated five stages of decision-making: appraising the challenge, surveying alternatives, weighing alternatives, deliberating about commitment to change, and adhering despite negative feedback. A critical element in their conception of the decision-making process is the decisional "balance sheet"—a multidimensional set of values, including favorable and unfavorable consequences, that anyone making a decision considers. These decision-making dimensions are considered critical in the process of change, both in taking action and in maintaining the new behavior.

Although it is difficult to see how decision-making quality can be the only relevant dimension in successful modification of addictive behaviors like alcoholism, the decision to enter treatment and follow through on intervention techniques is certainly relevant to treatment. Decision-making deserves more intensive and sophisticated research and should be addressed in any treatment model.

MULTIVARIANT APPROACHES TO A MANY-SIDED PROBLEM

A great deal of energy has been spent on identifying alcoholism, but anyone working with alcoholics knows that there is no typical alcoholic. The evaluation of individuals who have drinking problems must include major areas of functioning and establish profiles of impairment that are relevant to treatment. Logically, a useful treatment model must address the multivariant needs of the alcoholic population (27). Often this means availability of programs that address the varying needs of alcoholics in different stages of the illness. This approach is really identical to the subclassification approach, as the first task seems to be defining which types of alcoholics do best in which types of programs (16). Other researchers have attempted to develop integrated or comprehensive treatment packages that address the basic needs of the alcoholic patient (11,38).

Lazarus (18,19) provided a comprehensive model of therapy. He assesses seven basic modalities for each patient and designs interventions relevant to problems in each modality. His acronym, BASIC ID, represents the first letter of each area of functioning assessed: behaviors, affective processes, sensations, images, cognitions, interpersonal relationships, and drugs (biological functions). Since this comprehensive assessment is the beginning of effective therapeutic intervention, Lazarus proposed a true diagnostic treatment model. Yet his model does not explain interactions among these factors nor does it indicate where the initial or primary focus of treatment should be.

All attempts to develop multivariant models could be improved upon. What follows is a discussion of treatment issues as they apply to the older patient and a description of several aspects of a new comprehensive model being developed specifically to treat patients for alcoholism and other addictive behaviors.

AGING, ADDICTIVE BEHAVIORS, AND TREATMENT

Estimates of the number of elderly alcoholics vary tremendously, some considering 10 to 15% of the general elderly population as suffering from the disorder (29). Generally, drinking decreases with advancing age, however, this does not mean that there is no alcohol problem among the elderly (28).

Everyone bemoans the absence of accurate figures and the problem of the hidden elderly alcoholic. Even if our estimates were accurate, their projection into the future would be fruitless because the current cohort of elderly persons differs from other future groups. Those who grew up in the 1920s and 1930s have different attitudes from those who grew up later. Medical advances may be able to keep problem drinkers alive much longer than those in the past. Like the disintegration of the family, social problems may affect alcohol consumption more than is currently true. Thus, alcoholism treatment may be faced with an insoluble dilemma. Will the programs and interventions we develop from our current knowledge of the elderly be appropriate for future generations? Unless we get a more comprehensive picture of elderly alcoholics and their needs and problems, we will not be able to address these issues. This seems possible only with a relevant and flexible treatment model that can address generational and age differences.

TYPES OF ELDERLY ALCOHOLICS

Most researchers agree that basically there are two distinct types of elderly alcoholics, those who began drinking at an early age and those who turned to alcohol to cope with the problems of aging (24,29,34,42). This appears to be a simplistic solution to a complex problem because patterns of alcohol use across the life-span are so variable. Dunham (8), in an interesting retrospective analysis of drinking patterns over the life-span, identified six basic patterns of alcohol consumption. Some individuals began drinking heavily in their twenties, not decreasing alcohol consumption until their fifties. Others continued a pattern of heavy drinking from their teens, while still others who began light drinking in their thirties increased their consumption at age 70. Another pattern showed heavy drinking beginning in the middle fifties and continuing in the seventies. Other elderly individuals had patterns of abstinence, continued light drinking, or highly variable consumption rates. Although there are problems with retrospective self-reports and the sample was restricted, the variety of patterns challenges the simple two-type assumptions currently in vogue. Another interesting aspect of the study is that changes in drinking patterns seem to occur at points in the life cycle seen as critical stages in adult development (13,20). Many different patterns of alcohol use appear to occur during the life-span; however, they may be related more to issues of adult development than to coping with problems of old age (4).

Are elderly alcoholics and problem drinkers different from young adult alcoholics? The issue has been discussed at length (3,24), but a definitive answer is not possible. The major issue of the discussion often centers on case finding rather than case treatment. Elderly alcoholics do not always find their way to alcoholism treatment (34,41,42). The fact that aged alcoholics are more difficult to find indicates they are underserved, not necessarily different. Rosin and Glatt (34) examined a group of elderly patients, aged 65 to 92, found in psychiatric and geriatric clinical settings, who had alcohol problems. Women outnumbered men, and more of those in the psychiatric group lived alone, complained of loneliness, and were excessive drinkers of long-standing. Examining the precipitating causes of drinking problems, Rosin and Glatt identified three primary factors—dementia, inveterate drinking, and personality factors—and five reactive factors—bereavement, retirement, loneliness, infirmity, and marital stress. Psychiatric patients and geriatric medical patients did not differ greatly in their reports of precipitating factors. Although these findings support the distinction between primary versus reactive alcoholics that has been discussed in the general alcoholism literature, they do not support the view of elderly alcoholics as a distinct population group. Except for retirement, the reactive factors are like those found in younger adults. Thus, there is not much evidence that the elderly represent a special treatment population. Again, what seems to be needed is a comprehensive treatment model that could be used for both elderly and younger alcoholics to determine if any special needs support the demand for specialized or separate treatment programs (24).

AGING AND CHANGING

Are the elderly different in their ability to change? The assumption seems to be that children grow, develop, and change but that adults only grow older. How much does this pessimistic view color our stereotype of the elderly as either unable to change or too old to have valuable treatment resources wasted on them? Therapeutic nihilism with regard to alcohol treatment for the elderly has no foundation (24,28). Elderly individuals can and do change addictive and other behaviors. In fact, the growing awareness of health issues with age can increase the likelihood of successful modification of smoking (40) and alcoholic (42) behaviors. The few outcome studies that have a separate elderly population indicate that the elderly have as good or better rates of successful treatment outcome (24). The elderly alcoholic is not a fixed, immovable object but is capable of substantial behavior change. Some of the pessimism about change in the elderly may, in fact, be the result of low expectations and of the failure to promote change among elderly patients.

Our conclusions parallel those of Mishara and Kastenbaum (24). There seems to be no evidence that elderly alcoholics should be a separate treatment entity. No studies have attempted to look at differential treatment effects. To address the issue adequately, we must consider differences among elderly alcoholics and between older and younger alcoholics. It is highly unlikely that there is a "typical" elderly alcoholic or only two types of elderly alcoholics. Some way of assessing areas of impairment and their change with different treatment modalities is as important for the elderly alcoholic as for those of younger age. Finally, the possibility of change in alcoholic behavior is as relevant for the 70-year-old as for the 25-year-old.

A COMPREHENSIVE MODEL OF ADDICTIVE BEHAVIOR CHANGE

A comprehensive treatment model focuses on behavior change and addresses the psychological, biological, and social factors that may affect and be affected by the alcohol problems. This is critical for the elderly alcoholic about whom so little is known. Such a model provides a framework of assessment to reveal the direction of treatment: in addition to providing a means of evaluating individuals, it provides population data useful for designing successful interventions and for understanding population differences and needs.

STAGES AND PROCESSES OF CHANGE

Changing alcohol consumption patterns and life-styles are the primary goals of alcoholism treatment for patients at any age. Change is a complex phenomenon that has been treated simplistically by theorists and practitioners. Except for the behaviorists, theorists have described at length the dynamics, nature, and cause of problems, giving little attention to modifying, eliminating, or strengthening certain patterns of living. When they do focus on change, theorists often promote one method or process of change they consider critical for every type of change. Such simple concepts hinder effective intervention.

Several basic assumptions about change underlie the current model. That change is not an all-or-none phenomenon is especially true of addictive behaviors in which issues of decision-making and maintenance are so important. Change is a continuous event. Therapists who envision addictive behavior change as a discontinuous process often focus on active change only. They require, therefore, that individuals coming to treatment must want to change. Then, if the interventions that follow are powerful enough, they believe that the change in the patient should be stable enough to be noted at "follow-up" some 3 months, 6 months, or a year later. Treatment failures are attributed to lack of motivation, ineffective intervention, or the patient's inability to "maintain" the change. This perspective offers a narrow view of intervention and promotes an inadequate conceptualization of change.

To see addictive behavior change as continuous, as progressing in stages at which certain issues come to the foreground and require specific interventions, is more useful. Horn (14) discussed a model of health-related behaviors in an attempt to look at various stages of initiation, establishment, and change of the problem behavior, as well as of maintenance of new, healthier patterns. Our examination of smoking behavior change yielded a similar concept of stages of change (5). Addictive behavior change is more fruitfully envisioned as a process that has distinct, separable, but not totally separate, stages of change (31).

Table 1 enumerates seven stages of change an individual goes through to modify addictive behavior. Although these seven stages appear to cover all the relevant steps, their number is not absolute. McConnaughy et al. (21) found only four separable stages: precontemplation, contemplation, active change, and maintenance.

TABLE 1. *Progressive stages of addictive behavior change*

1. Immotive	5. Active change
2. Precontemplation	6. Maintenance
3. Contemplation	7. Relapse
4. Decision-making	

It is also possible that there are separate substages of active change or maintenance; these questions can be resolved only by further research with the model.

The linear progression of the stages is as follows. *Immotive* alcoholics are those who do not want to change, see no real problem, and avoid or deny any information to the contrary. Individuals on *precontemplation* are only a short distance away from being immotive. They may be slightly more receptive to information about their drinking and may be unable to deny its impact on their lives. They are not, however, seriously considering an effort to change. The *contemplators*, on the other hand, are beginning to weigh the pattern and consequences of their drinking and are seriously considering modification of their drinking behavior. Ideally, this would lead them to a firm decision to act and *decision-making* variables would be critical. The next logical step would be *active change*. Here individuals would take steps to disrupt their pattern of drinking: change their alcohol consumption, cut down, become detoxified, avoid favorite drinking spots.

One of the least understood and, until recently, undiscussed aspects of addictive behavior change is *maintenance*. Not a passive holding action, maintenance seems to represent continual learning (6,22,23,31). Long-term maintenance may be seen as termination of the process of change or, as in AA principles, continued awareness of the changed state and consciousness of the disease.

Relapse is a serious problem in addictive behavior change. Often, active change and maintenance do not result in long-term maintenance but in relapse, which is a separate stage and not simply the reverse side of maintenance. Relapse brings with it a distinct set of problems that have enormous implications for future modification of behavior.

Although the stages are represented as a linear progression from immotive to maintenance or relapse, movement through the stages can be quite erratic and circular (6,31). A person may regress as well as progress through the stages of change, and often the process of addictive behavior change looks like a revolving door rather than a successful linear movement. Individuals can also become stalled at various stages, spending months or years in contemplation or maintenance. Thus the stages are not time-determined. They are best defined by a combination of attitudinal or cognitive variables as well as by behavioral measures of the addictive problem.

The stages concept allows us to envision addictive behavior change in separable dimensions and to focus on the issues, problems, and challenges presented by individuals at each stage. Because the stages are separable but not separate, treatment considerations and relevant issues at the different stages are unique. Intervention should focus on movement from one stage to another rather than on unrealistic promotion of active change for an immotive alcoholic.

Research currently in progress explores the implications of the stages of change for treatment outcome (5,6), the change processes most useful for each stage of change (30,32,33), and the interventions or techniques to be used at a particular stage (7,22). Analyzing the stages, processes, and techniques of change offers great promise for using and creating more effective interventions for addictive behavior change.

The stages of change concept raises many treatment-relevant issues for the elderly alcoholic. What are the most effective ways of helping immotive elderly alcoholics to begin to think of changing their alcohol consumption? Currently, family intervention, employee assistance, and driving while intoxicated (DWI) prevention programs encourage younger alcoholics to move to precontemplation and contemplation. Do health concerns and social interactions give more leverage to those who would intervene with elderly alcoholics? Should the family of the older alcoholic be involved and at what stage? Are the processes of change that help younger alcoholics in active change the same as those used by the elderly? What are the most relevant decisional considerations for elderly alcohol-troubled individuals? Are maintenance and relapse significant problems for them? What are the most tempting relapse situations for elderly alcoholics? What kinds of coping skills does the aged alcoholic need to maintain sobriety? These are researchable, treatment-relevant questions important in designing programs that would promote lasting change in elderly people who have alcohol problems. For them, as for younger people, the stages and processes of change offer a way of looking at patient characteristics and processes that are relevant to treatment.

LEVELS OF PROBLEM INVOLVEMENT

Examining the stages and processes of change enables us to see how the elderly move through the process of change but does not reveal the unique problems of elderly alcoholics, nor does it allow us to subdivide the heterogeneous population of elderly alcoholics with regard to types of problems. To address this issue, the treatment model being proposed delineates four levels of a person's functioning in connection with the alcohol problem. By assessing problems at each level and their interaction with alcohol consumption in an antecedent and consequent manner, the intervenor can better determine the mode, type, and intensity of intervention needed at each stage of change.

The four levels of problem involvement are: symptomatic, interpersonal, systems, intrapersonal (Table 2). The focus is not on assessing every problem the patient may have because that would lead us to a general assessment of the individual's mental and physical health, some aspects of which may or may not be relevant to treatment of the alcohol problem. Levels are assessed in the light of their involvement with alcohol problems and their relevance to decision-making, active change, and maintenance. Using this problem involvement approach to evaluation, we give priorities to problems and focus on those most relevant to an individual. While these levels and the issues enumerated under them appear relevant to the treatment of all alcohol-troubled persons, we will examine them, paying particular attention to the areas that may be most useful in the treatment of alcoholism in the elderly.

The *symptomatic* level includes the patient's most immediate and relevant concerns. Alcohol consumption, quantity, frequency, and pattern are of primary concern

TABLE 2. *Levels of problem involvement*

A. Symptomatic level
  1. Alcohol consumption
  2. Anxiety
  3. Depression
  4. Lack of environmental support
  5. Physiological withdrawal symptoms
  6. Medical problems
  7. Coping skills
  8. Other psychiatric problems (symptoms)
 	
B. Interpersonal level
  1. Hostility
  2. Communication
  3. Interpersonal anxiety and fears
  4. Rejection-loss
  5. Intimacy
  6. Sexual functioning
  7. Passive-dependency
  8. Control and countercontrol
	C. Systems level
	  1. Family system (current)
	  2. Family system (origin)
	  3. Work-employment system
	  4. Social network system
	  5. Legal system
	
	D. Intrapersonal level
	  1. Identity-self
	  2. Identity-sexual
	  3. Independence (responsibility)
	  4. Basic needs (trust, self-esteem,
	     security)
	  5. Frustration/anger
	  6. Meaning in life (goals-value)
	  7. Personality disorder
	  8. Reality orientation

and a critical area of intervention. To develop a rational and effective treatment plan, however, other problems must be included. The elderly often have physical problems, and they often lack environmental support. Medical problems, alcohol-related and otherwise, lack of environmental support, mood, coping skills, and signs of organic brain dysfunction require priority attention for this age group. Problems at this level are frequently those that have the urgent concern of the patient and require initial attention. Excessive concern with these problems may, however, result in the neglect of other problems at other levels and may delay or prevent successful treatment.

The use of alcohol to ease the anxiety of social situations, to facilitate communication, and to handle interpersonal problems makes assessment of the *interpersonal level* essential. Often problems at this level are evident early in an evaluation, either from observation of interaction in the interview or from the patient's description of relationships. Anger, hostility, problems of intimacy, loss, and interactions with others are frequently involved in the elderly person's drinking behavior. Many reactive factors in alcoholism among the elderly, identified by Rosin and Glatt (34), can be classified at this level.

On the *systems level* it is recognized that the individual, with all his characteristics, talents, and deficits, not only is engaged in dyadic interaction but is one interactive part of a greater whole. Here the system itself may be seen as causing or contributing to alcohol problems. Assessment of the patient at this level views his or her interactions within various systems, such as family, employment, social, and legal. Occasionally a system's problem may require primary intervention before issues at the symptomatic level can be managed effectively. A family that gives conflicting messages to the elderly alcoholic, encouraging treatment yet providing the alcohol for home consumption, undermines effective treatment. The social networks of elderly alcoholics may promote drinking or be so limited as to make sobriety difficult if not impossible. Employment may not be as relevant an issue for older patients, yet termination of membership in the work force and diminished income, or inability to use skills and energy may be a major problem to be assessed at this level. These difficulties contribute to loneliness and ultimately to the drinking behavior. Assessment of the systems level for the elderly alcoholic is important both for treatment and for prognosis.

The fourth level, the *intrapersonal level*, includes problems that are basic, pervasive, and probably long-standing. Issues such as identity, dependence, basic trust, as well as character problems or deficits in reality orientation, are of initial interest to treatment. At this level many elderly alcoholics who have had a long-standing pattern of problem drinking may demonstrate serious difficulties related to drinking. This level is the most difficult one for intervention, especially for elderly patients whose problems at this level may be so ingrained and remote from their awareness that direct intervention is problematic. Medication may be needed to correct the patients' reality distortions. Yet, with the elderly alcoholic, awareness of problems at this level rather than direct intervention should generally be the focus of attention. This does not imply that using this level of assessment is relatively useless for the elderly alcoholic. Awareness of intrapersonal issues may be extremely important in deciding on treatment facility, on residential placement, or on type of intervention most appropriate to deal with problems at other levels.

This multilevel assessment of problems is useful for differentiating individuals with alcohol problems. Without losing perspective of the presenting problems at the symptomatic level, the assessment task is to examine how each of the other levels interacts with alcohol problems so that treatment programs and strategies may be developed. The geriatric alcoholic, as well as younger alcoholics, may be able to be managed simply with attention to problems at the symptomatic level. This would be most efficient, and changes in problems at other levels may follow symptomatic relief. Although attention to other levels is often necessary, one should not intervene needlessly in problems that are unlikely to produce early change in the patient's drinking behavior. Keeping in mind all the patient's problems, one must select and assign priorities to those for specific intervention. The levels of problem involvement can help us, conceptually and practically, develop effective interventions to move individuals through the stages of addictive behavior change and to monitor change at each level.

CONCLUSION

The stages and processes of change and the levels of problem involvement constitute the basic building blocks of a treatment model that is at once eclectic and integrative. The model is not concerned with the etiology or identification of alcoholism as a disease but rather with addictive behavior change. Concentrating on alcoholic behavior changes facilitates creation of a model that can direct diagnosis for intervention. Making this model operational and using it will increase our understanding of alcoholism treatment in general and address more effectively the issues of alcoholism treatment with the elderly.

ACKNOWLEDGMENTS

The authors would like to thank Jane Bemko for her invaluable assistance in our literature search, Lore Feldman for her considerable editorial help, and Becky Porter for her time and dedication in typing and revising this manuscript. Portions of the research reported in this chapter were supported by Grant CA27821 from the National Cancer Institute.

REFERENCES

1. Armor, D. J., Polick, J. M., and Stambul, H. B. (1976): *Alcoholism and Treatment*. Prepared for National Institute on Alcohol Abuse and Alcoholism under Grant 1739-NIAAA. Rand Corporation, Santa Monica, CA.
2. Baekeland, F., Lundwall, L., and Kissin, B. (1975): Methods for the treatment of chronic alcoholism: A critical appraisal. *Research Advances in Alcohol and Drug Problems*, Vol. 2, edited by R. J. Gibbons, Y. Israel, H. Ralant, R. E. Popham, W. Schmidt, and R. G. Smart, pp. 247–328. John Wiley and Sons, NY.
3. Barnes, G. M., Abel, E. L., and Ernst, C. A. S. (1980): *Alcohol and the Elderly: A Comprehensive Bibliography*. Greenwood Press, Westport, CT.
4. DiClemente, C. C., and Webb, L. J. (1982): Adult development and alcohol abuse. *Presentation at the Sixth Annual Conference on Alcoholism: Perspectives for the 80's*. El Paso, TX.
5. DiClemente, C. C., and Prochaska, J. O. (1982): Self-change and therapy change of smoking behavior: A comparison of processes of change of cessation and maintenance. *Addict. Behav.*, 7:133–142.
6. DiClemente, C. C. Prochaska, J. O., and Gordon, J. (1982): TRIMS alcohol treatment center. (Unpublished manuscript) Texas Research Institute of Mental Sciences.
7. DiClemente, C. C., and Gordon, J. R. (1982): Developing a self-efficacy scale for alcohol treatment: An abstract. *Alcoholism: Clinical and Experimental Research*, 6(1):140.
8. Dunham, R. G. (1981) Aging and changing patterns of alcohol use. *J. Psychoactive Drugs*, 13(2):143–151.
9. Edwards, G., Orford, J., Egert, S., Guthrie, S., Hawker, A., Hensman, C., Mitcheson, M., Oppenheimer, E., and Taylor, C. (1977): Alcoholism: A controlled trial of "treatment" and "advice." *J. Stud. Alcohol*, 381:1004–1031.
10. Emrick, C. D. (1975): A review of psychologically oriented treatment of alcoholism. II. The relative effectiveness of different treatment approaches and the effectiveness of treatment versus no treatment. *J. Stud. Alcohol*, 36(1):88–108.
11. Freedberg, E. J., and Johnston, W. E. (1979): Behavioral change in a short-term, intensive, multi-model alcoholism treatment program. *Psychol. Rep.*, 44:791–797.
12. Gibbs, L. E. (1980): A classification of alcoholics relevant to type-specific treatment. *Int. J. Addict.*, 15(4):461–488.
13. Gould, R. L. (1972): The phases of adult life: A study in development psychology. *Am. J. Psychiatry*, 129(5).
14. Horn, D. (1976): A model for the study of personal choice health behavior. *Int. J. Health Educ.*, 19(2):89–98.
15. Janis, I. L., and Mann, L. (1977): *Decision Making: A Psychological Analysis of Conflict, Choice and Commitment*. Free Press, NY.
16. Kissin, B. (1977): Theory and practice in the treatment of alcoholism. Treatment and rehabilitation of the chronic alcoholic. *The Biology of Alcoholism*, Vol. 5. Plenum Press, NY.
17. Layden, T. H., and Smith, J. W. (1973): Nonmetric pattern analysis of behavioral and biological disease symptoms in alcoholism. *Arch. Gen. Psychiatry*, 28:246–249.
18. Lazarus, A. A. (1976): *Multimodal Behavior Therapy*. Springer, NY.
19. Lazarus, A. A. (1981): *The Practice of Multi-Modal Therapy*. McGraw-Hill, NY.

20. Levinson, D. J., Darrow, C. N., Klein, E. B., Levinson, M. H., and McKee, B. (1978): *The Seasons of a Man's Life*. Alfred A. Knopf, NY.
21. McConnaughy, E. A., Prochaska, J. O., and Velicer, W. F.: Stages of change in psychotherapy: Measurement and sample profiles. *Psychotherapy, Theory, Research and Practice. (in press)*.
22. Marlatt, G. A., and Gordon, J. P.: *Relapse Prevention: A Self-Control Strategy for the Maintenance of Behavior Change*. Guilford Press, New York. *(in press)*.
23. Marlatt, G. A., and Gordon, J. P. (1979): Determinants of relapse: Implications for the maintenance of behavior change. In: *Behavioral Medicine: Changing Health Life Styles*, edited by P. Davidson. Brunner/Mazel, NY.
24. Mishara, B. L., and Kastenbaum, R. (1980): *Alcohol and Old Age*. Grune and Stratton, NY.
25. Noble, E. P., editor (1978): *The Third Special Report to the U.S. Congress on Alcohol and Health*. U.S. Department of H.E.W., Public Health Service. #017-024-00892-3.
26. Partington, J., and Johnson, G. F. (1969): Personality types among alcoholics. *Q. J. Stud. Alcohol*, 30:21–34.
27. Pattison, E. M., Sobell, M. B., and Sobell, L. C. (1977): *Emerging Concepts of Alcohol Dependence*. Springer, NY.
28. Petersen, D. M., and Whittington, F. J. (1977): Drug use among the elderly: A review. *J. Psychedelic Drugs*. 9(1):25–37.
29. Price, J. H., and Andrews, P. (1982): Alcohol abuse in the elderly. *J. Gerontol. Nurs.*, 8(1):16–19.
30. Prochaska, J. O. (1979): *Systems of Psychotherapy: A Transtheoretical Analysis*. Dorsey Press, Homewood, IL.
31. Prochaska, J. O., and DiClemente, C. C. (1982): Transtheoretical therapy: Toward a more integrative model of change. *Psychotherapy: Theory, Research and Practice*. 19(3):276–288.
32. Prochaska, J. O., DiClemente, C. C., Velicer, W. F., and Ginpil, S. (1982): Predicting self change movement through the stages of smoking cessation and relapse. (Unpublished manuscript) University of Rhode Island.
33. Prochaska, J. O., DiClemente, C. C., Velicer, W. F., and Zwick, W. R. (1981): Measuring the processes of change used in smoking cessation. Paper presented at the *Annual Meeting of the Internative Council of Psychology*, Los Angeles.
34. Rosin, A. J., and Glatt, M. M. (1971): Alcohol excess with elderly. *Q.J. Stud. Alc.*, 32:53–59.
35. Skinner, H. S., and Jackson, D. N. (1974): Alcoholic personality types: Identification and correlates. *J. Abnorm. Psychol.*, 83:658–666.
36. Smart, R. (1978): Do some alcoholics do better in some types of treatment than others? *Drug Alcohol Depend.*, 3:65–75.
37. Tuchfield, B. S., Simuel, J. B., Schmitt, M. L., Ries, J. L., Key, D. L., and Waterhouse, G. J. (1976): *Changes in Patterns of Alcohol Use Without the Aid of Formal Treatment*. Research Triangle Institute, Research Triangle Park, NC.
38. Vogler, R. E., Compton, J. V., and Weissback, T. A. (1975): Integrated behavioral change techniques for alcoholics. *J. Consult. Clin. Psychol.*, 43(2):233–243.
39. Wanberg, K. W., Horn, J. L., and Foster, F. M. (1977): A differential assessment model for alcoholism. *J. Stud. Alcohol*, 38:512–543.
40. West, D. W., Graham, S., Swanson, M., and Wilkenson, G. (1977): Five year followup of a smoking withdrawal clinic population. *Am. J. Public Health*, 67(6):536–544.
41. Zimberg, S. (1979): Alcohol and the elderly. In: *Drugs and the Elderly: Social and Pharmacological Issues*, edited by D. Peterson, F. Whittington, and B. Payne. Charles C Thomas, Springfield, IL.
42. Zimberg, S. (1978): Diagnosis and treatment of the elderly alcoholic. *Alcoholism: Clinical and Experimental Research*, 2(1):27–29.

Alcoholism in the Elderly, edited by
J. T. Hartford and T. Samorajski.
Raven Press, New York © 1984.

Future Directions for Alcohol Research in the Elderly

Thomas Crook and Gene Cohen

*Center for Studies of the Mental Health of the Aging, National Institute of Mental Health,
Rockville, Maryland 20857*

At the turn of the century, approximately 3 million people in the United States, or 4% of the population, had reached or passed the age of 65 years—that arbitrary point at which the individual is considered by many to have joined the ranks of the elderly. Today, elderly Americans number more than 25 million, or 11% of the population, and if present trends continue, the figure will reach 55 million, fully 20% of the population, within the next 50 years.

Although many individuals remain physically and emotionally healthy into and beyond the seventh and eighth decades of life, the prevalence of a broad range of physical and emotional disorders is increased in these years. For example, depression and suicide occur more frequently in the elderly than in any other age group, sleep disorders increase dramatically, and cognitive disorders such as senile dementia become tragic and dehumanizing threats to the individual.

Remarkable progress has been made during the past several years in understanding many of the major mental health disorders of late life. For example, senile dementia, which was once considered untreatable and even a "normal" consequence of old age, is now seen as resulting from quite specific disease processes that may very well be responsive to treatment. Similarly, it is now clear that depression in the elderly can often be treated quite successfully through either psychotherapy or judicious use of antidepressant medication.

In the case of alcohol-related problems in the elderly, the last several years have also witnessed a dramatic expansion in our knowledge, as demonstrated by the excellent foregoing chapters in this publication. On the basis of recent research, it is now possible to address the dual questions: "How serious is the problem posed by alcohol in the elderly?" and "What are the questions to which future research should be directed?"

HOW SERIOUS IS THE PROBLEM?

Although satisfactory epidemiologic data are not yet available, it appears that elderly individuals tend to drink less than young adults and that the incidence of alcoholism may decrease with age. Obviously, many early-onset alcoholics do not survive to old age and others stop drinking in adult life in response to treatment or to the harsh realities associated with alcoholism. On the other hand, alcohol-related problems develop late in life in an unknown proportion of individuals.

In terms of physiologic changes with age, it appears that the metabolism, absorption, and distribution of alcohol are not strikingly different in young and old adults. However, it also appears that because of dramatically reduced body water volume with age, and perhaps membrane and neurotransmitter system changes, relatively small doses of alcohol may produce profound and often toxic effects in elderly individuals. As illustrated in Chapter 7 by Ritzmann and Melchior, dependence liability also appears to increase with age.

Thus, although alcohol may not be used as extensively by the aged as by young adults, it may be a particularly toxic drug in older individuals. The higher local organ concentrations of alcohol per unit dose may threaten organs already compromised by disease or age and may induce or exacerbate medical illness. The total societal costs of such alcohol-related medical illness in the elderly are unknown but perhaps formidable. Apparently brain tissue from older organisms is particularly sensitive to alcohol, and the clinical consequences of this sensitivity may include memory loss, confusion, and disorientation even at extremely low doses, as well as loss of motor control resulting in possibly serious falls. One example of the societal costs of alcohol-induced or exacerbated impairments of brain function in the elderly is provided by studies of automobile accidents suggesting that the already extremely high collison rate among older males is increased dramatically following ingestion of even very small amounts of alcohol.

It would appear, then, that alcohol usage does pose a serious problem in the elderly, although it is clear that many questions remain unanswered. Several of the pressing issues to which future research might profitably be addressed are outlined in the following paragraphs.

ISSUES FOR FUTURE RESEARCH

Patterns of Use and Abuse

It is clear, as discussed by Blazer and Pennyback in Chapter 2, that the epidemiologic data currently available on alcohol use in the elderly are not satisfactory. Among the problems in obtaining reliable figures on use and abuse are that aged persons with problems related to alcohol are less likely to be identified in the workplace and are less likely to come to the attention of the legal system or to enter treatment programs. Also, alcoholism may go undiagnosed by physicians, since symptoms of the disorder may be confused with symptoms of aging. Research now underway will provide additional useful data on alcohol use in the elderly, but more studies are clearly needed to assess the full extent of usage among the elderly and within major demographic and sociocultural elderly subgroups. More studies are needed to identify the principal demographic and psychosocial factors related to usage, to assess the effects of sociocultural environment and change in environment on usage, and to examine the full range of interpersonal factors, including intergenerational relationships, associated with usage. It is important in all these studies that attention be directed toward examining factors associated with "successful" use of alcohol and abstinence as well as with alcoholism and problematic use among nonalcoholics.

Life Course of Alcohol Use and Abuse

Questions relating to onset or termination of drinking in mid- and late life may be of major importance not only in understanding alcohol-related problems in the elderly, but also in understanding alcoholism in general. Of particular interest are such questions as: Are there substantial numbers of persons for whom the onset of problem drinking is in late life, and, if so, what factors are associated with this onset? Are factors such as bereavement or other interpersonal losses of major significance? Is the loss of daily structure following retirement of importance? Is a genetically determined neurochemical change implicated? Are there genetic or early-life predictors of late-life-onset drinking?

Of at least equal importance are questions relating to persons with a life-long history of problem drinking who suddenly stop drinking in mid- or late adulthood. For example: How large is this group and what physiological, psychological, or sociocultural factors are associated with termination? If there is a genetic basis for alcoholism, what factors protect some individuals until late in life? Is there neurochemical support for the clinical reports that some persons who terminate drinking find that alcohol simply stops producing pleasure? As in the case of questions related to late-life onset, such questions appear to be not only of major significance for the elderly, but also of obvious relevance to the etiology and treatment of alcoholism in earlier life.

Relation to Normal Daily Functions

What are the effects of alcohol on sleep, appetite, sexual function, and other aspects of normal daily function in the elderly? Relevant questions include: How widely is alcohol used in the self-medication of sleep disorders in the elderly, and what are the differential effects on sleep physiology and daytime wakefulness in old and young individuals? What are the effects of alcohol on appetite and diet? Do "empty" alcohol calories diminish already generally reduced appetite for food in the elderly and lead to nutritional deficiencies? And with regard to sex, what are the long-term consequences of the testicular effects of alcohol in males? As noted in Chapter 10 by Bosmann, chronic alcohol consumption adversely affects female sexual function at the hypothalamic-pituitary level during reproductive years, but what is the effect in elderly women? In designing studies on the effects of alcohol on daily functions such as sleep, appetite, and sex in the elderly, it is important that investigators not preclude the possibility that effects at some dosage levels are therapeutic.

Relation to Physical Function and Disease

As described by Bosmann and by other authors in preceding chapters, the long-term effects of alcohol in the elderly are degenerative on the brain, heart, intestinal tract, pancreas, and especially on the liver. Long-term consumption may be associated with various chronic diseases in the elderly, including gout and osteoporosis. Also of importance in the elderly are possible life-threatening acute effects, such as precipitous urinary obstructions in elderly males with prostatic hypertrophy or respiratory arrest in patients with sleep apneas. Also, because of reduced body water, elderly individuals may reach lethal concentrations of alcohol at a much lower dosage level than young adults. Clearly, a great deal more research is needed to fully explore the association between alcohol and both chronic and acute physical disorders. Questions also arise concerning the extent to which physical damage is reversible in the elderly following termination of drinking, and, of particular importance, how physiologic damage can be minimized in elderly subjects who continue drinking.

Important questions also arise concerning the relationship between alcohol and trauma in the elderly. Falls resulting in hip fractures or other skeletal damage are a major problem in the elderly and a frequent factor necessitating institutionalization. Questions may be raised concerning how frequently falls and other nonvehicular accidents are related to alcohol in the elderly, and what steps can be taken to diminish the magnitude of the problem.

Of particular importance are the interactions between alcohol and other drugs prescribed for medical or psychiatric indications. As discussed in Chapter 9 by Garver and in Chapter 10 by Bosmann, alcohol interacts with many drugs that are widely prescribed to aged patients. For example, superadditive effects occur with concurrent use of alcohol and benzodiazepines. In fact, as illustrated by Bosmann, the interaction of nitrazepam and alcohol can be fatal. Adverse reactions may also be expected when alcohol is used in combination with tricyclic antidepressants, antihypertensives, anticonvulsants, and antibiotics. Among the possible life-threatening acute adverse drug interactions, as discussed by Bosmann, is the potentiation by alcohol of the anticoagulant property of aspirin, leading possibly to massive gastric hemorrhage. These and other possible alcohol-drug interactions in the elderly require detailed study aimed at examining the magnitude of the problem and the possible steps to diminish risk.

Relation to Other Mental Health Disorders

Relatively little appears to be known about the relationship between alcohol use and the other major health disorders of later life. The relationship would appear to be intimate; for example, in Chapter 15 Hartford and Thienhaus suggest that 30% of alcoholics have either a schizophrenic or major affective disorder but that many questions remain unanswered. For example, with regard to depression: What is the relationship between alcohol and depression in later life? Is heavy drinking a warning signal of impending depression in advanced age? Do elderly individuals use alcohol extensively to self-medicate in depression? Does alcohol exacerbate symptomatology in late-life depression? How does alcohol affect the course of depression? How intimately is alcohol related to suicide in the elderly? Numerous important questions can also be raised concerning the relationship between alcohol and late-life sleep disorders, anxiety disorders, and schizophrenia and related disorders. In the latter disease category, the role of alcohol in exacerbating paranoid symptomatology and dysocial behavior is of particular interest.

In the organic brain syndromes, including senile dementia, alcohol has frequently been observed to produce a marked exacerbation in symptomatology even at very low dosage levels. The effects of alcohol in elderly persons with mild signs of cognitive loss require examination, as do the effects in persons with the moderate and severe cognitive impairments seen in senile dementia.

Important questions are also apparent concerning the role of alcohol in the etiology of senile dementia. Although, as suggested in Chapters 8 and 10, alcohol is probably not associated with premature aging, chronic alcohol use may very well increase vulnerability to senile dementia and to other organic brain disorders in late life. This possibility is of both practical and theoretical importance and would appear to merit future research.

Treatment for Alcohol-Related Disorders

A great many important questions exist concerning the treatment of alcohol-related disorders in the elderly. Aged persons may underutilize available treatment services for alcoholism and alcohol-related disorders, although Hartford and Thienhaus point out in Chapter 15 that 34% of Alcoholics Anonymous (AA) members in North America are 50 years of age or older. Studies are clearly needed to determine if treatment services are, in fact, underutilized by the elderly and, if so, what steps can be taken to assure appropriate service delivery. Beyond that, critical questions concern the efficacy of established treatment approaches in elderly patients. For example: How effective is AA in the elderly? Are insight-oriented therapies indicated? How effective are group versus individual approaches to psychotherapy? Is behavior therapy a useful approach? And what is the role of psychotropic drugs in treating the elderly alcoholic? Samorajski and colleagues suggest in Chapter 4 that cholinomimetic agents may be useful in treating the recovering elderly alcoholic, and this possibility should be investigated.

A specific issue that requires attention concerns the utility of disulfiram (Antabuse®) treatment in the elderly. As discussed in Chapter 11 by Gambert and colleagues and in Chapter 15 by Hartford and Thienhaus, side effects of disulfiram may not be negligible in the elderly, and the toxic response to alcohol ingestion may actually be life threatening.

As discussed in Chapter 4 by Samorajski and his colleagues, hyperexcitability may increase with age on withdrawal from alcohol. In the compromised and frail aged individual, withdrawal may be particularly dangerous, and research on medical and psychiatric management merits consideration. A specific question relates to the utility of benzodiazepines in detoxification.

An issue that deserves careful attention before treatment studies are undertaken in the elderly is the question of therapeutic goals. In young adults the explicit goal of treatment may be abstinence whereas the implicit goals often involve resumption of employment and other earlier role functions and repair of damaged family and other interpersonal relationships. In aged alcoholics retired from the workplace and often socially isolated, resumption of earlier role functions and restoration of extensive interpersonal ties may be impossible. Thus, as argued by DiClemente and Gordon in Chapter 16, successful therapy for alcohol-related problems in the elderly may require much more than symptomatic treatment. In view of the possible special therapeutic needs of aged patients, it may be necessary not only to establish the relative efficacy of existing treatments, but also to develop treatment strategies tailored specifically to aged patients.

Therapeutic Uses for Alcohol

In addition to considering the clear problems associated with alcohol in the elderly, future studies might profitably consider possible therapeutic uses of the substance. Is it possible, for example, that in view of the sensitivity of aged organisms to alcohol, the drug is a more effective analgesic in aged than in young patients? Of course, use of alcohol in Brompton's mixture is recognized in terminally ill patients. Similarly, do small amounts of alcohol produce therapeutic cardiovascular effects in some elderly patients? With regard to psychological effects, do small amounts of alcohol produce useful sedative or anxiolytic effects in the elderly? Also, are the disinhibiting "cocktail party" effects of a small amount of alcohol advantageous in encouraging social interaction in some settings? Clearly such effects are ascribed to alcohol by many young adults, and in several nursing homes, "pub sociotherapy" has been shown to facilitate social interaction. In any case, it is important that researchers not preclude beforehand the possibility that alcohol may have therapeutic effects in elderly patients.

SUMMARY

Although the proportion of the elderly population affected by alcohol may not be extreme, the drug appears to be particularly toxic in the elderly and to exact a very high medical and social toll. For example, the aged driver under the influence of even a very small amount of alcohol may represent an extreme danger on the highways. Similarly, the direct medical effects of alcohol and the secondary effects resulting from falls and other traumas are clear. Thus, research into the problems associated with alcohol in the elderly is of clear and pressing public health significance. Only through efforts of researchers such as those who contributed to this volume will we come to understand and treat problems associated with alcohol in the elderly. Clearly the contribution of such knowledge to the welfare of our aged citizens would be immense.

Subject Index

ABO blood group, 13
Acetaldehyde, 155, 157, 163
  alcohol choosing animal strains and, 8
  chemical effects of metabolism of, 71
  levels in animal studies, 45–46, 53, 60–61
Acetate, 163
Acetylcholine (ACh), 50, 69, 72, 75, 232
Acetylcoenzyme A (acetyl-CoA), 163
Acyl chains, 141–142, 145
Addiction, 166–167
Addictive behavior change, 268–274
Adenosine monophosphate (AMP), 87,
  181–182
ATPase, 40–41, 139, 144–145, 148, 182
Adenylate cyclase, 87, 100
Adrenergic synapses, 73, 76–78, 165
Adrenocorticotrophic hormone (ACTH),
  127–128
Aged and aging
  ability to change and, 268
  brain membranes and, 142–143
  brainstem auditory evoked potentials,
    209–211
  cerebral blood flow, 236–238, 244
  changes in body distribution of alcohol,
    153
  decline in drinking with age, 19, 30
  development of tolerance to alcohol,
    117–133
  diagnosis of alcoholism and, 27, 254
  drug responsiveness and, 35, 43
  EEG and, 202–203
  effect on initial sensitivity to alcohol, 122
  effects of, 43, 149
  electrophysiological parallels with
    alcoholics, 201–218
  epidemiology of alcoholism and, 25–32,
    278–279
  ethanol related disorders in, 117
  fatal effects of alcoholism in, 166
  increase in the proportion of the population
    of, 35, 117, 277
  interaction of alcohol and, 43–44,
    105–106, 139, 149
  long latency evoked potentials and,
    213–214
  neuropathological changes in, 228–229
  neurotransmitter function and, 65–79

  nigrostriatal dopamine system and, 87–90
  norepinephrine system and, 98–101
  normal and cholinergic binding, 76
  nutrition, 39, 183–184
  pattern reversal evoked potentials and,
    211–212
  preference for ethanol and, 124
  premature aging model, 193–194
  psychological decline, 232–234
  sensory evoked potential, 206, 215–216
  serotonin and, 85, 103–104
  severity of withdrawal and, 123
  sleep and, 204
  synaptic function and, 67, 70–72
Alcohol
  absorption, 153, 162
  anthropological evidence of use, 10
  brain membranes and, 144–149
  distribution, 140–141, 153–155, 163
  effects on dopamine, 90–96
  effects on norepinephrine, 101–103
  effects on serotonin, 103, 105
  elimination rate, 123, 140, 157, 184
  increase in muscarinic receptors, 51
  membrane fluidization and, 72, 144–148
  metabolic effects, 163–166, 177–178
  metabolism, 140, 153–159, 163
  pharmacokinetics, 162–163
  preference for, 123–124
  therapeutic value, 161, 282
  usage rate by sex, 30
Alcohol dehydrogenase (ADH), 8, 13, 155,
  157, 163
Alcoholic dementia, 235–236; see also
  Dementia
Alcoholics
  assessment, 266, 271–273
  cognitive deficits in, 193
  electrophysiological parallels with aging,
    201–218
  elderly differ from young adults, 267
  immotive, 270–271
  motivation and treatment outcome,
    265–266, 269
  neurological differences, 13
  percentage diagnosed with mental
    disorders, 256
  serotonin reduction in, 103

283